ENERGETIC KINESIOLOGY – PRINCIPLES AND PRACTICE

To the memory of

Richard Utt (1950-2011)

Energetic Kinesiologist and originator of Applied Physiology

ENERGETIC KINESIOLOGY – PRINCIPLES AND PRACTICE

Charles T Krebs PhD

Applied physiologist, kinesiologist and research scientist; founder of LEAP
(Learning Enhancement Acupressure Enhancement Programme)

and

Tania O'Neill McGowan BSc Grad DipEd

Kinesiologist and Managing Director of O'Neill Kinesiology College,
Perth, Western Australia

Foreword by

James L Oschman PhD

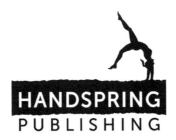

HANDSPRING
PUBLISHING

HANDSPRING PUBLISHING LIMITED
The Old Manse, Fountainhall,
Pencaitland, East Lothian
EH34 5EY, United Kingdom
Tel: +44 1875 341 859
Website: www.handspringpublishing.com

First published 2014 in the United Kingdom by Handspring Publishing

ISBN 978-1-909141-03-2

British Library Cataloguing in Publication Data
A catalogue record for this book is available from the British Library

Important notice
It is the responsibility of the practitioner, employing a range of sources of
information, their personal experience, and their understanding of the particular
needs of the patient, to determine the best approach to treatment.

Neither the publishers nor the authors will be liable for any loss or damage of any
nature occasioned to or suffered by any person or property in regard to product
liability, negligence or otherwise, or through acting or refraining from acting as a
result of adherence to the material contained in this book.

Commissioning Editor, Mary Law, Handspring Publishing Limited
Text design by Pete Wilder, Designers Collective
Cover design Bruce Hogarth, Kinesis Creative
Artwork by Rich Prime, Designers Collective
Typeset by Palimpsest Book Production Limited, Falkirk, Stirlingshire
Printed and bound by CPI Group (UK) Ltd, Croydon, CR0 4YY
Cover *Hand of Light* image by Seth Chwast sethchwastart.com

The
Publisher's
policy is to use
paper manufactured
from sustainable forests

CONTENTS

Foreword

There is this medicine and that medicine

and this method and that method

and there is the way the body really is.

Kerry Weinstein

The quote is symbolic of a monumental shift taking place in health care and introduces a book that makes an extraordinary contribution to that change. What is evolving is a better way to think about the techniques that support our health and that help us recover from injury and disease. Modern research and clinical experience are cutting through the morass of confusion inflicted on all of us, in which questionable science is used to 'prove' how the human body works, usually with a primary goal of selling something. The message is often a false view of our vulnerability rather than the optimistic perspective of the body's innate ability to heal itself.

In *Studies Show*, John H. Fennick describes how we are continually bombarded with the results of studies that purport to prove that this or that treatment or lifestyle or dietary ingredient is good or bad for us. The average person, the physician and even the seasoned researcher finds it challenging to evaluate these assertions, to the point that many people simply do not trust any health claim.

The way the body really works leaps from the pages of this book in the form of carefully documented information on the working together of nerves, muscles, movement and energy—concepts that have been validated through extensive research and clinical practice. No longer does the future of medicine rest mainly on experiments done in laboratories of biochemistry and molecular biology. Instead, we are learning that academic scientist-therapists such as Dr Charles Krebs and his colleague Tania O'Neill McGowan are at the cutting edge of biomedicine, the place where discoveries in alternative, complementary and integrative medicine join with the findings from basic research to provide real knowledge on how the body works, and to provide a vision of the successful health care system of the future.

Academic biomedicine is learning that a vast amount of important and reliable information is emerging from observations made by sensitive individuals who touch their patients every day and carefully observe, test and retest the subtle phenomena taking place under their hands. Delighted patients have direct experiences that enable them to validate the success of Energetic Kinesiology.

Charles and Tania are among the master therapists of our time. They have brought to modern medicine a series of insights and discoveries that could be achieved only by persons with a rigorous scientific background combined with experience of teaching and practicing an emerging and tremendously exciting field of therapeutics. Charles has studied with the great teachers and leaders of the previous generation of Energetic Kinesiologists (George Goodheart, Gordon Stokes, Bruce Dewe, Richard Utt and Sheldon Deal), who stood on the shoulders of the academic kinesiologists who preceded them (Robert and Charles Lovett, as well as Florence and Henry Kendall). Note the term *academic kinesiologists*, signifying that these individuals sought to find out and verify rather than prove; the mature scientist knows that even the best science leads only to approximations, not to proofs.

Charles has traveled the world, teaching, treating and researching, continually expanding the scope of his discipline and revealing his ongoing discoveries to a therapeutic community that is thriving, in part because of the advances he has made. Charles has also developed the Learning Enhancement Acupressure Program.

This method applies muscle biofeedback and acupressure techniques to correct specific learning problems. The result is much more than relief of aches and pains—it allows people to fulfill their destinies, the reason they sought help in the first place.

Charles's background is in research science and neuroscience. He has worked as a researcher and a university lecturer, and he has over 20 years of clinical experience. His intimate and virtually holographic understanding of the brain and its connections throughout the body provide detailed support for his unique therapeutic approaches.

Charles is also the author of two other remarkable and highly acclaimed books. *A Revolutionary Way of Thinking: From a Near Fatal Accident to a New Science of Healing* is the remarkable story of how Charles recovered from an accident that left him with quadriplegia. He was facing death, or at least a life sentence of physical and mental disability. With his deep knowledge of human anatomy and physiology, as well as an incredible will, Charles decided that he would walk again—and he did. In the process, he synthesized a vast amount of wisdom from ancient medical texts from the East to the latest discoveries of western neuroscience. The book proved to be a monumental contribution to the field of kinesiology. It includes the most thorough account of the history of this field available until publication of this book. A second important book, *Nutrition for the Brain*, revealed Charles's deep understanding of biochemistry and nutrition.

Tania has a background in physics and now owns and manages an Energetic Kinesiology college in Western Australia. The college offers fully integrated training, including one of the first programs to provide an Advanced Diploma of Kinesiology.

It is a major event when therapists of this caliber choose to document their life's work in a book such as this. I am honored to be one of their many friends and colleagues, and I am grateful for the privilege of writing the foreword for this masterful volume.

Students and teachers of every branch of complementary, alternative, integrative and energy medicine will find valuable insights and techniques they can use between the covers of this brilliant book. Anecdotes from the experiences of patients and remarkable healers met along the way make the book very readable and enjoyable. It is also extremely well-illustrated. Great illustrations are vital from my perspective and this book has a wealth of them.

Other highlights include the following:

- A comprehensive understanding of the structure and function of the ancient and modern energy systems of the body, which enables therapists to both apply new models from physics and quantum physics to healing and to explain their results to their delighted clients.
- A new understanding of homeostasis, chaos and stress, and how compensations accumulate, stabilize, and thereby resist change, as well as how to get around this dilemma.
- Practical applications of these understandings in the resolution of a wide range of physiological and emotional issues.
- A discussion of the remarkable biofeedback mechanism of muscle monitoring, which enables therapists to directly contact the subconscious and cause it to divulge its secrets.
- A critical scientific description of muscle monitoring, formerly called muscle testing—what it can do and what it cannot do.
- The recognition that the body knows how to heal itself but sometimes needs some gentle help from outside.
- The recognition that every person is unique and that every treatment must therefore be completely individual.
- An explanation of why randomized clinical trials are consequently of little value in studying Energetic Kinesiology, but how high-quality science and validation can nevertheless be done by critical scientists such as Charles and Tania.
- A description of the broader application of kinesiology beyond its use as a powerful resource for treating musculoskeletal issues; kinesiology can be used in the treatment of a wide range of disease issues, the reason being well-documented relations between the

musculoskeletal system, the lymphatic system and visceral functions.

- A history of how the connections with pathophysiology came about through the work of Chapman, Bennett and Goodheart, who made systematic studies of the links between weakness of specific muscles and specific disorders.
- A fearless venture by Charles and Tania into controversial concepts such as auras, the astral body and chakras, but in practical ways that make sense even to the most skeptical observer.
- Descriptions of the connections between ancient and modern conceptualizations of human energetics, which will be fascinating to all therapists.

With *Energetic Kinesiology* Charles and Tania leave a new, remarkable and indelible footprint for their field and for health care in general. This book is far more than a therapeutic manual. It is a book that will be studied by current and future generations of healers from every branch of therapeutics. I congratulate the authors and publisher for producing a volume that will help untold numbers of patients from around the world live more comfortable and fulfilling lives.

James L. Oschman, PhD
Author of Energy Medicine: The Scientific Basis
Dover, New Hampshire, USA

December 2013

References

1. Fennick, JH 1997, *Studies Show: A Popular Guide to Understanding Scientific Studies*, Prometheus Books, Amherst.
2. Krebs, C 1998, *A Revolutionary Way of Thinking: From a Near Fatal Accident to a New Science of Healing*, Hill of Content Publishing, Melbourne.
3. Krebs, C 2006, *Nutrition for the Brain: Feeding Your Brain for Optimum Performance*, Michelle Anderson

Preface

Overview of the book

Energetic Kinesiology is currently an emerging field internationally in the complementary health sciences, gaining more and more scientific support and recognition. The field of Energetic Kinesiology is growing rapidly and is increasingly being taught in professional colleges and schools worldwide; however, at present there is little published literature covering the principles and practices of this exciting field. Our goal in writing this book was to help fill this gap and begin to bring greater coherence into both its theory and practice.

The book is intended to bring together a vast array of information, research and clinical knowledge into a format that is accessible and immediately useful to kinesiologists, other health professionals and students of kinesiology. It includes a comprehensive treatment of the historical development of the field, as well as a description of the fundamental techniques employed in the field and the underlying physiological and energetic basis of these techniques. For those with some experience in kinesiology, this book will provide the theoretical background necessary to more deeply understand, and to explain to others, how the techniques are applied and why they are effective.

The concepts covered in this book are by their very nature rapidly changing, as this is a developing field. We have chosen the content of the book based on feedback from students and practitioners about the difficulty of finding comprehensive explanations of kinesiology techniques and the mechanisms on which they are based. It is important to understand that this textbook was not written to cover the entire field of Energetic Kinesiology but rather to be a first step in the exploration of this emerging field. Many of the concepts and clinical applications included in this book have not yet withstood the rigorous scrutiny of scientific investigation. However, they have been included on the basis of observations of their clinical efficacy by ourselves and thousands of clinicians around the world over the past three decades.

One aspect of this book that is unique is the historical content. Dr Charles Krebs knew most of the originators of Energetic Kinesiology techniques personally and has been privileged to have heard the stories of the development of these techniques firsthand, witnessed their development, or been actively involved in their research and development. The book has many historical anecdotes, which makes it a very interesting read for existing practitioners as well as those new to the field.

We have included a historical overview of the concepts relating to the development of emotions. This is because we have found that too often the connection between clinical sciences and the esoteric workings of the human mind become mutually exclusive in approaches to understanding how thoughts and emotions can influence all aspects of our function. Indeed, one of the unique attributes of Energetic Kinesiology is its holistic approach to the mind and body as an interactive unit influenced by not only our physical and physiological states but also our emotional and psycho-spiritual states.

In addition, there is a detailed discussion of the energetic structures of Man and how these interface with our physiological, emotional and psycho-spiritual functioning. This section, together with the final section outlining a scientific model for energetic healing, provides a valuable resource for all practitioners of energy medicine.

In writing this book, we had to make choices about which techniques and procedures are fundamental to the practice and application of modern Energetic Kinesiology. This book is not intended as an encyclopedic collection of *all* the concepts and techniques used in Energetic Kinesiology, as the modalities involved in this field are at present highly varied. We have attempted to include a core set of techniques and procedures that are used in Energetic Kinesiology worldwide and have consistently demonstrated clinical efficacy. If we have omitted techniques that others consider integral to their practice of kinesiology, it was unintentional, as we were constrained by both knowledge and a need to keep this book a manageable size.

We thank the many students and practitioners who read drafts and made suggestions for the order, content and clarity of this book. We extend our sincere appreciation to the giants of the field, who had the creative insights and persistence to lay the foundations of this work. It has been a unique pleasure working on this project, and we hope that readers find the content and ideas as exciting as we do.

How to use this book

This book has been written in an order that allows the reader to grasp the concepts necessary for understanding Energetic Kinesiology. However, the chapters also stand alone as reference points for specific topics.

It is envisioned that this book will be of interest to a variety of audiences. These audiences may include the following:

- students of kinesiology
- kinesiology practitioners
- chiropractors
- manual therapists
- psychoemotional therapists
- energy medicine practitioners.

The book is divided into a number of sections. Section I, *Understanding Kinesiology*, defines and introduces a historical context for the field of Energetic Kinesiology. Section II, *The Energetic Structures of Man*, begins with a historical perspective of Man's view of health and healing. It then discusses in detail the multidimensional bodies and the primary energetic systems of the body: the chakra–nadi system, the acupuncture meridian system and the Tibetan figure 8 energy system. Section III, *Understanding and Applying Muscle Monitoring*, provides an in-depth discussion of muscle physiology, including the control of muscle function, states of muscle imbalance and the emotional control of muscle response. It concludes with the various types of muscle monitoring and the validity of muscle monitoring. Section IV, *Core Kinesiology Tools*, discusses the fundamental techniques that are essential for the practice of modern Energetic Kinesiology.

Section V, *Client Assessment*, outlines the processes that need to be employed when working with clients to ensure effective kinesiology treatment. Section VI, *Set-up: Information Gathering*, outlines a series of techniques used to access conscious and subconscious information as well as ancillary factors needed to effectively define a client's issue. Section VII, *Core Correction Techniques*, covers a variety of correction techniques commonly used in modern Energetic Kinesiology. Section VIII, *Concluding Sessions*, includes the factors that are necessary to effectively complete the kinesiology treatment, including ongoing support for the client. Finally, section IX, *A Model for Energetic Healing*, provides a scientific model for energetic healing, including the role of the practitioner in healing.

Kinesiologists and students of kinesiology will most likely utilize all the sections contained within this book. However, practitioners trained in other health modalities may choose to access specific sections of this book to gain a better understanding of particular topics.

Explanations of terminology used in this book

We have presented this material using terminology that is common to the field of Energetic Kinesiology. When discussing muscle monitoring in a general rather than a clinical context, the term *monitor* is used to identify the person doing the muscle monitoring. However, when discussing the people involved in the therapy, the *practitioner* provides treatment to the *client*.

The term *muscle monitoring* will be used throughout this book rather than *muscle testing*, which has been used since the beginning of kinesiology. The rationale for this change in terminology is explained thoroughly in chapter 8, *The physiology of muscle monitoring*.

We have used the term *core kinesiology tools* when discussing the non-verbal mechanisms used in treatment, such as holding specific hand positions (hand modes) and touching specific acupoints. This group of techniques is used together with muscle monitoring to provide kinesiology treatment and can be thought of as the tools used in this field. In contrast, the section covering *core correction techniques* describes the procedures used to resolve the imbalances discovered using these core kinesiology tools.

A kinesiology balance has distinct phases, but these have not always been taught explicitly in kinesiology training programs. In this book, we have given these phases distinct names: 1, setting the context; 2, set-up: information gathering; 3, applying correction techniques; and 4, challenging corrections. We elaborate on each of these phases throughout the book.

Warning to the general public

There is currently a wide variability among practitioners in this field. Just because a practitioner calls themselves a kinesiologist or kinesiology practitioner does not mean they have been trained in or can competently apply all the techniques outlined in this book. If you are seeking kinesiology treatment, you need to do your research and question prospective practitioners to ensure you find a kinesiologist who is properly qualified in your country and who is able to competently apply their skills to achieve long-term clinical results.

Charles T Krebs
Cambridge, Massachusetts, USA

Tania O'Neill McGowan
Perth, Western Australia

December 2013

SECTION I

Understanding kinesiology

Energetic Kinesiology is a powerful healing modality that combines ancient eastern energetic healing arts with western physiological healing sciences. The main tool used in Energetic Kinesiology is muscle biofeedback, which makes the subconscious stresses and imbalances within the body observable. Further sections of this book will discuss muscle monitoring and the physiological mechanisms involved in this process of using subconscious muscle response as a feedback tool, while this section outlines the features that define Energetic Kinesiology to provide an introduction to this emerging health care field.

In order to understand Energetic Kinesiology, it is also necessary to have an overview of the historical development of the field. This section therefore goes through the full development of the field from academic kinesiology in the early 1900s, to Applied Kinesiology in the 1960s, then finally to Energetic Kinesiology, which developed in the late 20th century and is still developing today. The history presented here is a summary of the development of Energetic Kinesiology modalities, which has led to the kinesiology tools and techniques presented throughout this book.

Chapter 1

UNDERSTANDING KINESIOLOGY

What is Energetic Kinesiology?

Kinesiology literally means 'the study of movement,' and in its original form it was indeed an academic discipline studying the movement of the body and how the body moves. Several academic kinesiologists then focused on how the muscles causing movement could be assessed for their integrity of function using manual techniques that, while not being quantitative, can provide qualitative information.

In the 1940s, Florence Kendall and Henry Kendall, a wife-and-husband team of academic kinesiologists, began the study of muscle movement and how this may be assessed by manual muscle testing. Their research culminated in *Muscles: Testing and Function*, first published in 1949.[1] This now classic work was last revised in 2010 and remains one of the standard references in academic kinesiology.[2]

In 1964, Dr George Goodheart brought manual muscle testing into the chiropractic field, and then in the late 1960s made the linkage between muscle testing and the energy systems of Chinese acupuncture. Goodheart called his system *Applied Kinesiology*. Other chiropractors trained in this system went on to develop creative applications, effectively shifting the emphasis from more mechanical applications to more energetic applications, thus planting the seeds for what has now become the field of *Energetic Kinesiology*.

From an investigation of its origins, it can be seen that Energetic Kinesiology is both a science and an art. Although it has method, rules, principles and logical techniques, it also involves direct interaction between practitioner and client. This interaction involves intuition and feel as a major component of its application, both characteristics of an art form.

A far-reaching healing science

Kinesiology is a potent and remarkable system that enables a practitioner to work with a wide range of issues. While it can work exceedingly well with the defusion of emotional stress, it may work equally well with the elimination of muscular pain and weakness. It can also be effective in the elimination of allergies and food sensitivities, as well as loosening the grip of self-destructive habits such as obsessions and addictions.[3]

The reason kinesiology can have such wide-ranging effects is based on several factors. First of all, it is an energetic model that states that energy reflects physiology, and that energy effects physiology. Second, it is based on a model of health in which the body–mind seeks an innate sense of balance, but sometimes this body–mind needs assistance to re-establish this balance. Third, the body–mind actually leads the practitioner to the source or origin of the problems creating stress. It is through the remarkable biofeedback mechanism of muscle monitoring that the subconscious can be directly contacted and just as directly divulge its secrets.[4]

Thus, the kinesiologist is not the dispenser of healing knowledge to the client but rather the facilitator of the body's own wish to be healed and whole. One of the most fascinating aspects of being a kinesiologist is that every person is unique and every treatment is utterly individual. Each treatment is a personal journey for both the practitioner and the client.

Therefore the practitioner operates more as a detective than as a diagnostician. In fact, in kinesiology we do not diagnose at all; we simply follow the trail of clues that the body provides us through the muscle response. What is even more significant is that the person's muscle response not only directs us to the cause of their problems but also directs the practitioner to the therapy that will most effectively resolve these problems.

With the advent of Energetic Kinesiology in the late 20th century, the healing arts have come full circle. Ancient eastern energetic healing arts have melded with western physiological healing sciences. Mind and body are being reunited, and the person who seeks healing is empowered with the responsibility for their own health.

The future of kinesiology seems to hold boundless promise. At the moment, kinesiology is still a developing health science that holds great promise to treat numerous conditions in a holistic, non-invasive way. The major tool used in kinesiology is muscle monitoring, a form of direct biofeedback.

A biofeedback system

Kinesiology is a biofeedback system that uses subconscious muscle response as a feedback tool. Biofeedback is the provision of information about the state of a biological system back to that system in order to regulate the system. For instance, when your body temperature becomes too cool, this triggers the hypothalamus to release thyroid-stimulating hormone–releasing factor, which through a cascade of hormones increases the production of energy in every cell of the body, causing the body's temperature to rise. However, once this cellular energy production has re-established normal body temperature, the hypothalamus turns off this cascade of hormones. Over time, the body temperature decreases, and through biofeedback this cycle is reinitiated. See Figure 1.1.

In muscle monitoring, the biofeedback takes the form of a change in muscle response to varying types of inputs. The muscle response can indicate both the type of information that is needed and the factor or factors blocking this information flow. Information feedback can take the form of verbal content, structural imbalance, nutritional imbalance, energetic imbalance, psychoemotional imbalance and even spiritual imbalance.

Perhaps the most powerful component of muscle biofeedback is that it can make the subconscious stresses and imbalances within the body observable both at the physical and psychoemotional levels. That is, the change in muscle states is both felt and observed by the person experiencing kinesiology as well as the practitioner. Indeed, most of our physical, emotional and mental processing occurs outside our consciousness, and therefore imbalances within these systems remain largely unknown to our conscious

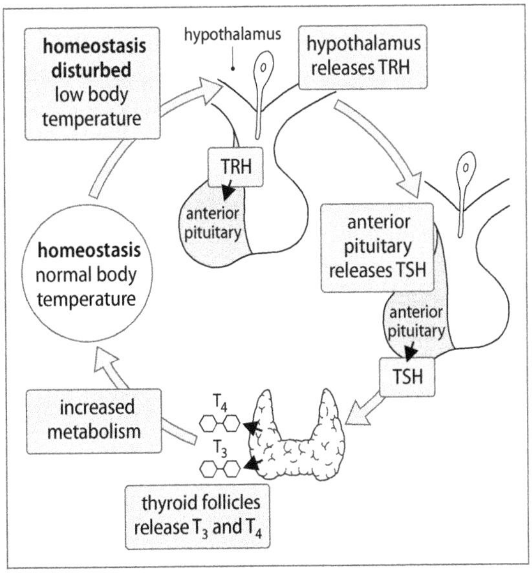

Figure 1.1 An example of a negative biofeedback system: the control of body temperature. Temperature sensors in the hypothalamus detect a decrease in body temperature; thyrotropin-releasing hormone (TRH) is released to the anterior pituitary gland; it releases thyroid-stimulating hormone (TSH); TSH travels via the blood to the thyroid gland; it releases tri-iodothyronine (T_3) and thyroxine (T_4) into the blood; stimulated by T_3 and T_4 the thyroid gland then releases thyroxine that travels to the cells of the body and increases cellular metabolism, generating heat; this increases overall body temperature until the hypothalamic temperature sensors detect that the body is too hot; this turns off the release of TRH; then turns off the release of TSH; which in turn turns off the release of T_4 by the thyroid gland; this slows down cellular metabolism, leading to the initial condition (the body temperature is too low); initiating the whole negative feedback cycle to be repeated.

mind.[5] Thus, kinesiology provides a tool to bridge this gap between the conscious and the subconscious, making subconscious stresses overtly observable.

There is no more direct biofeedback than muscle response, because the muscles are run first and foremost by a series of subconscious systems that interface at many different levels within your being. Clearly, muscle function is a major component controlling our structure, which is directly affected by our nutritional status. Although less well understood, the energetic systems of the body also interface directly with muscle function, and imbalances within these energetic systems can directly alter muscle function.

Likewise, our emotional states directly affect our muscle function such that changes in emotional state result in changes in muscle tone and tension. Muscle biofeedback can also provide direct information about our mental processing and even our level of spiritual awareness, although the mechanisms are not currently well understood. Because of this unique multifactorial interface with the major systems of the body, muscle biofeedback provides the keys to the kingdom of understanding physical level phenomena, such as musculoskeletal problems, as well as emotional, mental and spiritual issues.

The philosophical basis of kinesiology supports the Hippocratic principle of 'doing no harm' by applying only non-invasive techniques as directed by the client's own biofeedback. Hippocrates perceived the flow of *physis*, the natural vital force flowing within each person, to be a 'healing power' or 'self-adjusting power' within the body that 'though untaught and uninstructed, does what is proper to preserve a perfect equilibrium'.

However, at times this self-adjusting or healing power is reduced because of blocks in the normal flow of physis via events that create a breakdown in the normal feedback needed to provide the data for these healing powers. Therefore some external system is necessary to provide this information

feedback to the system, with which it can then self-correct. We know of no better biofeedback system than muscle monitoring as applied in Energetic Kinesiology!

Client-based therapy

Kinesiology is inherently a client-based therapy, because it is totally reliant on biofeedback from the client to direct the therapy. For instance, once a stress issue has been identified by muscle biofeedback, the nature of the factor creating this stressor is then identified by further muscle biofeedback, and finally the actual therapy to be applied is also identified by muscle biofeedback. Therefore the client totally directs the therapy by the feedback they provide via muscle monitoring.

When a kinesiologist begins a session with the client, they have the information the client has provided regarding their presenting issue, but they do not know *a priori* the causal factors underlying this issue. However, quite quickly the client's muscle biofeedback can identify the type of stressor involved and the therapeutic techniques required to effectively address this stressor. Thus, each session is unique to the individual being treated, rather than based only on practitioner knowledge and application of a standard technique or protocol.

A kinesiologist does not 'heal' or 'fix' their client by application of their knowledge; rather, they participate with their client in a journey of exploration to discover the factor or factors creating the symptoms that they presented with. The kinesiologist does need to have considerable knowledge and skills to both uncover these factors and then apply effective therapies to resolve the presenting issue. That is, the more in-depth knowledge and skills the kinesiologist has, the more effectively they can understand the information that muscle monitoring provides and the more techniques they will have at their disposal for this feedback to select as therapy.

References

1. Kendall, HO & Kendall, FP 1949, *Muscles: Testing and Function*, Williams & Wilkins, Baltimore.
2. Kendall, FP, Kendall McCreary, E, Provance, PG, McIntyre Rodgers, M & Romani, WA 2010, *Muscles: Testing and Function With Posture and Pain, Fifth Edition*, Lippincott Williams & Wilkins, Baltimore.
3. Holdway, A 1995, *Kinesiology*, Element Books, Shaftesbury. Levy, SL & Lehr, C 1996, *Your Body Can Talk*, Hohm Press, Prescott. Scott, J & Goss, K 1988, *Cure Your Own Allergies in Minutes*, Health Kinesiology Publications, San Francisco.
Barton, J 1983, *Allergies—How to Find and Conquer, Third Edition*, Biokinesiology Institute, Shady Cove.
Stokes, G & Whiteside, D 1985, *Structural Neurology*, Three In One Concepts, Burbank.
Dewe, BAJ & Dewe, JR 1992, *Professional Kinesiology Practice, Volumes I–IV*, Professional Health Publications International, Auckland.
4. Levy, SL & Lehr, C 1996, *Your Body Can Talk*, Hohm Press, Prescott.
5. Noback, CR, Strominger, NL & Demarest, RJ 1991, *The Human Nervous System, Fourth Edition*, Lea & Febiger, Philadelphia.

Chapter 2

THE HISTORICAL DEVELOPMENT OF KINESIOLOGY

Academic kinesiology

Kinesiology has an interesting lineage. The science of manual muscle testing was first developed in the early 20th century by a Boston orthopedic surgeon, RW Lovett, who also invented the first turnbuckle brace for treating scoliosis. Lovett used his muscle testing to analyze disabilities resulting from polio and nerve damage. He applied muscle testing to trace spinal nerve damage, because muscles that tested weak often had a common spinal nerve.

The system of muscle grading that Lovett developed was first published in 1932, and it introduced the five levels of testing muscles that remain the basic formula used in today's physical therapies. At first, he used only three levels of testing muscles against gravity, but he later added the more subjective levels four and five to include pressure from the therapist in addition to gravity.[1]

Henry and Florence Kendall, also working with people recovering from paralytic polio myelitis, modified and systematized Lovett's ideas and in 1949 published their pioneering book *Muscles: Testing and Function*.[2] Muscle testing became a new science in the field of Academic Kinesiology, the in-depth analysis of the exact motion of muscles and the way they move joints.

Each muscle has a unique job to do, which it can do best only in its position of greatest mechanical advantage. Basically, muscles, joints and bones are lever systems that use the mechanical advantage of a fulcrum to magnify the mechanical force of muscle contraction. This allows a short muscle contraction both to be powerful and to produce a large range of motion. When the muscle is in the position of its maximum mechanical advantage, it is called the *prime mover* or the *agonist*.

When a muscle is isolated by its testing position

as the prime mover then manually monitored and can develop its full integrity of function and 'lock' firmly, it is rated a *plus five* response. If, however, firm pressure is applied and the muscle gives in the direction of the pressure, then it is a *plus four* response. If only medium pressure is applied and the muscle gives way, then it is rated *plus three*.

If the person can move the muscle into the test position against gravity, but only slight pressure results in the muscle giving way, then it is rated *plus two*. If there is difficulty just getting the muscle into the monitoring position against gravity or maintaining the muscle in this position against gravity, it is rated *plus one*. Zero on the scale is when the muscle cannot move the limb against gravity, a condition known as *flaccid paralysis*. Because the strength of individual muscles varies in different people, the scale is not an absolute measure of strength but rather a measure of the relative integrity of muscle function.

Dr George Goodheart, a Detroit-based chiropractor, took an interest in the work of Kendall and Kendall. A very keen observer, he was one of those rare people who are able to make fantastic discoveries by looking at research from a different perspective and synthesizing the information in a different way. It is often not just seeing new things but rather seeing things already known in new ways that leads to discovery.

As Goodheart began to increasingly use muscle testing in his practice, he found that some clients had specific muscles that would test weak, were hypotonic, when certain types of disease conditions were present. For instance, he found the clavicular division of the pectoralis major (the pectoralis major clavicular, PMC), the chest muscle that connects to the collarbone, would generally be hypotonic in clients who complained of stomach ulcers. He would then apply certain procedures for the treatment of ulcers and reassess the strength of the PMC. After treatment, the muscle would suddenly be strengthened. This confirmed both the relationship between ulcers and the muscle response, and the efficacy of the treatment. The change in muscle response was immediate and visible.

An eclectic reader, Goodheart was interested in all sorts of different areas of knowledge, and while he found that his techniques worked to strengthen the muscles of some individuals, many others were not helped at all. He started looking for other answers. He came across the work of early American osteopaths Frank Chapman and Charles Owen, who had postulated that many types of pathologies, or the symptoms of diseases, had their origins in sluggish lymph flow. Lymph is the bodily fluid that carries nutrients to tissues and organs and carries toxins away. Sluggish lymph flow means that over time, tissues became more toxic and less functional.[3]

Chapman worked out that there were many points on the bodies of individuals who were showing various symptoms of disease that, when palpated or massaged, would be tender. Chapman discovered that with continuous massage these tender points or areas would become less tender, with tenderness often disappearing. When next assessed, the tenderness was absent, and this was associated with improvement in the disease condition. Chapman and Owen postulated the existence of new, previously unrecognized reflexes that they called the *neurolymphatic reflexes* and published their findings in the 1930s.[4]

Through trial and error, Goodheart correlated some specific muscles to the neurolymphatic reflex points of Chapman and noticed on testing that a moderately weak muscle seemed to be associated with a malfunctioning organ. From these initial observations, Goodheart recognized that many of the disease conditions described by Chapman as being associated with a specific Chapman reflex point were similarly associated with a specific muscle weakness, and conversely, every time he observed a weak or dysfunctional organ, there was a corresponding weak muscle. He now began to systematically investigate the relationship between Chapman reflex points and the muscle weaknesses he had found to be associated with the same disease conditions. He established that rubbing the reflex point Chapman had assigned to a disease would often strengthen the muscle associated with the same pathology. *The master synthesizer was at work.*

Despite the great success of his newly discovered Chapman reflex points, some conditions and their associated weakened muscles failed to respond to these techniques. Therefore Goodheart kept looking. In the 1930s, another American chiropractor, Terrence Bennett, had come up with his own model for restoring health based on proper blood flow. Like the lymph system, when blood flow becomes congested tissues do not get the right amount of oxygen and nutrition. Bennett reasoned that this set up the prime conditions for diseases to take hold. Like Chapman, Bennett had worked out his own set of reflex points. He called these *neurovascular reflexes*, and his body of work *neurovascular dynamics*. Most of Bennett's reflex points were on the head, but there were also a number of points on the trunk and legs.

Bennett found that applying light pressure to these points would stimulate increased blood flow to the associated tissues and organs. As with Chapman's work, stimulation of these Bennett reflex points would often result in major improvement in the conditions being treated. In the 1930s, Bennett formed the Neurological Research Foundation to teach his technique. Bennett found that applying light pressure to these points would stimulate increased blood flow to the associated tissues and organs, and organ function was enhanced or restored.

The dangers of radiation were little known in Bennett's day, so some of his experiments involved procedures that would not be considered safe today. One was to inject volunteers with radiopaque dyes that make the blood visible to X-rays. Volunteers then lay down beneath a full-length fluoroscope that emitted X-rays, and by holding different reflex points he could observe change in blood flow. While his volunteers were thus exposed to X-rays, which would not be permitted today, it allowed Bennett to develop a valuable body of knowledge that became known as the Bennett reflex points.[5]

As he had done with the Chapman reflex points, Goodheart began to systematically investigate the relationships between Bennett reflex points and those muscles that would not strengthen with his other techniques.[6] He was delighted to note that in many cases it constituted the missing link. Working primarily with the Bennett reflex points on the head and upper chest, he was able to assign specific Bennett reflex points to specific muscle weaknesses. He found that by 'tugging' on these neurovascular points, 'stimulation occurred and muscles would regain normal function'.

The origins of the Applied Kinesiology diagnostic and treatment method can be traced to 1964, when a 24-year old man Goodheart was treating asked for help with a long-term problem. The young man could not pass pre-employment physicals that required him to press in a forward direction with his arms because his scapula would just poke out at almost a 90° angle from his back, a condition called winged scapula. However, Goodheart's examination revealed no abnormalities associated with his winged scapula, even though the patient had complained of this condition for 15–20 years, and surprisingly, there was no atrophy.

Goodheart remembered reading in Kendall and Kendall's book that a lifted scapula related to a muscle called the anterior serratus, which originates from the upper ribs under the arm and inserts along the middle border of the scapula. When the anterior serratus contracts, it pulls the scapula onto the back, and therefore the protruding shoulder blade suggested that the anterior serratus muscle was weakened. During a busy day in his clinic, Goodheart set aside time to work on this client and, as predicted, found the anterior serratus weak. He then began to palpate or firmly massage the beginnings (origins) and ends (insertions) of this muscle, and in so doing found a series of hard little beads or muscle knots. As he palpated more firmly, the knots disappeared. Goodheart went along both ends of the muscle (the origin

and the insertion) and pressed all the knots until they disappeared. Then he again had the man push against the wall. This time, the scapula sat correctly. Further, when the anterior serratus muscle was manually retested it could now develop a plus five lock. Even more significantly, the function of the muscle seemed to be permanently restored.[7] In short, muscle testing was proving not only to be a diagnostic tool but also to have therapeutic value.

It had become evident to Goodheart that a relationship between organs and muscles existed, but the exact mechanism of this relationship eluded him. A friend gave him a book about acupuncture written by Felix Mann, M.D., and he was intrigued by Mann's description of the relationship between the visceral organs and acupuncture points. Goodheart researched the relationship between the sedation and tonification points of acupuncture and muscle function, and how these acupoints could be used to restore normal muscle function. He published a paper on this in 1966, at a time when there was little interest in the subject. Goodheart saw that this was another diagnostic and therapeutic tool that could be verified by muscle testing, and observed that while the Chinese practiced acupuncture, there were other Asian practitioners, notably those practicing Japanese acupuncture, who did not use needles but rather a variety of means to stimulate the acupoints, including finger pressure. Goodheart then proposed that digital pressure was adequate stimulation for the diagnosis and treatment of various conditions, as he established the relationship of acupuncture point stimulation using muscle testing.

By integrating the acupuncture meridian system and its organ–meridian relationship into a muscle-testing context, Goodheart made the seminal breakthrough that remains the centerpiece of all Energetic Kinesiologies: the muscle–meridian–organ (and later from his research, –gland) matrix. Thus, the tried-and-trialed thousands-of-years-old system of the Chinese was integrated into modern western physiology and now accessed through the unique feedback of muscle testing.

By synthesizing his discoveries, Goodheart

pioneered a system that brought together work done by his predecessors: Chapman's points (for lymphatic function); Bennett's points (for vascular function); his own origin–insertion technique (for muscular problems); cranial bone manipulation, after William Sutherland, D.O.; the work of upper cervical specialist Leon Lewis Truscott, D.C., Ph.D., on which he based his article *Vertebral challenge methods*, published in 1972; and his work on the muscle–acupuncture meridian–organ relationship using muscle testing feedback for both diagnosis and therapeutic efficacy. This marked the beginnings of the new science of Applied Kinesiology.

Applied Kinesiology

As interest in Applied Kinesiology expanded from George Goodheart's lectures, Applied Kinesiology study groups led by his best students formed throughout the USA. Initially, there were six of Goodheart's protégés who would gather at his practice, and over time they set up study groups. In 1973, there was a gathering of these study group leaders, who became known as the Dirty Dozen. As time passed, they grew to 28 but strangely continued to be called the Dirty Dozen.[8]

In the late 1960s, when the West was just beginning to explore the ideas filtering through from Asia, he began to read the Chinese medical literature that detailed the ancient knowledge of the acupuncture meridian system, the system the Chinese claimed mapped the flow of energy through the body.[9]

Goodheart found that when muscles did not respond either to origin–insertion stimulation or to Chapman's or Bennett's reflex points, by holding specific acupuncture points the weakened muscles would often strengthen. Again, there was a relationship between a specific muscle response and a specific meridian. In 1966, he wrote a research manual on strengthening muscles by holding finger contacts on acupuncture points called *tonification points*.[10]

Goodheart began to recognize that there is an extraordinary complex of inter-relationships linking muscle response with imbalances in the muscular system, the lymphatic system, the vascular system, and even the more esoteric energy systems of Chinese medicine. Because each muscle and reflex point reflects the state of balance of a particular organ system (such as the PMC relating to the stomach), and because the Chinese had named their meridians after the organ with which they were associated, Goodheart, in a flash of insight, realized that the organ was the key in this relationship.

When an organ system is stressed (diseased), the muscle may develop an imbalance (weakness), the Chapman reflex point may become tender, the Bennett reflex point may become active and the associated meridian flow may be disturbed. The brilliant melding of all these observations became the muscle–organ/gland–meridian complex, the core concept of Applied Kinesiology.

Essentially, Goodheart had started at the most physical level of knotted muscles and tender reflex points and moved to more subtle responses of reflex points that needed only light touch. Then, he had entered the more esoteric domain of energy. At this level, it is possible to effect change merely by touching the meridian.

The Chinese system had given Goodheart a layout of thousands of years of empirical observations about the energetic system and the principles by which it works. To this body of knowledge Goodheart added the muscle response correlation, which meant that the energy balance of these meridians and their associated organs could be quickly and consistently ascertained by direct muscle feedback. According to Goodheart, it remains one of the West's few contributions to the East in terms of the application of energetic techniques.

The Chinese method of accessing energy imbalances in the body was written down in the *Huang Di Nei Ching* or *Yellow Emperor's Inner Classic of Medicine* between the first century BC and the early first century AD, based on a thousand years of accumulated knowledge.[11] Yet as the system was based on reading subtle energetic states of the wrist pulse, it was very intuitive and took many years to master as a diagnostic art. Goodheart had tapped into the same energy systems but now could access these systems very quickly through the instant biofeedback afforded by using muscle testing as the diagnostic tool.

Touch for Health

Another member of the Dirty Dozen was chiropractor Dr John Thie, who saw the synthesis of western and eastern knowledge as very exciting. It strengthened his belief that people should be able to take care of their own health, and that the West should change the foundation of its health system from crisis management to prevention. He also versed himself in the Chinese system and realized that if everyone could balance their own energy on a regular basis, they might be able to maintain their own health more effectively. Thie took the basic techniques that had been worked out in Applied Kinesiology and developed a new system that he called *Touch for Health*.[12]

Thie's view was that too seldom in western society are we touched for health, because generally touch is seen to have negative or sexual connotations. In fact, touching is one of the most healing things one human being can do for another. If I sit across a room and listen to your story or your problems, I can empathize with you. But how much more secure will you feel, and how much more will you feel my empathy, if I am holding your hand? When I touch you, you can feel the sincerity of my words. You can feel my empathy and energy. Everyone knows that touch is a real experience. In fact, today it is recognized that touch is healing and releases oxytocin, the healing hormone.[13]

Within the constructs of western medicine that prevailed when Thie was introducing his system, doctors were supposed to be cool, analytical, technical, white-coated and separate. They certainly were not supposed to touch someone in a feeling way, because that would potentially detract from their ability to diagnose objectively. Touch for Health was therefore seen as a fringe therapy of the early 1970s.

Despite considerable opposition, Thie wanted to teach lay people so that they could balance their own health as well as the health of their family and their close friends. So he started to teach the basic principles of Touch for Health in workshops that could be taken over a couple of weekends. In essence, he taught the procedure known as the 14 Muscle Balance, which assesses the balance of energy in the 14 major meridians that are related to specific organs.

In the 14 Muscle Balance procedure, a muscle, representative of each meridian, was manually assessed for its state of balanced function. If the muscle was found to be weak, the basic techniques developed by George Goodheart (origin–insertion, Chapman and Bennett reflex points and meridian tracing), were then employed to strengthen the weakened muscle. Once all 14 muscles were balanced, meridian energies were also balanced, restoring the balance of yin and yang in the body. Often, this very simple system could produce profoundly positive health outcomes.

Thie started teaching his system in California. It quickly spread throughout the USA and from there to many other countries across the world. Now there are millions of people in more than 50 countries who know about Touch for Health and who can practice it with great effect. Not only that, but Touch for Health made the basic techniques of Applied Kinesiology available to ordinary people.

Clinical Kinesiology

One of George Goodheart's most brilliant protégés, Dr Alan Beardall, made several crucial discoveries that added additional tools to the developing field of kinesiology. While treating a famous marathon runner, Beardall discovered that individual muscles did not all function as one unit, but rather that many muscles had functionally unique divisions. He found that although a muscle may test strong, when one or a combination of its divisions were monitored, individual divisions of this strong muscle might test weak or 'unlock'.[14]

From 1975, through extensive anatomical study, clinical observation and testing procedures, Beardall identified these functional divisions within muscles, developed specific muscle tests for each division, and also isolated reflex points that differentiated these muscle divisions as unique functional units. He discovered more than 250 specific muscle tests isolating divisions of the major muscles of the body, and published his exciting findings in 1980.[15] He was eventually to publish five volumes of muscle testing instruction books,[16] and from this body of knowledge Beardall developed a new kinesiology modality he called *Clinical Kinesiology*.

Beardall was also the originator of the concept of the body as a 'biocomputer'. This concept has proven to be a powerful model for many aspects of the subconscious functions that can be tapped into by muscle monitoring.[17] The subconscious appears to process data in a binary way. Indeed, neurons running the muscles can only fire or not fire, lock or unlock. A lock in a muscle test thus indicates 'Yes, I am in balance; there is not enough stress to impede my function', while an unlock response indicates 'No, I am unbalanced; there is too much stress for me to work properly'.

More importantly, this simple 'yes' or 'no' response of the muscle is the summation of *all* the factors influencing the brain and central nervous system, from the level of your structural alignment to your nutritional and emotional status. In addition, the subconscious readout of muscle function is the interface with the other energy systems of the body, including the meridian systems. As such, these 'yes' or 'no' responses can also indicate states of energetic balance.

Beardall also developed several other innovative concepts that have become fundamental in the application of all the Energetic Kinesiology systems developed to this day. In 1983, he discovered what the yogis called *mudras* and what he termed *hand modes*. When the thumb is held to specific fingers and specific places on individual fingers, the yogis claimed it created a frequency related to a specific psychoemotional state.

Beardall found that hand modes related specific thumb-and-finger combinations to specific types or domains of imbalance within the physical body. His research found that each finger, when held pad to pad with the thumb, represented a major domain of energy flow: thumb to index finger responded to structural stresses, thumb to middle finger responded to nutritional stresses, thumb to

ring finger responded to emotional stresses, and thumb to little finger responded to energetic stresses such as meridian ch'i imbalances.

Beardall also developed another technique central to current Energetic Kinesiology, a means of retaining energetic information over time based on the sensory output of sensors in the hip joints. While he originally called this procedure *lock and advance*, it is now called *pause lock*, *retaining mode*, *circuit mode* or simply *putting an imbalance in circuit*. A description of this mechanism will be provided in chapter 13.[18]

So now, whenever Beardall discovered an imbalance through testing a muscle, he could quickly ascertain the nature of the problem causing that imbalance by using his new hand mode system. Was it emotional, nutritional, structural or energetic? Beardall's hand modes, often called *finger modes* in other kinesiology modalities, along with the complementary technique of retaining energetic information over time by putting it into circuit, are some of the most important tools used in modern Energetic Kinesiology systems.[19]

Once the muscle tests, reflex points and concepts developed in Applied Kinesiology and Clinical Kinesiology, both chiropractic fields, reached the public through Touch for Health, there was a great flurry of creative activity as new kinesiology systems were developed by innovative individuals from a diverse range of backgrounds.

Energetic Kinesiology

From these beginnings, kinesiology has blossomed to become a diversity of different types of kinesiology-based treatments. These new systems were developed by people who saw the incredible potential of the techniques, because they were not generally locked within the rigid western medical and physiological models.

While in Academic Kinesiology you are indeed testing a muscle for strength, in the more recently developed kinesiology systems the muscle response is used primarily as a form of biofeedback. Hence, in these systems you are monitoring, not testing, muscle function. The redefinition of the term *muscle testing* to *muscle monitoring* is to denote that we are now accessing only the integrity of the muscle response, and not its strength.[20]

The truly amazing aspect of muscle monitoring is that the response can indicate a wide variety of possible stressors. The muscle being monitored may respond by unlocking because of a physical factor (a sore muscle, for example), because of a disturbance in the function of its related organ system (blocked or restricted lymph or blood flow), because of a disturbance in its associated meridian (blocked energy flow), or because of a disturbing emotion or thought.[21]

If we monitor a muscle and it is strong and locks, and then ask a person to think about their mother, the muscle may suddenly give or unlock. This indicates to the kinesiologist that something has interfered with the integrity of the neurological flow between the muscle and the central nervous system, preventing normal muscle function. This interference may have come from whatever stress mother set up within this person's mind and body.

Your conscious brain may tell you that you and your mother get on famously. But when you consider that a stressor is not always conscious, and may often be held within the subconscious, which is also wired directly to the muscles, this previously undetected subconscious stress can be the factor that blocks neurological flow, disrupting the integrity of muscle function. This informs both the practitioner and the client that there is a stress around the client's mother, most probably related to an unresolved issue that occurred when the client was growing up, most often in early childhood.

This access into the usually inaccessible realms of your subconscious is one of the most powerful aspects of Energetic Kinesiology as it is now practiced. Something that you think can be instantly detected as a stressor within your physical–emotional being, and it may be something your conscious brain was never aware of until the muscle response made you aware of it. Further, the use of finger or hand modes allows a kinesiologist to identify the exact nature of that subconscious stress. Thus Energetic Kinesiology allows us to eavesdrop on our subconscious.

Biokinesiology

One of the first people to recognize this aspect of Energetic Kinesiology was a health practitioner in Southern California, John Barton. After the death of one of his children, Barton realized that western medicine did not hold all the answers, and he turned down a scholarship to the Massachusetts Institute of Technology. Instead, he launched into a career in holistic health, studying foot reflexology, acupressure, herbs and natural childbirth.

In the mid 1970s, Barton saw a demonstration of Applied Kinesiology on television and was hooked. Kinesiology became his tool to determine how the body could be balanced through massage, acupressure, position-releasing postures, nutrition and emotions. Out of this vast body of research developed another new field: Biokinesiology.[22]

Edu-K and Brain Gym

Another person in the 1970s whose life was changed by kinesiology was Dr Paul Dennison, a very dyslexic individual who was incapable of learning in the traditional educational system. Like so many others, he started innocently enough by attending a Touch for Health course.

The instructor showed him *cross-crawl* or *cross-patterning*, which is marching on the spot, moving opposite arms and legs in unison. He then demonstrated *homolateral crawl*, or marching on the spot with the same side arm and leg moving in unison. Dennison gained great benefit from these techniques and from the application of another Touch for Health technique called *Emotional Stress Release* (ESR).

In ESR, while the subject thinks of a stressful issue, gentle finger pressure is applied to the frontal eminences, the broad bumps on the forehead above the eyes. This appears to help return blood flow to the frontal lobes, which are our centers of thinking and new learning. When a person is stressed, blood flow is largely withdrawn from these regions and redirected to the subconscious survival centers. But when touch is applied to these points until subtle pulses are felt beneath the fingertips on the forehead, the emotional charge in the previously stressful situation is usually reduced or eliminated.

At the time, Dr Dennison was working with children with learning disabilities, and when he employed these same techniques with his students, he discovered that their learning abilities also improved. Inspired by these changes, Dennison developed further applications of kinesiology to create a kinesiology system that he initially called Educational Kinesiology and was later called Edu-K, or Edu-Kinesthetics, for working with children and adults with learning problems.[23]

Dennison perceived that learning problems lay in improper coordination of brain activity, and he developed a series of movement exercises, many of which were based on standard yoga *asanas* or postures, to reintegrate brain function. To these movement exercises he added several acupressure techniques and several standard remedial education techniques. He called his synthesis Brain Gym.[24] When Brain Gym exercises were practised regularly, they stimulated integrated brain function and thus greatly improved learning potential.

Three In One Kinesiology

In the cascade of discovery, Dennison's system spawned yet another form of kinesiology, created by Gordon Stokes, Candace Callaway and Daniel Whiteside. Stokes had been instructor–trainer for Touch for Health in the USA, and in an inspired collaboration with Callaway and Whiteside produced a creative amalgamation of concepts from a number of other kinesiology modalities including Edu-K, Touch for Health, Applied Kinesiology, Applied Physiology and psychotherapeutic practices. The partners called their system Three In One or One Brain Kinesiology and applied it to dyslexia, learning problems and emotional stress that had not been resolved by other methods.[25]

In the One Brain model, unresolved emotional stress was the basis of most learning problems, as unresolved emotions were shown to have the ability to block our learning as well as our personal growth and emotional and spiritual development. The threesome went on to develop much more in-depth emotional defusion techniques based on

ESR but which they named *Emotional Stress Defusion.*

The name change was important, because it indicated that the new method was not just the release of emotions but served to defuse and then reintegrate unresolved emotions into our lives. What was vital about this technique was that it facilitated greater choice. To get even deeper and be more precise about the nature of unresolved emotional issues, the group also added age recession techniques, as many of our deepest unresolved emotional issues originate in childhood, especially between 18 months and 5 years of age.

Applied Physiology

In the early 1980s, Richard Utt, an expert in electronic aircraft guidance systems, added to the growing number of kinesiology systems by developing Applied Physiology. Applied Physiology was based on an in-depth understanding of both western physiology and the Law of Five Elements of Chinese acupuncture. Utt developed a kinesiology-based acupressure application of the Law of Five Elements and the acupressure based technique called the Seven Ch'i Keys, to correct imbalances in the energy centers that the yogis called the *chakra* system.[26]

Utt's system allows the practitioner to determine which of two equally valid energy pathways within the Five Element system would most effectively equalize the energy and release stress, and thereby promote healing for the client. Utt also formulated the Seven Element Hologram, which is based on the holographic supertheory proposed by physicist David Bohm and neuroscientist Carl Pribram.[27] This is a single integrated kinesiology system capable of accessing all levels of the human hologram from the physical level, including the muscles, individual cells and subcellular functions, all the way through the levels of emotion and thought to the level of our attitudes, our essential beliefs.

Other types of kinesiology

As you can see by the incredible trajectory of this healing science, many other types of kinesiology have been developed and are still developing throughout the world. It is an incredible blossoming of knowledge. This science, which is a unique marriage of ancient eastern esoteric sciences with the modern physiology and physics of the West, is now in a stage of tremendously exciting fermentation. Kinesiology provides access to the holographic or whole body: the mind, the spirit, the emotions and the physical being—in essence, all the realms of being that can impact on our health. As such, it is a truly remarkable healing tool.

The Energetic Kinesiology modality tree

In the years following the initial development of Energetic Kinesiology, beginning with Touch for Health and Clinical Kinesiology, there was an explosion of different types of kinesiology modalities based on energetic techniques. Today, there

are over 40 different kinesiology-based modalities. Many of these kinesiology modalities have rigorous foundations. However, that is not the case for all of them.

While many kinesiology modalities continue to be taught in an informal workshop system, there is an increasing trend toward more comprehensive multiyear integrated trainings. At this time, kinesiology is a developing profession, and the trend toward more rigorous training is essential if kinesiology is to take its place as an effective health care modality.

The kinesiology modality tree presented in Figure 2.1 is the core set of Energetic Kinesiology modalities that evolved from Dr Goodheart, Dr Thie and Dr Beardall's original work. This tree is not meant to be a comprehensive presentation of all the current kinesiology modalities, as there are many other limbs and branches that are continually being added.

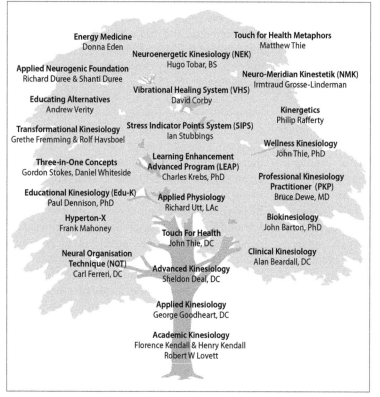

Figure 2.1 The Energetic Kinesiology modality tree. Since George Goodheart did the first kinesiology muscle test linking muscle biofeedback to the Chinese acupressure meridian system in the mid 1960s, Energetic Kinesiology as a field has grown rapidly, with new modalities of Energetic Kinesiology being developed over time. The modality tree we present here is not meant to be a comprehensive list of all the current Energetic Kinesiology modalities, but rather is a selection of core Energetic Kinesiologies from which the majority of other Energetic Kinesiology modalities originated.

Energy Medicine
Donna Eden

Touch for Health Metaphors
Matthew Thie

Neuroenergetic Kinesiology (NEK)
Hugo Tobar, BS

Applied Neurogenic Foundation
Richard Duree & Shanti Duree

Neuro-Meridian Kinestetik (NMK)
Irmtraud Grosse-Linderman

Vibrational Healing System (VHS)
David Corby

Educating Alternatives
Andrew Verity

Kinergetics
Philip Rafferty

Transformational Kinesiology
Grethe Fremming & Rolf Havsboel

Stress Indicator Points System (SIPS)
Ian Stubbings

Wellness Kinesiology
John Thie, PhD

Three-in-One Concepts
Gordon Stokes, Daniel Whiteside

Learning Enhancement
Advanced Program (LEAP)
Charles Krebs, PhD

Professional Kinesiology
Practitioner (PKP)
Bruce Dewe, MD

Educational Kinesiology (Edu-K)
Paul Dennison, PhD

Applied Physiology
Richard Utt, LAc

Biokinesiology
John Barton, PhD

Hyperton-X
Frank Mahoney

Touch For Health
John Thie, DC

Clinical Kinesiology
Alan Beardall, DC

Neural Organisation
Technique (NOT)
Carl Ferreri, DC

Advanced Kinesiology
Sheldon Deal, DC

Applied Kinesiology
George Goodheart, DC

Academic Kinesiology
Florence Kendall & Henry Kendall
Robert W Lovett

References

1. Legg, AT & Merrill JB 1932, Physical therapy in infantile paralysis. In: Legg, AT & Merrill JB, eds. *Principles and Practice of Physical Therapy, Volume II*, Mock Pemberton & Coulter, Hagerstown, p. 45.

2. Kendall, HO & Kendall FP 1949, *Muscles: Testing and Function*, Williams & Wilkins, Baltimore.
   Kendall, HO & Kendall, FP 1938, Case during recovery period of paralytic polio myelitis, *US Public Health Bulletin*, no.242.
   Kendall, HO & Kendall, FP 1946, Physical therapy for lower extremity amputation, *War Department Technical Manual*, Government Printing Office, Washington, pp. 8–293.

3. Guyton, AC 1991, *Textbook of Medical Physiology, Eighth edition*. WB Saunders, Philadelphia, pp. 170–184.

4. Owen, C 1937, *An Endocrine Interpretation of Chapman's Reflexes, Based on Chapman and Owen's Research at the Kirksville College of Osteopathy and Surgery*, privately published.
   Walther, DS 1981, *Applied Kinesiology, Volume I: Basic Procedure and Muscle Testing*, Systems DC, Pueblo, pp. 220–223.

5. Martin, RJ, ed., 1977, *Dynamics of Correction of Abnormal Function from Terence Bennett Lectures*, privately published, RJ Martin DC, Sierra Madre.

6. Goodheart, GJ 1981, *Applied Kinesiology, Fourth Edition*, privately published, Detroit.
   Walther, DS 1981, *Applied Kinesiology, Volume I: Basic Procedure and Muscle Testing*, Systems DC, Pueblo, pp. 234–239.

7. Goodheart, GJ 1986, *You'll Be Better: The Story of Applied Kinesiology*, AK Printing, Geneva, pp. 2.
   Walther, DS 1988, *Applied Kinesiology: Synopsis, Second Edition*, Systems DC, Pueblo.

8. Gin, RH & Green, BN 1997, George Goodheart, Jr., D.C., and a history of Applied Kinesiology, *Journal of Manipulative and Physiological Therapeutics*, Vol. 20(5), pp. 331–337.

9. Mann, F 1962, *Acupuncture: The Ancient Chinese Art of Healing and How it Works Scientifically*, Random House, New York.

10. Goodheart, GJ 1966, Chinese lessons for Chiropractic, *Digest of Chiropractic Economics*, Vol. 8(5), pp. 10–11.

11. Chang, ST 1976, *The Complete Book of Acupuncture*, Celestial Arts, Berkeley, p. 3.
    Xinnong, C, ed., *Chinese Acupuncture and Moxibustion*, Foreign Language Press, Beijing, pp. 1–2.

12. Thie, JF 1979, *Touch for Health*, De Voross, Marina del Rey.

13. Siegel, B 1990, *Love, Medicine and Miracles*, HarperCollins Publishers, New York.

14. Levy, SL & Lehr, C 1996, *Your Body Can Talk*, Hohm Press, Prescott, pp. 4–5.

15. Beardall, AG 1980, 'Differentiating the muscles of the lower back and abdomen', *selected paper of the International College of Applied Kinesiology*, International College of Applied Kinesiology.

16. Beardall, AG 1985, *Clinical Kinesiology, Volumes I–V*, Beardall, DC, Lake Oswego.

17. Beardall, AG 1982, *Clinical Kinesiology, Volume III: TMJ, Hyoid Muscles and Other Cervical Muscles Including Cranial Manipulation*, Beardall DC, Lake Oswego, pp. 2–4.

18. Utt, R 1997, *Stress: The Nature of the Beast*, Applied Physiology Publishing, Tucson, pp. 43–44.
    Dickson, GJ 1990, *What is Kinesiology?*, IHK Publishing, Melbourne, p. 58.

19. Beardall, AG 1982, *Clinical Kinesiology, Volume III: TMJ, Hyoid Muscles and Other Cervical Muscles Including Cranial Manipulation*, Beardall DC, Lake Oswego, pp. 2–4.
    Dickson, GJ 1990, *What is Kinesiology?*, IHK Publishing, Melbourne, pp. 58–60.

20. Walther, DS 1981, *Applied Kinesiology, Volume I: Basic Procedure and Muscle Testing*, Systems DC, Pueblo, pp. 1–5.
    Utt, R 1997, *Stress: The Nature of the Beast*, Applied Physiology Publishing, Tucson, pp. 23–28.

21. Krebs, CT 1997, 'The emotional control of muscle response: why your arm goes weak when you think a negative thought' in *Proceedings of the Fourth International Kinesiology Conference*, Zurich.

22. Barton, J 1986, *Encyclopedia of Mind and Body, Volumes I–VI and VIII*, Biokinesiology Institute, Shade Cove.

23. Parker, A & Cutler-Stuart, J 1986, *Switch on Your Brain*, Hale & Ironmonger, Petersham.
    Hannaford, C 1995, *Smart Moves*, Great Ocean Publishers, Arlington.

24. Dennison, P & Dennison, GE 1994, *Brain Gym, Teachers' Edition, Revised*, Edu-Kinesthetics,Ventura.
    Hannaford, C 1995, *Smart Moves*, Great Ocean Publishers, Arlington, pp. 108–129.

25. Stokes, G & Whiteside, D 1984, *One Brain: Dyslexia Learning Connection and Brain Integration*, Three in One Concepts, Burbank.
    Stokes, G & Whiteside D 1985, *Structural Neurology*, Three in One Concepts, Burbank.

26. Utt, RD 1989, *The Law of Five Elements*, International Institute of Applied Physiology, Tuscon.
    Utt, RD 1985, *The Seven Chi Keys*, Applied Physiology Printing, Tucson.

27. Wilber, K, ed. 1982, *The Holographic Paradigm and Other Paradoxes*, New Science Library, Massachusetts, pp. 68–79.
    Talbot, M 1991, *The Holographic Universe*, Grafton Books, London.

SECTION II

The energetic structures of Man

In order to understand Energetic Kinesiology, it is necessary to have an overview of the major energy systems of the body and how these interface to produce our physiology, feelings, thinking and higher states of spiritual awareness. Indeed, every aspect of our experience is expressed in each of these different levels. For instance, when you have a thought it automatically generates a feeling state that is expressed as an emotion, which at the same time creates a physiological state that may then alter your muscle tone and even your posture.

In the modern western perspective, human beings are considered to be purely physical beings possessing a physiology, emotions and thoughts that are generated by our complex nervous system. While it is recognized that people have spiritual beliefs, these are considered to be outside the realm of scientific investigation. In contrast, older western traditions and all eastern traditions continuing to the present day perceive Man to be a multidimensional being consisting not only of the physical body but also of energetic bodies that interpenetrate and extend beyond the physical body. This multidimensional being is considered to be Man.

Traditionally, this multidimensional body is composed of a very dense energetic body called the *etheric body*, which is then fully integrated with our physical body. Interpenetrating this physical–etheric body and extending beyond it is the *astral body*, the body that is most affected by emotions and emotional states. Interpenetrating and

extending even further beyond the physical body is the *mental body*, the body most affected by our thoughts. In the eastern and older western traditions, there is even a more expansive energetic body called the *causal* or *spiritual body*, which while penetrating the physical body extends well beyond our physical being. Depending on the specific tradition, the layers of our multidimensional body are subdivided and grouped in various ways. What we are presenting in this section is a simplified but cohesive model of the multidimensional bodies of Man, which collectively are called the *aura*.

Many traditions recognize that these various bodies have a coherent structure that is supported by various energy systems of the body. In the ayurvedic tradition developed on the Indian subcontinent, the primary energy system recognized was the *chakra–nadi system*, which interpenetrates all the auric bodies. In contrast, in China the focus was predominantly on the energetic system of the etheric body, called the *acupuncture meridian system*. The Tibetans recognized the acupuncture system of the Chinese and practiced their own unique form of acupuncture; they also recognized another traditional energetic system called the *figure 8 energy flows*. Figure 8 flows are an interface between the etheric and the higher energy bodies of Man. Each of these energetic structures and systems will be discussed in greater detail in this section.

The first of these energy systems introduced to kinesiology was the Chinese acupuncture meridian system. In Applied Kinesiology, Dr Goodheart introduced the meridian alarm points as a mechanism for locating which organ system and its related muscles may be involved in a particular imbalance by using muscle monitoring. In Applied Kinesiology, kinesiologists also introduced a way of applying the Law of Five Elements, the primary rules for energy flow within the meridian system, by using muscle biofeedback rather than the use of pulse points, as in traditional Chinese acupuncture. Over time, those developing various kinesiology modalities focused more and more on the interface of muscle monitoring with these various energy systems, and they established mechanisms of detecting stressors affecting these energy systems by using muscle monitoring.

Indeed, what makes Energetic Kinesiology *kinesiology* and *energetic* is the combination of muscle monitoring and various techniques for accessing these traditional energy systems of the body. Therefore in this section we provide a concise overview of these traditional energy systems and the rules and principles by which they work. This background is necessary to understand the techniques and the mechanisms underlying their use in future sections of the book.

Chapter 3

A HISTORICAL PERSPECTIVE

Man has long sought an understanding of how the world works, and all cultures have developed a perspective or worldview, now called a *paradigm*. The ancient worldview from approximately 150,000 years ago began with the rise of modern man, *Homo sapiens*. This view still persists in many indigenous cultures today: that our world is alive with energy; that all things have an energetic aspect, not only plants and animals but also the earth and air.

Early western view

The western view of our world has two distinct phases: the early view and the modern view. The early western view, like the eastern view, was largely phenomenological and based on observation of the natural world. It was clear to our ancestors that the world is full of forces that cause actions to occur and that a special vital force animates living organisms, hence the term *animism*. However, in the western view Man always stood apart and to a degree separate from the other animals and plants, as only he appears to be able to possess sophisticated communication of speech and be conscious of himself, and thus be able to control the environment in ways no other living organism appears capable of. Most importantly, only he appears to be able to have a personal relationship with a higher power, or powers, that control him and the world.

Initially in the western view, there were many gods with fairly human personalities but possessing superhuman powers, whom mankind had to appease so as not to experience the wrath of these often vengeful and angry gods lurking in an unseen world. However, these gods had a hierarchy, with normally a supreme god more powerful than the rest; for the Greeks, this was Zeus, and for the Romans, Jupiter. This was a largely mysterious world populated by powerful unseen forces that controlled mankind. In Europe and the Middle East, these polytheistic views gave way to a mono-theistic view with the life of Jesus Christ and then later, Muhammad.

The early Greeks developed the pondering on the nature of the world and Man's place in it into a science called *philosophy*. Then all further western thinking was based on the work of these early Greek philosophers and their deductive intel-lectual process. One of the most famous of these philosophers was Plato, and Platonism reigned from antiquity until well into the early Renaissance. The core belief of Platonism was that the world of form, the material world of the five senses, is an imprecise material representation of ideal forms, or *plata*, that exist in a non-material and timeless dimension.

The immaterial plata in Plato's view are the source of the *real* things in our world, because the shape of material objects is dependent on the information contained in the plata, of which the physical object is but an imperfect copy. If couched in more modern terms, you could say that the plata provide the energy template guiding the construction of the physical object or thing.

A later contemporary of Plato, the great healer and philosopher Hippocrates, developed vitalism to its highest form in the ancient world. The Hippocratic school saw healing arising from natural adaptive powers within the organism, the *physis*. In Hippocratic thought, the physis was perceived as a healing power or self-adjusting power within the body that 'though untaught and uninstructed, it does what is proper to preserve a perfect equilibrium'. Physis is also the root of the word *physician*, and in Hippocrates' view, as a guardian of the physis, the physician had a clearly supporting role: 'Not a ruler or violator of nature ... he stands ready to aid the healing power that is inherent.'[1]

In more recent schools of the early view in

western thought, the physis was called vital energy, life energy, *élan vital*, etc., all denoting that this property is essential for life. When there is sufficient physis or vital energy, health is maintained; lack of health is caused primarily by a diminished supply of this essential substance. Again, the non-material, energetic physis was seen to provide an energetic template necessary to maintain physiological health, with blockage of this 'body energy' the primary cause of ill health.

Early eastern view

In the East, the worldview was also phenomenological and based on observation, with a tendency to see the world from a more intuitive, holistic perspective. Like their western counterparts, the earliest eastern views saw Man surrounded by mysterious forces that control people's lives, and as in the West, these forces were usually raised to the mythical status of gods. With the rise of an integrated Chinese society, the emperor was now seen as divine, an earthly representative of a higher force with power over all people. However, this was not so much a monotheistic belief, as in the West, but a unified cosmology in which Man is an important part but not separate from the world; rather, he reflects this world. This is clearly stated in the ancient Chinese adage 'In the macrocosm is the microcosm, and in the microcosm is the macrocosm.'

In the eastern view, the world was seen as being filled with energy, but this energy extends into mankind himself, and in fact it is these flows of energy coursing throughout his physical body that maintain his physical structure and function. And like the early western view, it is these energy flows that maintain health and need to be balanced when sickness invades. Sickness in this model was seen as resulting from a disturbance of the energy flows caused by unknown forces but ascribed to perverse energies and demons.

There were two great eastern traditions—the yogic system, based on flows of pranic energy through the chakra–nadi system, and the ch'i flows through the acupuncture meridian system—which together control what we now call in the West *physiological homeostasis*. In the eastern view, the world of the five senses was not considered primary, as in the West, but rather only an illusion created by our senses, while the primary world was represented by the flows of energy that became manifest as the physical matter we see and feel and the physiology of living organisms.

Therefore, when the physiology becomes disturbed, as evidenced by patterns of disharmony, the proper thing to do was find where the energy underlying these patterns is blocked. Then techniques from the use of foods and herbs to more direct energetic techniques such as needle acupuncture would be employed to release these blockages. Once the energetic block is gone, the energy flows sustaining normal harmonious function are quickly re-established by the natural order, as in the Hippocratic model!

Therefore, the basis of both the eastern view and the early western view of Man and the universe was that the physical world of our senses becomes manifest from unseen energies of the universe, and once manifest as matter they follow natural laws with respect to its structure and function. The human body follows these natural laws that control the manifestation of matter from these underlying energetic systems. Disease results where these manifesting energies are blocked, and healing in these models results from removal of these blocks, allowing the energies to flow according to the natural laws that 'though untaught and uninstructed, do what is proper to preserve a perfect equilibrium.'

The primary differences between the eastern and early western views of Man in the universe were the different perspectives of Man in relationship to the universe, and Man's role in the universe based on the place of Man in relationship to theology and cosmology. In the East, the interpretation of phenomenological observations was based on inductive reasoning from patterns of harmony and symmetry in which Man is firmly embedded in the structure of the universe. But Man also reflects the structure of the universe and is controlled by the natural laws governing the universe. This eastern view, although not analytical, was no less logical than the western view, as it was very rule-based and internally consistent.

From the cosmological perspective of the East, Man was seen as an integrated unit comprising immaterial spirit and mind together with its material manifestation, the physical body, which are linked by the continual flows of energy into body–mind–spirit. Disease was thus perceived as distortions or blocks in the flows of the energies linking the body to its mind and spirit, therefore healing is best accomplished by restoring these flows of energy to their former harmonious patterns.

Development of the modern western view

In contrast, from the time of the Greeks to the present day, in the West the original phenomenological observations of our universe were evaluated from a deductive reasoning to understand how these natural laws might work to produce the world and universe we see. So the dominant view of the universe and how our world contained within it worked was based on logic. From this deductive linear perspective, the world follows mathematical rules and laws that can explain not only how it works but also make predictions about that which is not yet observed or known.

At the same time, the immaterial mind was considered separate from the material, physical body, permitting the body to be taken apart and understood from the deductive perspective of ever smaller pieces making up the whole. Disease was increasingly seen as being caused by specific identifiable disease entities which we now call germs (bacteria and viruses), or the physical disruptions of the microsystems making up a human body. Healing was the application of treatments considered logical and rational based on the current medical model.

From the western theological perspective, Man was created separate from the universe by his personal creator. Mankind's destiny is then to rule over the world created for him, and control not only his own fate but the fate of the world around him. With the separation of mind and body at the end of the medieval era, the immaterial mind and soul became the providence of organised religions and the body the providence of the physical sciences.

Sometime between the 13th and 15th centuries, the deductive principles of science were increasingly applied to understand our world. By the 17th and 18th centuries, the increasing application of the developing sciences of physics and mathematics to solve practical problems began the industrial revolution. Technology and science were increasingly used to solve physical problems of the production and harvesting of food and the manufacture of material goods, as well as the transportation of both food and goods to markets far from their source of origin. Then, in 1687, Isaac Newton, foreshadowed in the preceding century by Copernicus, Kepler and others, had his glorious insight: the universe is governed by a few physical, mechanical and mathematical laws. With these advances, the early western view gave way to the developing modern western view of the world and universe in which we live.

This new view was based on two things: 1, that the secrets of the universe could be unravelled by Man because they had been implanted by a reliable and all-powerful God whose perfect creation only awaited Man's discovery of the rules governing this creation, including Man himself; and 2, that the creator had given Man rational reason and science to understand the universe. This instilled tremendous confidence that everything made rational sense, everything should fit together, and everything could be proved and improved by science.

The reason this arose so rapidly in the West was precisely because Christianity provided the rational God who created an understandable universe and gave Man the ability to understand His natural laws, unlike other religions in other areas of the world, in which there was no consistently rational creator and the universe remained inexplicable and unpredictable. Over the course of the next two centuries, following Newton's discoveries and the further development of modern science, the modern western scientific view of the universe developed to the point that by the end of the 19th century physicists were making the statements that there was nothing left to discover and all that remained was working out the details!

This smug view of Man's understanding of the universe rapidly unravelled in the beginning of the 20th century, first with Einstein's discovery and mathematical proof of the law of relativity, making strange and almost incomprehensible predictions about the behavior of the universe at the macro level, and second, with the development of quantum mechanics, which described an ever more puzzling micro level ruled by mystery hypothetical subatomic particles, uncertainty and chance. The highly rational and understandable clockwork universe of Newton was replaced by a universe that is not only stranger than we think but stranger than we *can* think![2]

Table 3.1 summarizes the development of Man's perspective and understanding of himself and the universe in which he lives. It is interesting to note that both the eastern view and the early western views arose from the unified primitive view of a world full of unseen forces in a universe that is both unpredictable and incomprehensible. They also maintained similar perspectives on the structure of this world: 1, the physical world is manifest from immaterial energetic templates representing the perfect form of things; 2, the harmonious functioning of Man results from energy flows following natural laws, and disruptions of these energy flows lead to disease and physiological dysfunction, which can be eliminated by the re-establishment of these flows; and 3, human consciousness and intent are an important component in affecting the re-establishment of these healing flows of energy.

Beginning with the development of western science and mathematics at the end of the medieval era, the modern western view of a physical world governed by rational laws and models that predict how the world worked rapidly displaced the early western view of Man as an energetic being sustained by immaterial energy flows and the innate wisdom of the body. In its place was Man as a physical, mechanical being based purely on measurable physiological parameters that needed to be fixed from the outside, often in the modern medicine view by the addition of drugs and the mechanical alterations of surgery.

Interestingly, the modern quantum view of the forces and operations of the universe are beginning to sound more and more like the original eastern view, just using different words and concepts in their expression. A major difference is that the quantum view is based on western mathematical models that have been tested experimentally rather than the more intuitive 'knowing' of the models developed in the East.

References

1. Maxwell, H & Selwyn, S 1947, *A History of Medicine*, Alfred A. Knopf, New York, p. 178.
2. Heisenberg, W 1975, *Across the Frontiers*, Harper & Row, New York.

Table 3.1 Summary of different worldviews: paradigm of Man and the universe[a]

	Early western view (~5000 BC to 1200 AD)	Eastern view (~5000 BC to present)	Modern western view (~1200 AD to early 1900 AD)
Worldview paradigm	Phenomenological view based on observation, with tendency to see world from a more logical, causal perspective. Man apart from other living things, with relationship to personal gods. Vital force animates living things: animism or vitalism. Greek philosophers' view based on the concepts of ideal forms and flows of the physis or vital energy. This view developed from 500 to 400 BC and was codified in the writings of Plato, Aristotle, Hippocrates and Democritus between 400 and 100 BC. In the West, the Platonic and Hippocratic beliefs dominated the worldview until the Renaissance.	Phenomenological view based on observation, with a tendency to see the world from a more intuitive, holistic perspective. Cosmology reflected in Man: 'In the macrocosm is the microcosm.' • Yogic view: based on the flows of prana (cosmic energy) from the air. This view developed between 5000 and 1500 BC and was codified in the sutras of Patañjali by approximately 1500 BC. • Chinese view: based on the flows of ch'i, Shen and Jing from cosmic energy. This view developed between 3000 and 300 BC and was codified in the *Nei Ching* between 100 BC and 100 AD.	Based on observed physical objects and their properties. The world is seen as being derived from physical matter alone and not incorporating any subtle energetic components. Living organisms, including Man, are just an extension of these physical dimensions, and life is maintained by biochemical systems. This view started with the Renaissance and the development of the scientific method. From repeated observations of a limited number of factors (reductionism), models were created (described by mathematics) and from these models predictions were made of future outcomes (using mathematics). When outcomes match predictions, the model is valid.
Basis of the paradigm	There exist non-physical and non-mental forms, ideal forms, that are an absolute and eternal reality of which the phenomena of the world are an imperfect and transitory reflection.	These ancient models of a physical world manifesting from consciousness was confirmed using inductive reasoning from the whole to understand the pieces. This system of using qualitative standards persisted in the East into the past century, with a revival in this century.	Based on the atomic concept of Democritus that there are only physical atoms and empty space. The physical sciences developed following the deductive rules and principles of rational reasoning, using precise measurement to understand how the pieces created the whole.
Origins of the material world	Platonic view: material world originates from the plata or ideal forms that exist only in the non-material world yet manifest as imperfect copies in the material world.	The material world is maya (yogic) or illusion (Zen) and manifests from energetic templates. Yogic view: the material world originates from pure consciousness or the Logos as monads that then manifest as matter. Zen view: the material world originates from No Form (Clear Light Mind) and via the interaction of the two great polarities, yin and yang, that follow the Law of Five Elements manifesting and sustaining physical matter.	Democratic view: there exist only the smallest indivisible units of physical matter in the form of atoms and empty space. During the Renaissance, this view eclipsed the Platonic view, which had dominated since the time of the early Greeks. Newtonian view: describes the sensory world of 'real' physical matter that follows the basic Newtonian linear and logical laws of motion and gravity. In the late 1600s, Newton proposed his three laws of motion.

	Early western view (~5000 BC to 1200 AD)	Eastern view (~5000 BC to present)	Modern western view (~1200 AD to early 1900 AD)
Philosophy of health and healing	The physical world was seen as the representation of the non-material plata or energetic templates, with the physical body maintained by the flow of physis. Physis was perceived as a healing power or self-adjusting power within the body that 'though untaught and unin-structed, does what is proper to preserve a perfect equilibrium'. Physis is the root of the word *physician*. When there is sufficient physis or vital energy, health is maintained; lack of health is caused primarily by a diminished supply of this essential substance.	The physical body was seen as a manifestation of the underlying flows of energy that structure and maintain its coherence, homeostatic function. Yogic view: pranic flows through the chakra–nadi system maintain homeostasis via control of the endocrine and autonomic nervous systems. Chinese view: flows of ch'i through the acupressure–acupuncture system maintain homeostasis via control of the organ systems and secondarily via control of the endocrine and autonomic nervous systems. Health is maintained by the nutritive ch'i or prana distributed via these energy systems.	Believe only in the three-dimensional world of our five senses. Everything is based on solid atoms and electrons and space, which is an empty vacuum. Health and disease are related only to physical anatomy and physiology and the pres-ence or absence of disease enti-ties. When disease entities are present, only physical elements are considered in the creation and treatment of the ailment.
Relation-ship of body and mind	The physical world was seen as the representation of the non-material plata or energetic templates. The physical body is maintained by the flow of physis, an unseen healing power within the body.	Both the yogic and Chinese views held immaterial mind and consciousness the origin of the material world, with no separ-ation; there is only body–mind–spirit.	Descartes solved the body–mind problem by arguing that the mind is immaterial and the realm of the soul, whereas the body is material and therefore an object for experimentation.

[a]The ancient worldview from approximately 150,000 years ago with the rise of modern man, *Homo sapiens*, and still persisting in many indigenous cultures today is that the world is alive with energy: all things have an energetic aspect, not only plants and animals, but also the earth and air. For approximately 700–800 years, the modern western view has prevailed; however, since the 1900s relativity and quantum mechanics have begun to alter the western view.

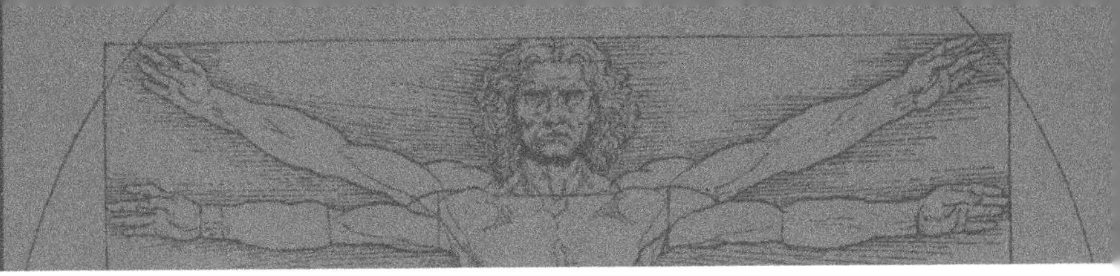

Chapter 4

THE LAYERS OF THE AURA AND OUR MULTIDIMENSIONAL BODY

The physical body

While the physical body is obvious to our physical senses as it can be seen, touched and felt both by ourselves and by others, the subtle bodies creating the layers of our aura are not detectable by our five physical senses. However, many subtle effects can be measured that appear to have no physical source, such as the healing energy of a healer's hands or the instantaneous psychic flow of thoughts from one person to another.

Once we incorporate the subtle bodies of Man into his physical body, we begin to see a multidimensional being. While the physical body is the only body currently recognized in western thought, in the East the subtle bodies associated with this physical body have been very well defined.[1]

In the East, it is generally recognized that humans have a physical body that is surrounded and interpenetrated by at least four other subtle bodies.[2] The other subtle bodies exist at different frequencies of subtle vibration. For instance, as electromagnetic radiation exists over a spectrum of frequencies from microwaves to gamma rays, the magnetoelectric radiation also exists over a frequency range of vibrations, from the lowest vibrations of the etheric to the highest vibrations of the causal or spiritual body. As an analogy, you can think of the piano keyboard with low C, middle C and high C; all are C notes but at very different frequencies. When a high C string is activated strongly, the low C string will also vibrate because of frequency resonance. However, if you are measuring the energy of vibration at the low C frequencies, you are perceiving only a small amount of the energy originally put into the high C string.

Figure 4.1 illustrates the four primary subtle bodies beyond the physical. It should be recognized that this is a highly simplified presentation, in that each of the subtle bodies may have a

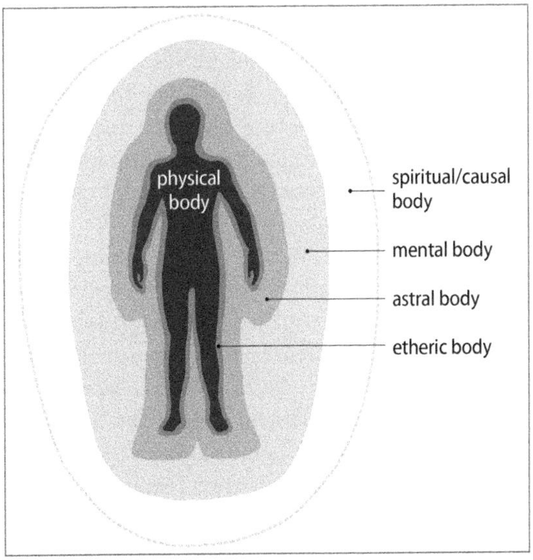

physical body
spiritual/causal body
mental body
astral body
etheric body

Figure 4.1 **The multidimensional human body.**
Interpenetrating and extending beyond the physical body are several subtle energy bodies of Man. The etheric body fits the physical body like a glove fits a hand, while the astral body extends well beyond the etheric body but has a less distinct shape and the mental and spiritual bodies become progressively egg-shaped fields surrounding the other subtle bodies.

number of layers, each with its own unique properties. Also note that while each layer extends beyond the lower, it does not exist just as a layer around the body but rather interpenetrates all the layers below it and then extends further from the physical body than the preceding subtle body.

The etheric body

Interpenetrating and surrounding the physical body like a glove on a hand, the etheric body is the densest of all the subtle bodies.[3] The etheric body is the realm of the acupuncture meridian system and also the subtle body that most directly interfaces with the physical body. In fact, it is within the acupuncture system that the magnetoelectric energy flows such as ch'i are transduced (changed in form) into the electromagnetic energy of the physical body. This forms a primary interface between the electromagnetic flows of the physical body and the subtle energy flows of the other subtle bodies. While acupoints have real electrical properties, they are also the portals and controllers for the flow of vital ch'i in the etheric body.

The astral body

Interpenetrating the physical body and extending beyond the etheric body is the astral body, which is the realm of the emotions.[4] The subtle matter of the astral body is at a higher frequency than the etheric body, and at the level of these frequencies 'like attracts like'. Have you ever noticed that when you are angry it attracts more anger, and that when you are joyful you are likely to notice more joy around you? This emotionally magnetic tendency is the basis of many truisms, including 'misery loves company', 'everybody loves a lover' and 'like minds attract'. Opposites attract only at the physical level.

At the level of astral matter, emotions exist as vibrational patterns that are then proposed to interface with the brain. This is thought to occur via transduction to the electromagnetic–electrochemical energy of nerve conduction in the survival centers of the brain, the periventricular survival system and the amygdala, which is the emotional control center for our survival and subconscious processing. Traditional yogic texts and Descartes both proposed that the pineal gland is the major site of transduction of our thoughts. These sites are proposed because the amygdala is the emotional center that controls our subconscious emotions, and the pineal gland secretes hormones that control both our moods and our physiology.[5]

These emotions then become physical feelings via nerve signals from the amygdala to the hypothalamus, which controls the autonomic nervous system and the pituitary, the master gland of the endocrine system. In other words, feelings are the physical body's way of experiencing what is really a subtle body vibrational pattern in the astral body.

The mental body

Interpenetrating the physical and extending beyond the astral body and consisting of even higher and more subtle vibrational energies is the mental body, the realm of thoughts.[6] This is the vehicle in which *self* or *ego* manifests and where our concrete intellect is expressed. Intellect is the ability to draw abstractions about physical reality and to make decisions. The word *intellect* itself means 'choice'.

Like the other subtle bodies, the mental body itself has several layers. The lower mental body dwells on mental images obtained from direct sensory experience and analytically reasons about purely concrete objects. The higher mental body is concerned with more abstract representations and concepts, often relating to other thoughts. Higher abstract reasoning and conceptualization are a property of this realm.

While the astral body generates emotions, the mental body generates thoughts as vibrational patterns that can be called *thought forms*. These thought forms can create patterns within the astral body that may then be transduced into neural activity that is experienced as feelings: 'I just had a very pleasurable thought.' Similarly, unpleasant thoughts can create unpleasant feelings.

Thus thought forms are the means by which the lower mental body can create and transmit concrete ideas to the brain for expression and manifestation. These ideas may then be turned into action, as the areas of the brain controlling movement are activated by conscious intent. Likewise, the higher mental body, through contact with your spiritual body, can create abstractions such as transcending self and direct healing intention to another person, but these remain highly subjective and internalized states.

It is also at the level of the higher mental body that we can contact and thus express our transcendent emotions: acceptance, compassion, empathy, altruism and the highest and most transcendent of all, unconditional love and forgiveness. We call these *transcendent* emotions because to access them you must transcend the ego. At the level of the lower mind, the self is seen as a separate *I* or *ego*. This ego self can never move past your own needs for those of another; your ego needs are always more important than another person's needs. From the level of your ego, you can never forgive, as 'they' did you wrong and must pay for it; vengeance and getting even always trump acceptance and heartfelt forgiveness. But from the perspective of your higher self, you can truly forgive another, no matter what they have done to you, through the higher mind and access to unconditional love. In true heartfelt forgiveness there is freedom.

In an interesting set of experiments, William Tiller, professor emeritus, Stanford University, and his coworkers have shown that by using just intention, people can alter their physical world in measurable ways. For instance, their intention can raise or lower the pH of water a whole pH unit or by a factor of 10, and do so repeatedly with very high statistical significance. Directed intent can also increase or decrease the speed of enzymatic reactions, and increase or decrease the rate of development of fruit fly larvae, again with strong statistical significance.[7]

Research by both the Institute of HeartMath and William Tiller has shown that by using the higher mental body to direct thoughts of love and compassion, the heart activates a pathway that 'locks' the heart rate, breath rate, and brain waves into a pattern similar to meditation. This greatly alters the physiology of the body, lowering the stress hormone cortisol and generally relaxing the body.[7]

Linda Russek and Gary Schwartz of the University of Arizona have also shown that just by focusing love and compassion on another person, the electrocardiogram of the sender appears in the electroencephalogram of the receiver, even though they were seated two meters apart without any type of physical contact.[9] All these experiments and techniques require focusing conscious intent, the activation of the higher mental body in eastern thought, to produce these results, which defy explanation in the current western scientific paradigm.

The causal or spiritual body

Interpenetrating the physical body and extending beyond the mental body, and consisting of the highest subtle vibrational energies, is the causal body.[10] This is the realm of spirit, of higher self and of your connection to God, whatever you conceive that to be. This body deals with the essence of things and the true causes that lie behind the illusion of appearance. This is the site of transcending consciousness.

It is also the realm from which *will* originates and provides us with the power to achieve goals in our life. In the esoteric traditions, will is said to originate at a very high level within the causal body. When activated, it causes transduction to thought forms of action, which the mind then uses to activate the physical body: 'Thy will be done.'

It is also the realm of devotion, of establishing a connection with the universal consciousness that some call God. At the level of the mental body, the self is manifested. At the level of the causal body, the soul is manifested and the limitations of physical time and space cease.

One of the reasons the yogis called the spiritual body the *causal* body is because in their view much of what happens in the physical body originates in this body, so it is the true *cause* of what is experienced. The transduction of our soul purpose generates thought forms, which in turn generate astral states of emotion, which in turn generate etheric patterns of ch'i and pranic flows that are then transduced into the physiological states of our physical bodies.

Many people believe that when we are in tune with our soul purpose, our life flows more harmoniously and we are healthier in mind and body. Likewise, the *real* cause of much physical illness and disease from a higher perspective is the blocked flows of ch'i and prana created by not following our soul's purpose, which then create distress in our mental, emotional and physical bodies.

The metaphysical and physical worlds

The limits to the physical world and lower mind

From the perspective of the lower mind, which houses the intellect, all that exists is that which our five senses can perceive, which now also includes all that electronic instruments can measure. It also houses the ego or perception that 'I am separate from the world and need to survive in this separate world.'

Physiologically, the lower mind is connected to our fight-or-flight survival reactions, elicited and controlled by fear. When people deny that anything except the physical world truly exists, they are operating only out of their lower mind. While these same people as scientists may be able to access the ability to use great powers of abstraction and conceptualization, properties of higher mind, they do not access the higher abilities of higher mind, which acts as an interface with the causal or spiritual body and the information this contains (see Figure 4.2).

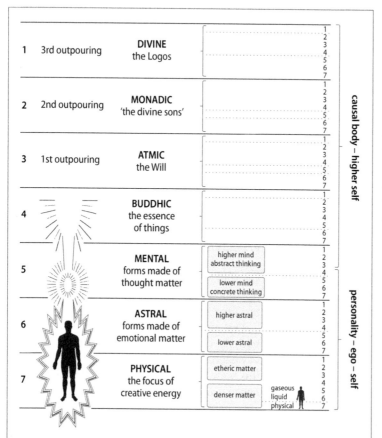

Figure 4.2 **The layers of Man.** When layers of the aura are perceived as a vertical stack, it can be clearly seen that the physical body is only a small part of who we are. In traditional systems of the East, the physical and etheric bodies are considered your temporal vehicle to which the other non-temporal subtle bodies are attached. Consciousness can be expressed either through the lower mind of sensory experience and intellect, the realm of our personality, or through the higher mind of abstraction and conceptualization, encompassing our higher self.

The continuity in the metaphysical world and higher mind

To move beyond the limitations of the physical world, you need to activate the higher levels of higher mind, which then accesses directly your connection to your spiritual body and all the information it contains. It is through the interface of higher mind that the spirit and the soul and the divine can be manifest to our consciousness (see Figure 4.2).

One of the primary energies accessed by every person through higher mind is will. The will is activated by conscious intention but originates beyond your physical, even though it may empower your physical to reach beyond its former physical limits. Another is compassion, when you truly *feel* from the heart for another person or animal, and of course the greatest is love, when true fusion with another and even your universe is possible, and separateness disappears.

It is only through the portal of higher mind that we have direct, personal connection to our divinity and can experience spiritual transcendence in which all sense of separateness disappears to leave a sense of oneness, of continuity with the universe. This is the timeless space of Zen and the endpoint of all meditative systems, where 'all is one' and the appearance of separation disappears.

References

1. Lockhart, M 2010, *The Subtle Energy Body: The Complete Guide*, Inner Traditions, Vermont.
2. Gerber, R 1996, *Vibrational Medicine*, Bear, Santa Fe.
   Brennan, BA 1988, *Hands of Light: A Guide to Healing Through the Human Energy Field*, Bantam Books, New York.
   Bailey, AA 1953, *Esoteric Healing*, Lucis, New York.
   Saraydarian, T 1981, *The Psyche and Psychism (2 Volume Set)*, Aquarian Educational Group, Cave Creek.
   Tiller, WA 1997, *Science and Human Transformation: Subtle Energies, Intentionality and Consciousness*, Pavior, Walnut Creek.
   Swanson, C 2010, *Life Force, The Scientific Basis*, Poseidia Press, Tucson.
3. Gerber, R 1996, *Vibrational Medicine*, Bear, Santa Fe.
   Brennan, BA 1988, *Hands of Light: A Guide to Healing Through the Human Energy Field*, Bantam Books, New York.
   Bailey, AA 1953, *Esoteric Healing*, Lucis, New York.
   Saraydarian, T 1981, *The Psyche and Psychism (2 Volume Set)*, Aquarian Educational Group, Cave Creek.
   Tiller, WA 1997, *Science and Human Transformation: Subtle Energies, Intentionality and Consciousness*, Pavior, Walnut Creek.
   Swanson, C 2010, *Life Force, The Scientific Basis*, Poseidia Press, Tucson.
   Powell, AE 1997, *The Etheric Double*, Theosophical Publishing House–Quest Books, Wheaton.
4. Gerber, R 1996, *Vibrational Medicine*, Bear, Santa Fe.
   Brennan, BA 1988, *Hands of Light: A Guide to Healing Through the Human Energy Field*, Bantam Books, New York.
   Bailey, AA 1953, *Esoteric Healing*, Lucis, New York.
   Saraydarian, T 1981, *The Psyche and Psychism (2 Volume Set)*, Aquarian Educational Group, Cave Creek.
   Tiller, WA 1997, *Science and Human Transformation: Subtle Energies, Intentionality and Consciousness*, Pavior, Walnut Creek.
   Swanson, C 2010, *Life Force, The Scientific Basis*, Poseidia Press, Tucson.
   Powell, AE 1996, *The Astral Body*, Theosophical Publishing House–Quest Books, Wheaton.
5. LeDoux, J 1996, *The Emotional Brain: The Mysterious Underpinnings of Emotional Life*, Simon & Schuster, New York.

   Tortora, GJ & Grabowski, SR 1996, *Principles of Anatomy and Physiology, Eighth Edition*, Harper Collins, New York.
   Pert, CB 1997, *Molecules of Emotion: Why You Feel the Way You Feel*, Scribner, New York.
6. Gerber, R 1996, *Vibrational Medicine*, Bear, Santa Fe.
   Brennan, BA 1988, *Hands of Light: A Guide to Healing Through the Human Energy Field*, Bantam Books, New York.
   Bailey, AA 1953, *Esoteric Healing*, Lucis, New York.
   Saraydarian, T 1981, *The Psyche and Psychism (2 Volume Set)*, Aquarian Educational Group, Cave Creek.
   Tiller, WA 1997, *Science and Human Transformation: Subtle Energies, Intentionality and Consciousness*, Pavior, Walnut Creek.
   Swanson, C 2010, *Life Force, The Scientific Basis*, Poseidia Press, Tucson.
   Powell, AE 2004, *The Mental Body*, Theosophical Publishing House, Wheaton.
7. Tiller, WA, Dibble, WE & Kohane, MJ 2001, *Conscious Acts of Creation*, Pavior, Walnut Creek.
8. Childre, DL & Martin, H 2000, *The HeartMath Solution*, HarperCollins, New York.
   Tiller, WA 1997, *Science and Human Transformation: Subtle Energies, Intentionality and Consciousness*, Pavior, Walnut Creek.
9. Schwartz, GE & Russek, LG 1999, *Living Energy Universe: A Fundamental Discovery that Transforms Science and Medicine*, Hampton Roads, Charlottesville.
10. Gerber, R 1996, *Vibrational Medicine*, Bear, Santa Fe.
    Brennan, BA 1988, *Hands of Light: A Guide to Healing Through the Human Energy Field*, Bantam Books, New York.
    Bailey, AA 1953, *Esoteric Healing*, Lucis, New York.
    Saraydarian, T 1981, *The Psyche and Psychism (2 Volume Set)*, Aquarian Educational Group, Cave Creek.
    Tiller, WA 1997, *Science and Human Transformation: Subtle Energies, Intentionality and Consciousness*, Pavior, Walnut Creek.
    Swanson, C 2010, *Life Force, The Scientific Basis*, Poseidia Press, Tucson.
    Powell, AE 2003, *Causal Body and the Ego*, Theosophical Publishing House, Wheaton.

Chapter 5

THE CHAKRA–NADI SYSTEM

The chakras

Chakras are subtle energy structures recognized in many esoteric traditions but most intensively studied and described by the yogis of India over the past five millennia. While there is considerable variation in names and details, there is broad agreement about the essential structure and function of chakras and their related energy system, the nadis system.[1]

The name *chakra* is the last five letters of a Sanskrit word 25 letters long that means 'spinning wheel of light'. When viewed from the front, they appear as spinning wheels or disks of light to clairvoyants and yogis and have been ascribed various colors.[2] From the side, they are said to appear as cones of light that project outward from a point on the skin.

The chakra system is one of the primary subtle energy systems of the body. This system consists of seven primary chakras and many minor chakras. In fact, each joint has a minor chakra associated with it, and there may be more than 360 individual chakras in the human body.[3]

There are seven primary chakras. The crown chakra is located at the top of the head and projects upward. The brow chakra projects forward from the point between the eyebrows. The throat chakra projects forward from the notch of the throat. The heart chakra projects forward from the bottom of the sternum. The navel or solar plexus chakra projects forward from the navel. The sacral or sexual chakra projects forward from just above the pubis, and the root or base chakra projects downward from the perineum at about an 80° angle forward. Smaller chakra cones also project from the back of the body at a point opposite the entry point of each of the major frontal cones (see Figure 5.1).[4]

Each chakra cone is made up of many smaller cones, all of which constantly oscillate clockwise and counterclockwise. However, because each cone in each of the major chakras rotates more clockwise or more counterclockwise, the large chakra cone is often said to spin. Each chakra has a characteristic spin starting at the crown and alternating first clockwise then counterclockwise, the direction depending on your sex and psycho-emotional state.

Chakras penetrate all levels of the subtle body from the causal to the etheric, and act to transduce the energies of the subtle bodies into electromagnetic energy for use at the physical level. This transduction of ordering or organizing energy is one of the primary mechanisms that maintains the coherence of the etheric template, which in turn maintains the functions of the physical body.

Chakras act as subtle energy step-down transformers, stepping down the higher frequency vibrations of the causal to the mental body, the mental frequencies to the lower vibrations of the astral body, and the emotional vibrations of the astral body to the densest subtle energy of the etheric body.[5] The energetic vibration of each layer can affect the subtle body above or below it, and the chakras are therefore one of the major integrating sites of the subtle bodies.

Via the chakras, subtle energy changes in any of the subtle bodies can become manifest as physiological events at the cellular level. In this way, the various subtle bodies interact with and affect the structure and function of the physical body. At the level of the etheric body, the chakra and acupuncture systems interact and together create the energetic template that then manifests as the physical body.

The nadis

Interconnecting the primary and secondary chakras are numerous subtle energy channels called *nadis*, which distribute the pranic energy

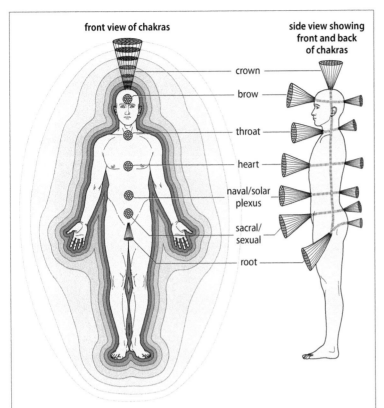

front view of chakras

side view showing front and back of chakras

crown
brow
throat
heart
naval/solar plexus
sacral/sexual
root

Figure 5.1 Location of the major chakras. Note how there is a central channel (sushumna) that connects the crown chakra with the root chakra, to which all the chakras are also connected. The primary cone of each chakra is made up of many smaller cones. Each primary cone projects from the front of the body and the back of the body, with the front cone being the larger of the two. Note also that each primary chakra penetrates all layers of the human body from the physical to the spiritual.

taken in by the chakras. Not only do the nadi channels connect the chakras to each other, but also to specific parts of the physical cellular structure.

Nadis can be considered fine threads or minute channels of subtle energetic matter that are similar to the meridians of the acupuncture meridian system. Like the meridian system, there are bigger and smaller nadi channels associated with physiological structures within the body (see Figure 5.2).[6]

Various sources have described up to 72,000 nadis that are interwoven within the physical body, particularly the nervous system. Some of these nadis connect directly to the endocrine glands, while others are interconnected with the autonomic nervous system, especially the autonomic nerve plexuses.[6] Because of these direct connections with the endocrine autonomic nervous systems, the chakras may directly affect the physiological function of the body (see Figure 5.3).

The chakra–nadi system and physiological functioning

Each chakra is associated with a particular endocrine gland and a specific nerve plexus at the level of the location of each chakra within the physical body (see Table 5.1).[7]

The chakras provide an influx of cosmic energies that the yogis term *prana*, their term for the life force or *élan vital*. Prana is said to originate as cosmic energy or free energy of the universe that is conducted into the body via the chakra cones. This could be termed the *primary outpouring*. Once it enters the chakra cones, prana is then distributed to the associated endocrine organs and nerve plexuses via the nadi system.[6]

The primary role of the chakras is to act as a step-down transformer to transduce cosmic energy into pranic energy, which is then

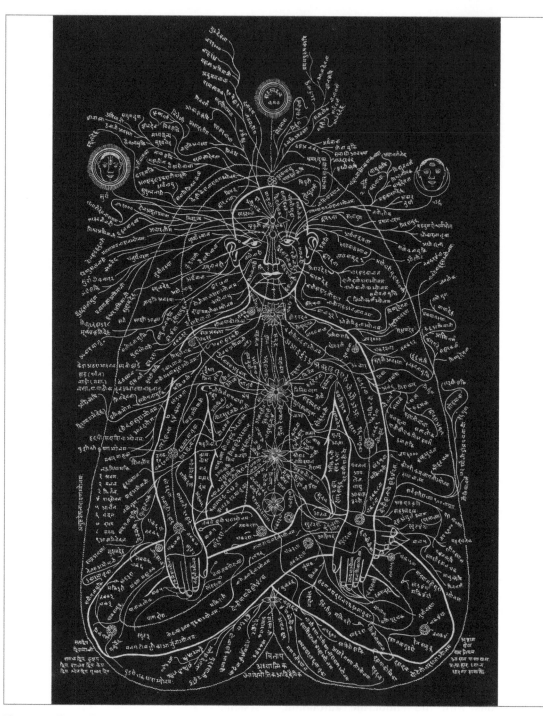

Figure 5.2 The nadi system. Original drawing of the chakra–nadi system from the yogic literature, showing the chakras as an energy center along the midline of the body, with bigger and smaller nadi channels that surround our physical body. The bigger nadi channels, called *marmas*, have greater influence on our physiology and function than the smaller nadi channels. Reproduced from Mookerjee, A 1975, *Yoga Art*, Thames & Hudson, London, plate no. 9, with permission.

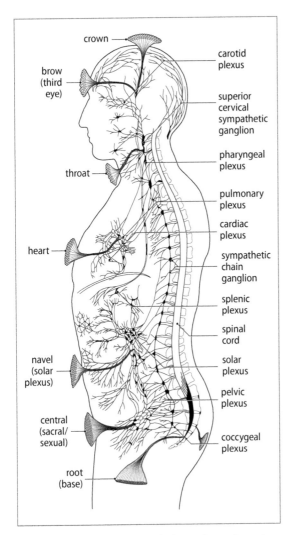

Figure 5.3 Chakra locations relative to the major autonomic nerve plexuses. Each of the seven major chakras is associated with one of the major autonomic nerve plexuses. In this way, each chakra may have a direct influence over the autonomic functions controlled by each nerve plexus. After Leadbeater, C 1927 *The Chakras*, Theosophical Society Publishing House, Wheaton, pp. 40–41.

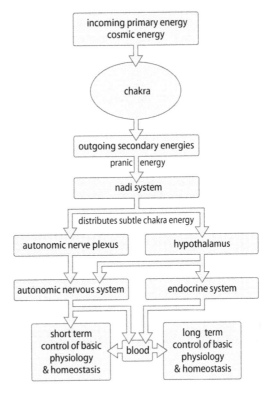

Figure 5.4 Source of pranic energy in the chakras and mechanism of their physiological effect. Cosmic energy entering the chakras is stepped down to physiological usable pranic energy as it transits the chakra cone, and is then distributed via the nadi system to both the autonomic nerve plexuses and their associated endocrine glands to assist in both short-term and long-term maintenance and regulation of physiological homeostasis.

distributed through the nadi system. This is then transduced once again into physiology in the autonomic nervous and endocrine systems to maintain homeostasis. One of the major sites of transduction of subtle flows of pranic energy into physiological function is the hypothalamus. In turn, both the autonomic nervous system and

the endocrine system are under the control of the hypothalamus, which maintains our basic homeostasis.

The autonomic nervous system controls our short-term homeostasis by allowing rapid neural response to varying external conditions, while the endocrine system is involved with maintenance of long-term homeostasis via the release of hormones that maintain longer-term physiological adaptations (see Figure 5.4).

Thus, when the chakra pranic energy is stepped down to the level of etheric flows in conjunction with the etheric acupuncture system, these etheric flows are transduced into electromagnetic and electrochemical energies that modulate and regulate our physiological function. The yogis observed that the pranic energy provided a source of self-organizing energy that helps maintain the etheric template. And it is the etheric template that ultimately sustains physiological function.

References

1. Leadbeater, CW 1927, *The Chakras*, Theosophical Publishing House, Wheaton.
   Swami Satyananda Swaraswati 1985, *Kundalini Tantra*, Yoga Publications Trust, Bihar.
   Brennan, BA 1988, *Hands of Light: A Guide to Healing Through the Human Energy Field*, Bantam Books, New York.
   Gerber, R 1988, *Vibrational Medicine*, Bear, Santa Fe.
   Judith, A 2004, *Eastern Body, Western Mind: Psychology and the Chakra System As a Path to the Self*, Random House, New York.
   Myss, C 1996, *Anatomy of the Spirit*, Crown, New York.
   Bruyere, RL 1989, *Wheels of Light*, Simon & Schuster, New York.
   Dale, C 2009, *The Subtle Body: An Encyclopedia of Your Energetic Anatomy*, Sounds True, Boulder.
2. Leadbeater, CW 1927, *The Chakras*, Theosophical Publishing House, Wheaton.
   Swami Satyananda Swaraswati 1985, *Kundalini Tantra*, Yoga Publications Trust, Bihar.
   Brennan, BA 1988, *Hands of Light: A Guide to Healing Through the Human Energy Field*, Bantam Books, New York.
3. Gerber, R 1988, *Vibrational Medicine*, Bear, Santa Fe.
   Tansley, DV 1972, *Radionics and the Subtle Anatomy of Man*, CW Daniel, Saffron Walden.
4. Swami Satyananda Swaraswati 1985, *Kundalini Tantra*, Yoga Publications Trust, Bihar.
   Brennan, BA 1988, *Hands of Light: A Guide to Healing Through the Human Energy Field*, Bantam Books, New York.
5. Gerber, R 1988, *Vibrational Medicine*, Bear, Santa Fe.
6. Swami Satyananda Swaraswati 1985, *Kundalini Tantra*, Yoga Publications Trust, Bihar.
   Gerber, R 1988, *Vibrational Medicine*, Bear, Santa Fe.
7. Leadbeater, CW 1927, *The Chakras*, Theosophical Publishing House, Wheaton.
   Gerber, R 1988, *Vibrational Medicine*, Bear, Santa Fe.

Table 5.1 Endocrine and autonomic nervous system plexus and physiological system associated with each chakra

Chakra	Endocrine system	Nerve plexus	Physiological system
Root	Gonads	Sacral–coccygeal plexus	Reproductive
Sacral	Leydig cells	Sacral plexus	Genitourinary
Navel	Adrenal glands	Solar plexus	Digestive
Heart	Thymus gland	Heart plexus	Circulatory
Throat	Thyroid gland	Cervical ganglia medulla	Respiratory
Brow	Pituitary gland	Hypothalamus pituitary	Autonomic nervous system
Crown	Pineal gland	Cerebral cortex pineal	Central nervous system (central control)

Chapter 6

THE ACUPUNCTURE MERIDIAN SYSTEM

A Brief History of Chinese Acupuncture

The second of the primary subtle energy systems of the body is the acupuncture meridian system recognized by the ancient Chinese and developed as part of traditional Chinese medicine. The practice of needle acupuncture pre-dates written Chinese history, as stone and bone acupuncture needles similar to needles still used today have been found in archaeological sites throughout China dating from several thousand years BC.[1]

The Chinese method of accessing energy imbalances in the body began to be written down between 300 and 100 BC, when 161 bilateral points were recognized.[2] Thousands of years of accumulated acupuncture knowledge was codified and written down in the *Huang Di Nei Ching* or *Yellow Emperor's Inner Classic of Medicine* between the first century BC and the early first century AD.[3] By this time, classical theory recognized about 360 acupoints on the surface meridians; 54 were located along the midline of the body, comprising the Governing and Central Vessels or meridians; and 308 were located along 12 bilateral vessels or lines of acupoints on both sides of the body. The midline and bilateral acupoints together give a total of 670 meridian acupoints.[4] By 1100 AD, the Chinese had anatomically accurate figurines showing these acupoint locations.[5]

The concept of energy points on the skin that direct the flow of an invisible force the Chinese called *ch'i* or *qi* was long considered a primitive superstition or belief system by western science, because there was no way to verify the existence of the energy points or any way to prove that this mysterious force was real. Then about 50 years ago it was discovered that acupoints have a unique electrical property: they are null points electrically.[6] Null points are points on the surface of the skin of least electrical resistance. Skin normally has a very high electrical resistance, so once this discovery was made it was easy to develop a meter to electrically locate these null points. Whenever the probe makes contact with an acupoint, because of lower resistance the increased electrical flow is converted to sound or light. These electrical null points became called *electrodermal acupoints*.

Even more remarkably, the electrical mapping of these electrodermal points was very highly correlated with maps of the Chinese acupoints.[7] Not only are acupoints the points of least electrical resistance on the surface of the skin, but the acupoints have been shown to have a unique histological microstructure and the cells directly beneath them have a slightly different structure to that of their neighbors.[8] Most acupoints are situated in small surface depressions, identifiable by palpation, and are often hypersensitive. Beneath these surface depressions, the epidermis is thinner and has a characteristic structure with modified collagen fibers.[9] Senelar claims that more than 80% of the known acupoints examined have this unique structure.[10]

But why are only more than 80% of the acupoints correlated with electrodermal acupoints? Because there are two quite different types of acupoints: electrodermal points and needling points. Electrodermal acupoints are the points of least electrical resistance, as determined by electrical measurement, and indeed are needled. Needling points, on the other hand, are points on the skin used to access the deeper meridian energy flows but are not located exactly on an electrodermal point. It happens that in some cases the electrodermal point is immediately above a small artery or nerve, and to needle the electrodermal point would either cause bleeding or pain. Because the actual meridian pathways run beneath the surface of the skin, they are connected to the electrodermal point via a small channel of varying length, depending on how deep the meridian channel is below the surface of the skin.

To avoid the problems associated with these electrodermal points, the Chinese established the needling points away from the actual electrodermal point, but to be needled at such an angle and a depth that the tip of the needle would intersect the vessel or meridian below the electrodermal point at the junction with the channel to the electrodermal point on the skin (see Figure 6.1). In this way, satisfactory stimulation was effected without the problems of bleeding or pain. But of course this now means that the electrodermal point no longer coincides with the needling point.

The nature of ch'i

The Chinese claimed that the subtle energy they called ch'i or qi circulated through a series of vessels or channels, later named *meridians* by the French, who initially studied acupuncture in the late 1800s and early 1900s.[11] The Chinese proposed that this ch'i was a dynamic force, in constant flux, that circulates throughout the body, following the specific meridian pathways and obeying specific rules.[12] Acupuncture or acupressure therapy consists of either stimulating or dispersing the flow of ch'i via activation of specific acupoints on the surface of the body. One of the premises of both the energy medicine of the West and traditional Chinese medicine is that for every energetic imbalance there are corresponding or related symptoms, or disturbance in function, at one or all levels of the body.[13]

Western science does not yet have the instruments to directly measure what the Chinese call ch'i but for which the best western translation is 'energy'. But ch'i does not directly equate to the western concept of energy as being a force something like electricity. Ch'i has a different quality from the coarser physical energy and is aligned more with the early Greek and Roman concepts of the *élan vital* or vital energy and the subtle energy of current vibrational energy models.[13] While in the West the notion of subtle invisible forces running through the body had been in constant use for several thousand years, these concepts were totally eclipsed in the western world by the end of the medieval era.

Western science may claim that ch'i does not exist, and that it is a hypothetical force the Chinese created to explain how acupuncture could affect the physiology of the body, but this statement cannot be made 'scientifically'. The only statement that can be made scientifically is that western science is ignorant of the existence of ch'i, because western science cannot measure ch'i. Until you can measure something you cannot say it is not there, and indeed, it does not make it *not there* just because you cannot measure it! As an analogy, people got just as sunburned before science could measure or detect ultraviolet radiation; science's ignorance of the existence of ultraviolet radiation did not make it non-existent!

Although western science currently does have the instrumentation to measure the existence of the acupoints of the Chinese meridian system, at least their electrical properties, the actual flows of

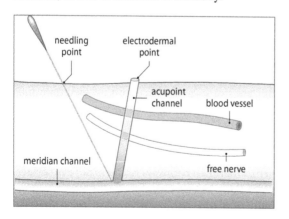

Figure 6.1 Electrodermal points versus needling acupoints. All acupoints are electrodermal points, the points of least electrical resistance on the surface of the skin. Electrodermal acupoints are linked to their deeper primary meridian pathway by a short acupoint channel. If small blood vessels and/or free nerve endings pass through the acupoint channel, needling this electrodermal point may cause bleeding or excessive pain. To prevent this, needling points are offset from the electrodermal acupoint but needled at such an angle and depth that the needle tip can activate ch'i flow in the meridian pathway.

ch'i along the subtle energy pathways called meridians have not yet been unequivocally detected. Richard Gerber in his excellent book *Vibrational Medicine* cites several studies that do show that some type of subtle energy flows along pathways on the surface of the skin similar to the meridians of Chinese acupuncture.[14]

In fact, in the 1960s a team of researchers led by Dr Kim Bong Han did extensive experimental work with the acupuncture meridians of rabbits and other animals. These studies included injecting radioactive phosphorus-32 (^{32}P, an isotope of phosphorus) into acupoints; its uptake into tissues was then followed using microautoradiography. Much to the researchers' surprise, they discovered that the ^{32}P was actively taken up along a fine duct-like tubule system that followed classical acupuncture meridians. In contrast, concentrations of ^{32}P in tissues immediately surrounding the meridians or injected near acupoints were negligible. When ^{32}P was injected into nearby veins, little to no ^{32}P could be detected in the meridian network, suggesting the meridian system is independent of the circulatory system.[15]

More recent work by French researchers confirmed Kim's finding in humans using radioactive technetium-99m (^{99m}Tc) injected into the acupoints of humans, with the isotope's uptake followed by gamma camera imaging. The technetium-99m migrated 30 centimeters in 4–6 minutes along the meridian pathway, a speed of migration not seen when the technetium-99m was injected into random points on the skin.[16]

Furthermore, Kim found that the ductiles of the meridians branched out to ever smaller ductiles until the terminal ductiles reached the tissue cell nuclei. This could provide a mechanism for how alterations in ch'i flow may effect gene expression, and may indeed be one of the epigenetic factors affecting our development and function. Kim's further research showed that there are two duct systems. There is an *external duct system*, comprising a superficial tubular meridian system that parallels the traditional meridian system of the Chinese, as well as a deep tubular system called the *internal duct system*, which is associated with the organs. These two systems are linked as one continuous system connecting the organs of Chinese acupuncture with the meridians.[15]

More recently, using infrared thermography Schlebusch and colleagues have shown the presence of very specific pathways of heat following acupuncture treatment of specific acupoints.[17] These pathways of heat ran exactly down meridian pathways, with many of the acupoints on that meridian being 'hotter' than the pathway itself. Figure 6.2 demonstrates this visually. As far as we know, there are no neurological or physiological mechanisms that could produce this pattern of temperature distribution.

There is, however, still some controversy with regard to the meaning of heat pathways that light up when recorded by infrared thermography. For instance, Litscher refutes the contention that infrared thermography of stimulated acupoints or meridians can reveal evidence of meridian

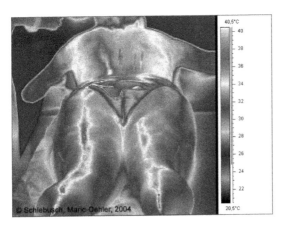

Figure 6.2 Infrared thermography of acupoint stimulation by acupuncture. The illustration shows pathways of light that form along the surface of the skin when specific bladder acupoints are needled for several minutes. These infrared light pathways exactly follow the bladder meridian from the mid lower back up to the shoulder and down from the sacrum to the feet. Bladder acupoints light up even more strongly than the pathways themselves, the darker spots long the leg pathways. After Schlebusch.[17]

structures, and stated in his 2005 paper that 'these infrared patterns represent only technical reflection artifacts.'[18] Despite his conclusions, there are inconsistencies in his interpretation of his data that he fails to address. First of all, he failed to report infrared thermographs of his subjects before acupoint treatment with moxibustion, and therefore no control infrared images are available for comparison with the unexpected bilateral heating of both legs and feet when the application of moxibustion or heat was to only one leg or foot. Hence, the cause of the bilateral increase in temperature in infrared thermographs on both legs and feet given in Litscher's paper is unknown.[18] The application of heat to one leg or foot should have no effect on the temperature of parallel areas on the opposite leg or foot, nor create 'technical reflection artifacts' on both sides of the body, unless there is a connection between the two areas. In Popp and coworkers' paper on light piping, this is exactly what was observed.[19] Application of moxibustion to acupoints on one leg caused parallel pathways of light recorded as biophoton flows to appear on the other leg.

In Chinese acupuncture, the meridians are bilateral and connected by horary channels that provide a mechanism for the transfer of energy, including heat, from one side of the body to the other, and could account for the bilateral increase in temperature of identical areas on the opposite side legs and feet observed in the study by Litscher, who also applied moxibustion to the same or nearby acupoints. Second, Litscher's finding that needle or laser needle acupuncture activation of acupoints did not create observable infrared pathways is in direct contrast to the findings of Schlebusch's group[17] and Popp's group,[19] who showed observable infrared pathways that correlate with acupoint activation by cupping, needle acupuncture and moxibustion. Two other studies also report infrared images of meridian-like structures including hotspots at the correct locations for acupoints along the corresponding meridian pathway following needle acupuncture or acupressure activation.[20] In contrast to Litscher's results, Schlebusch and colleagues showed whole body infrared images of two subjects when they were asymptomatic for headache and backache, and then again when these conditions were active.

When asymptomatic, there was no evidence of infrared images or technical reflection artifacts along meridian pathways, but once subjects were symptomatic and experiencing these conditions, infrared images clearly revealed relevant meridian-like structures. Therefore it is likely that in the absence of overt meridian activation by either a physical–physiological condition or a treatment such as cupping, acupuncture, acupressure or moxibustion, there are indeed no obvious infrared pathways observable on the body. But once acupuncture or acupressure therapy activates flow within the meridians, this activation then develops observable meridian-like infrared structures and pathways on the body.

In another example from Schlebusch and coworkers, when the subject was experiencing a headache in her temples, the infrared images displayed intense warming specifically on the side of the head and along the length of the gall bladder meridian down the body. Indeed, in traditional Chinese medicine temple headaches are correlated with over-energy, or excess heat, in the gall bladder meridian.[21] In fact, in all Litscher's figures the technical reflection artifacts were not randomly oriented but rather oriented in the same direction and aligned with the structures of the meridians in those areas of the body. For instance, the infrared reflection artifacts in his 2005 paper align with the bladder meridian on either the front or the back of the leg, not in just random directions as would be expected if they represent only reflection artifacts. This is despite the fact that in Litscher's study moxibustion was applied for only 5 minutes, rather than the traditional 15–20 minutes that would have more fully developed these meridian-like heat pathways.

Likewise, in the study by Schlebusch and colleagues, when the subject with the lower back pain was asymptomatic the infrared images showed no heat pathways; or in Litscher's terms, no technical reflection artifacts. However, when the same subject *did* have lower back pain and was receiving treatment by either cupping or needle acupuncture, infrared images demonstrated extensive meridian-like artifacts that exactly correspond to the bladder meridian structure including hotspots at specific bladder acupoints. In fact, these pathways extended from the upper back to the ankles, a distance of more than a meter from the source of stimulation.

Litscher's blanket statement that every apparent infrared image of heat flows on the body following acupoint stimulation represents only a technical reflection artifact, and therefore meridian-like structures do not exist, is not supported by more recent studies using infrared images that both confirm and extend the findings of Schlebusch's group on the existence of pathways of energy flow suggestive of meridian-like structures in the human body.[20]

In summary, there appear to be pathways indicative of meridians on the surface of the body that are observable by activation of acupoints and infrared thermography, or measurable by electrical recording of impedance. Furthermore, these pathways and their associated acupoints are said to have electrical properties of lower impedance and lower electrical resistance than the surrounding skin. However, the electrical specificity of the meridians and acupoints has been controversial, with studies that show specificity of meridians and acupoints and others that do not.[22]

Ahn, in his systematic review of the properties of acupuncture points and meridians contends that claims for acupoint specificity have been viewed with considerable skepticism by the conventional scientific community because of confounding factors such as skin moisture, electrode pressure and a number of other factors. Any distinct electrical characteristics are attributable to external factors and/or artifacts and not to the acupoints or meridians.[23]

Nevertheless, Ahn concluded that although there is not yet unequivocal evidence, the majority of the evidence does support the claim that acupuncture points and meridians are electrically distinguishable. Indeed, in his 2011 paper Litscher studied the electrical properties of acupoints and meridians using very sophisticated measurements, and found that acupoints did appear to be points on the skin of low impedance and connected to other acupoints via pathways of lower impedance.[24]

In fact, in a review of acupoint specificity Choi and colleagues state that acupoint specificity is controversial because many acupuncture studies on the effects on pain using control points have found that sham points have similar effects to those of verum acupoints. In addition, the results of pain-related studies based on visual analog scales have not supported the concept of acupoint specificity. In contrast, hemodynamic functional magnetic resonance and neurophysiological studies evaluating the responses to stimulation of multiple acupoints on the body surface have shown that acupoint-specific actions were present. In the conclusion of her review article, Choi confirms that brain-imaging studies have shown that stimulation of different acupoints elicits unique brain patterns, even though these studies do not show the pathways through which these changes occur.[25]

Despite the lack of absolute proof of the existence of the meridian system and ch'i flows, the remarkable correlation between the acupoints mapped by the Chinese thousands of years ago with the location of these same points, as detected by modern electrical instrumentation, isotope tracing and infrared thermography, would suggest that the Chinese had a reliable technique to detect and verify the acupoints. And if they could accurately detect the location of the acupoints, why would you not believe them when they state that these acupoints control and direct a force that flows through these points?

At first, western science said there were no acupoints and no flows of ch'i. Then, 'Oops! There are acupoints after all and exactly where the Chinese said they were', but science still holds that there are no flows of ch'i. Because there are no flows of ch'i to produce effects, then either acupuncture is ineffective or it works only via the nervous system, for instance the Melzack–Wall gate theory of acupuncture anesthesia or the placebo effect.[26]

However, recent brain-scanning studies using functional magnetic resonance imaging have shown unequivocal correlation between specific acupoint stimulation on the surface of the body and highly specific patterns of cortical and subcortical activation.[27] Of considerable interest is the fact that the patterns of cortical and subcortical activation have no known nervous system connection to the points on the skin being stimulated, and further, stimulating different acupoints shows different patterns of cortical and subcortical activation. In addition, there are now a number of studies showing that activation of sham points do not show any consistent patterns of brain activation.[28]

So how did the ancient Chinese know the location of all 670 acupoints that make up the integrated acupuncture meridian system? And why did they state that there were flows of ch'i controlled by these points?

The short, if unscientific, answer is that some of the monks and Chinese medical practitioners who had spent many years in meditation developing extremely subtle levels of perception were able to actually see or sense these acupoints and the movement of ch'i through the body. For instance, the *Ling Shu* states with regard to the longitudinal luo vessels, 'The meridians that are floating and that often remain visible to the naked eye are the linking meridians.'[29] Charles Krebs also has a friend who spent seven years as a Zen monk in Asia and India, and three years in a Chinese monastery becoming a master of acupuncture. After two years in the monastery training in acupuncture, he could suddenly see not only acupoints but also the ch'i energy flowing in the meridian vessels connecting the acupoints.

These subtle energies and vessels were as clear to the monks, Chinese medical practitioners and Krebs's friend as if they were looking at a pattern on a piece of cloth. Interestingly, even in a monastery training 300 students and dozens of instructors, the ability to see the acupoints and ch'i flows was not common. At the time Krebs's friend was there, only he, the abbot of the monastery and the head acupuncture teacher could do so!

In the West, if you suddenly could see acupoints and meridian flows only observable to a few other people, this would not constitute a valid source of knowledge on which to build a healing system. But because the people doing the seeing had attained a level of enlightenment, it was accepted in the East that you may have the ability to reliably see what is unseen by people who have not yet developed these subtle levels of perception.

Because these masters could see the patterns of energy, they could perceive which patterns were harmonious and balanced, indicating wellness, and which patterns were disharmonious, indicating imbalance or disease. From this knowledge came the Law of Five Elements, one of the central tenets of acupuncture.

The Law of Five Elements

The Law of Five Elements states there are certain directions of energy flow and acupoints on the body that when activated cause the movement of energy from one point to another.[30] Everybody has only a specific amount of energy or ch'i flowing through them, so an over-energy in one place by definition means that there has to be an under-energy in another place. Because the Chinese diagnosticians were using inductive reasoning (looking at the whole), they did not name diseases as such; rather, they were interested in a complex of patterns that made up the whole. It was from these patterns that they were able to diagnose imbalances.[31]

Chinese medicine is not less logical than the western system, just less analytical.[31] All the information the Chinese needed to know to re-establish balance was where the over-energy and under-energy existed. With that knowledge, they could employ the Law of Five Elements to locate the correct acupoints to stimulate. Stimulation of these acupoints would remove the block to energy flow. Once unblocked, the excess energy would naturally flow to where it was deficient. When energy was in balance, theoretically health was restored.

One of the reasons why the West found the Chinese view of the body so confusing for so long had a lot to do with the ancient language in which Chinese medical information was couched. The Chinese explanations related to the cosmology of a Taoist and then Confucian agrarian society of over 2000 years ago. An inductive, lyrical language written in allegory and metaphor, it evokes the experience of a largely rural world. Energy flows were thus compared to rivers, flooded rice paddies and overflow channels. Organs were called Emperors or Ministers, and the laws were called Grandmother–Son or Mother–Son Laws. The Five Elements are described as having qualities of Earth, Fire, Metal, Wood or Water. Was it any wonder that when the West first came across these ideas, the lack of technical language and use of metaphors made the information inaccessible at best or nonsensical at worst?

Despite our confusion with their system and the lack of attention paid by the Chinese to internal anatomy, they were well aware of organ function. They called the meridian flows by organ names not because they referred to the organs themselves, but because part of the energy flow of each meridian sustained the function of a specified organ.[32] Thus they talked of lung energy, heart energy and kidney energy, and what they meant was the complex energy structure of which the physical organ was but one small part.

To the western mind, such a description immediately designates only a physical organ with a specific function. But the Chinese descriptions did not mean a heart as a muscular organ pumping blood. Rather, it talked about a concept of heart: the Emperor, as the source of power in the system that not only drives the blood but is also the power behind the emotions of love, hatred and anger.

And when the Chinese describe a meridian, they are not describing a static physical unit but a matrix of dynamic energetic interactions that affects all planes of the being. The Chinese do not see a physical body and a mind as being separate structures. They see a body–mind–spirit that creates an integrated being.[33]

To quote the great chronicler of Chinese history Joseph Needham, 'In accord with the character of all Chinese thought, the human is an organism, neither purely spiritual nor purely material in nature.'[34] Mind and emotions are no less influential in their view of health than the state of the physical body, that part of us which can be seen, touched and felt.

What ties the body to the mind and spirit is the etheric energy of ch'i, which is the interface between the physical body and the subtle energy bodies of mind and spirit.[35] These subtle bodies have been recognized for millennia in the esoteric traditions of China, India and Tibet. An ancient Chinese adage held that 'There is nothing between Heaven and Earth except ch'i and the Laws that govern it.'[36]

Interweaving yin and yang

Early Chinese thought developed the concept that there are two fundamental properties of the universe: yin and yang. These polar opposites are perceived to be present in all things and interconnected by ch'i. As the *Nei Ching* states, 'The entire universe is an oscillation of the forces of yin and yang.' Although yin and yang are complementary opposites, they are neither specific forms of energy nor material things; rather, they are qualities used to describe how things function in relation to each other and the universe.[37]

Yin and yang really represent a way of thinking in which all things are but a part of a whole. No thing can exist in and of itself but can only be defined by its opposite. For instance, hot is the absence of cold, dark is the absence of light, wet is the absence of dry and so on. Yin and yang are thus opposite properties that define each other.

In the original metaphor, yin was 'the shady side of the mountain' and yang was 'the sunny side of the mountain'. Yin is associated with the qualities of cold, dark, matter, passivity and rest, and considered feminine. Yang is associated with the qualities of heat, light, energy, activity and movement, and considered masculine.[38]

In yin–yang theory, these two properties are in constant interaction and relation. All things have two aspects, a yin aspect and a yang aspect, and yin and yang mutually create each other and control or balance each other. Boiling water exemplifies these abstractions. As water heats, it becomes more yang (hot), but as each water molecule escapes into the air as vapor, it cools or becomes yin because of water's latent heat of evaporation. This is why sweating, yang, makes you cool, yin.

The famous *tai qi* or yin yang symbol, shown in Figure 6.3, represents the relation and

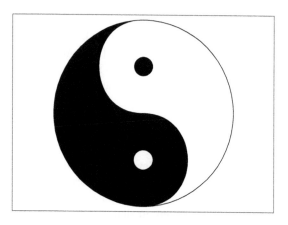

Figure 6.3 *Tai qi* **symbol of the interaction of yin and yang.** The symbol represents the dynamic interaction between the two complementary properties or polarities that comprise all things. The white dot in the black and the black dot in the white show that nothing can be entirely yin or yang, and the curved line between yin and yang shows that yin is always transforming into yang and yang into yin, with the state of harmony represented by a balance of yin and yang.

interdependence between yin and yang. The white dot in the black and the black dot in the white signify that in yin (black) there is always the seed of yang (the white dot), and vice versa. No thing is, or can be, all yin or all yang. Yin and yang are complementary properties that compose the whole, and the curved line between them expresses the movement of yin transforming into yang and yang transforming into yin. The fact that the black and white sides are equal demonstrates the balance of yin and yang when there is harmony.

What is most interesting is that there are a set of equations in calculus called *limit cycle equations* that describe the interaction of two dynamically interacting factors, such that the expression of one factor alters the expression of the other factor in a synchronous way. Figure 6.4 is a graphic representation of a limit cycle. Notice any similarities to the yin yang symbol?

It could be said that the whole of Chinese medicine—its physiology, its pathology, its diagnosis and its treatment—can all be reduced to the fundamental theory of yin and yang. This theory serves to explain the organic structure, physical function and pathological changes in the human body, and in addition guides the clinical diagnoses and treatment.[39] Ch'i flowing through the meridians and following the Law of Five Elements is the mechanism by which yin and yang are expressed within the body.

When the Chinese talk about a meridian or vessel, they are describing conduits made of subtle matter through which ch'i flows. Ch'i has various properties or qualities that connect the body–mind–spirit into a dynamic integrated organism, an idea that western medicine is only now beginning to entertain.

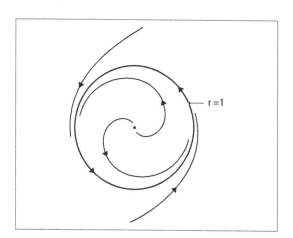

r = 1

Figure 6.4 Calculus of limit cycles expressed graphically. The similarity to the *tai qi* symbol developed millennia before the invention of calculus and the graphical representation of a limit cycle would seem prescient, as both describe the dynamic interaction of two dynamically interacting factors, such that the expression of one factor alters the expression of the other factor in a synchronous way. After Yanchi Liu, 1988, *The Essential Book of Traditional Chinese Medicine, Volume 1: Theory*, Columbia University Press, New York, p. 46.

The cardinal or primary meridians

The Chinese say that there are 14 major meridians in the body, each of which has its own acupoints. Two of these vessels, the Governing and Central Vessels, flow up from the region of the groin. Central Vessel runs up the midline of the front of the body from a point on the perineum to a point just below the bottom lip. It carries yin energy. Governing Vessel runs from the tip of the tailbone, up the spine and over the top of the skull to a point on the frenulum of the upper lip. It carries yang energy. The other 12 vessels are bilateral, with one running up or down the right, and one up or down the left side of the body. Of these bilateral meridians or vessels, six are yin and six are yang.[40]

In the Chinese anatomical position, the arms are raised above the head, and thus all yang meridians (except Governing) run from Heaven toward Earth, and all yin meridians run from Earth toward Heaven. Via the Law of Five Elements, the yin flowing from the Earth is thus integrated with the yang flowing from Heaven. The old adage may therefore be restated as 'There is nothing between yang and yin except ch'i and the Law of Five Elements that governs it.'

To make this simpler, the 12 major meridians, Cardinal Vessels, can be visualized as a series of 12 tall cylinders arranged in a circle and filled to a certain level with fluid (ch'i), as shown in Figure 6.5. Note that the Central and Governing Vessels, while part of the extended meridian system, are not part of the Law of Five Elements. Each of the 12 cylinders is directly connected to the next

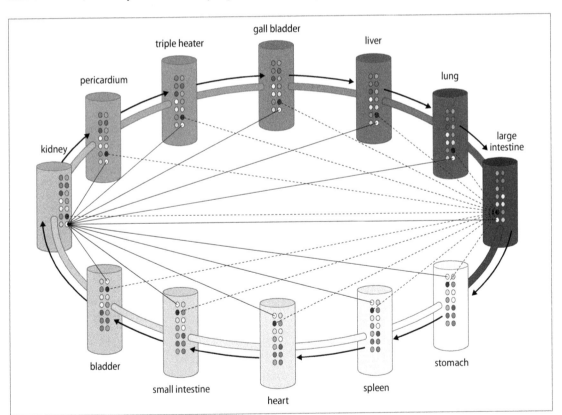

Figure 6.5 Meridian–cylinder analogy. When each meridian is represented as a cylinder with the flows between its command points to other meridians, these pathways of flow create a web or matrix. Note: these connections are shown only for two meridians; if all connections had been drawn, it would truly form a web or orb of interconnections.

cylinder in the circle by big pipes. However, each cylinder is also connected to every other cylinder by smaller secondary pipes called *command vessels*, which begin and end with a command point of the Law of Five Elements (see the numbered circles in Figure 6.6). These are called command points because they act as the valves on these secondary channels or meridians controlling the flow of ch'i between meridians.

These cylinders (meridians) are in turn connected by a myriad of pipes of varying diameters (primary, secondary, tertiary, etc.) through which the fluid circulates. Some of these pipes only connect to other pipes, but every time a pipe joins a cylinder or another pipe, there is a valve, the acupoint (see Figure 6.7). A force impels the fluid to circulate constantly in a clockwise direction. Provided all the valves are adjusted correctly, the fluid in all the cylinders will remain at the same height, containing the same amount of energy, or a balance of yin and yang.

However, rather than the meridians being

arranged in a circle as shown, the Chinese envisioned the meridians to be grouped into Five Elements, each Element being represented by a coupled pair with one yang meridian and one yin meridian. Each element represented a primary quality, and these qualities were named with reference to elements in the natural world that to them represented these qualities. Thus you have the Fire element, Earth element, Metal element, Water element and Wood element (see Figure 6.6).

These five elements were linked together by the energy flow of ch'i that flowed through complex pathways they called *channels* or *vessels*, but which were translated by the French as *meridians*. The vessels or meridians have primary pathways of flow along which are distributed the acupoints. The acupoints can be visualized as valves that control or redirect the flow of ch'i so that the ch'i may be evenly distributed throughout the body. A tenet of acupuncture theory is that all imbalances in bodily function are related to unbalanced ch'i flow. So when one system has too much energy and it has

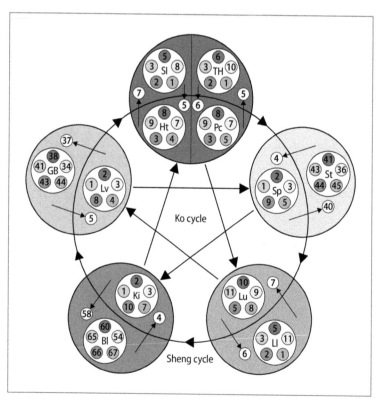

Figure 6.6. **Law of Five Elements of acupuncture.** The figure shows the flow of ch'i through the meridian system. Each element is a yin meridian coupled with a yang meridian, and two primary flows that balance each other: the yang Sheng or promotion cycle, a clockwise flow from element to element, and the yin Ko or control cycle regulating or controlling the ch'i flow from the meridian that proceeds this meridian in the flow of the Sheng cycle. Bl, bladder; GB, gall bladder; Ht, heart; Ki, kidney; LI, large intestine; Lv, liver; Lu, lung; Pc, pericardium; SI, small intestine; Sp, spleen; St, stomach; TH, triple heater.

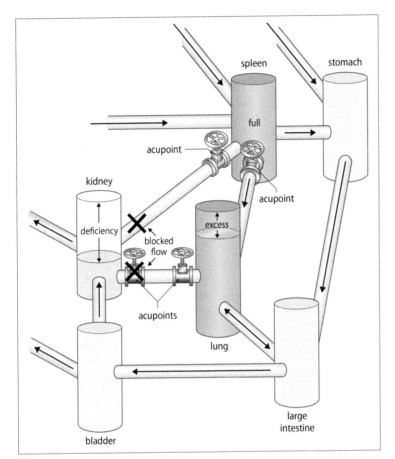

Figure 6.7 The meridian–blocked valve analogy. Each primary meridian is visualized as a cylinder in a ring of cylinders in the Law of Five Elements pattern. Each time a pipe meets a cylinder, there is a valve, the acupoint that controls the flow of the fluid (ch'i). The levels of fluid in the kidney and lung cylinders represent the classic over-energy–under-energy problem in acupuncture; the answer is to adjust the valves in the direction of flow, and the fluid levels will equalize following natural laws.

an excess of energy, this results in physiological disturbances that in western physiology we term *inflammatory*. When there is too little ch'i energy in a system it is deficient in energy; these physiological disturbances in the western system would be called *congestive*.

Each of the acupoints is an entry or exit point for the connection of the primary vessels or meridians to each other or to secondary, tertiary vessels directing the ch'i flow to specific physiological structures. And while only the primary meridians are normally shown in acupuncture books, there are a number of levels of vessels interconnecting these primary meridians to each other as an interconnected web of energetic structure. The flow of ch'i energy is thus regulated by activation or stimulation of the acupoint valves.

But what happens if a valve is turned down, restricting or blocking the flow of fluid? The level will rise in the cylinder upstream because fluid is flowing in faster than it can now flow out. This cylinder will gain an excess of fluid (ch'i) relative to other cylinders. Because each meridian is either yin or yang, one part of the system will now have an excess of yin or yang (see Figure 6.7).

The level in the downstream cylinder will fall compared with the others, as fluid is being lost faster than it is being replenished. This part of the system will become deficient in either yin or yang. In the Chinese medical system, the proper thing to do is to find the valve that is blocked and adjust it. Once the blockage to flow is removed the fluid will seek its own level automatically to re-establish a balance of yin and yang.

In the body, once the energy block is removed and the balance restored, the physiological function that was affected by the previous energy or ch'i disturbance suddenly disappears. In the

Chinese system, pain is only a sign of over-energy in a particular place, and if you drain the excess energy away the pain will also drain away. This is something acupuncture and acupressure practitioners see demonstrated daily in their clinical practices, with clients often stating 'The pain was right here!' as they desperately poke around trying to find pain that appears to have simply vanished as if by magic!

It is an effective, eloquent system whose principles are simple but whose applications can be complex, and the effects of this application can be far-reaching! Indeed, it was the application of this ancient knowledge integrated with the western technology of direct subconscious biofeedback from muscle monitoring that really allowed kinesiology to take off.

It should be noted that in traditional Chinese thought there are really Seven Elements, but the first Element, Governing Fire, represented by two of the Eight Extraordinary Vessels, Governing and Central Vessels, is more in the domain of Spirit, equating more to our *soul* than our physiology, and hence is not a part of the Five Element system of acupuncture, which deals with the physiology of the body.

The Five Elements are traditionally (at least in western presentations) shown as five elements, but with the Fire Element composed of four, not two, meridians, like the other four elements. The Chinese always saw the Fire Element as having two aspects represented by two coupled pairs of meridians: Sovereign Fire Element (heart and small intestine meridians) and Ministerial Fire Element (pericardium and triple heater). Together, these two coupled yin–yang pairs covered all aspects of the qualities the Chinese related to Fire.

Structure of the acupuncture meridian system

While most people think of the meridian system as being a two-dimensional system of lines drawn on the surface of the body, this represents only the major energy pathways of this great system (see Figure 6.8). As noted above, the Chinese recognize 14 major meridians or vessels with their own unique acupoints that distribute ch'i around the body. These 14 major meridians are called the Cardinal or primary meridians, but they represent just the most obvious energy flows. Each of these major meridians has a number of specialized acupoints that regulate and direct the energy flow through these conduits by interconnecting these 14 major flows via a myriad of smaller vessels of varying size. An in-depth discussion of the complete structure of the acupuncture meridian system is well beyond the scope of this textbook, so for an excellent discussion of these secondary vessels you are referred to Royston Low's book *The Secondary Vessels of Acupuncture*.[41] For an accessible presentation of Chinese thought underlying Chinese Medicine, you are referred to Ted Kaptchuk's book *The Web That Has No Weaver*.[42]

Secondary vessels

After the primary meridians, the next most important meridians are the secondary vessels that provide the main channels interconnecting these primary meridians and the primary meridians to various aspects of bodily function. Because in the western literature the French name *meridian* has been most commonly used, as a convention we will use the term meridian only when referring to

Figure 6.8 **The 14 major meridians of the Chinese acupuncture system.** The *Central meridian* has 24 acupoints, and the meridian pathway runs up the midline of the front of the body from Central Vessel 1 on the perineum to the inferior labial groove (the midline point under the center of your lower lip), Central Vessel 24. The *Governing meridian* has 28 acupoints and runs up the midline of the back from Governing Vessel 1 at the tip of the coccyx (tailbone) over the head and down the forehead and nose to the frenulum of the upper lip (the strip of skin that connects the upper lip to the midline gum), Governing Vessel 28. The *stomach meridian* has 45 acupoints and runs from stomach 1 on the infraorbital foramen (the dent in the center of the lower bone of the orbit), up and then back down the side of the face, then down the front of the torso on either side of the midline, and down along the lateral surface of the leg and foot all the way to the tsing point on the little toe side of the second toenail, stomach 45. The *spleen meridian* has 21 acupoints and runs from the tsing point next to the medial side of the big toenail spleen 1 up the inside of the leg and continues up the torso to an

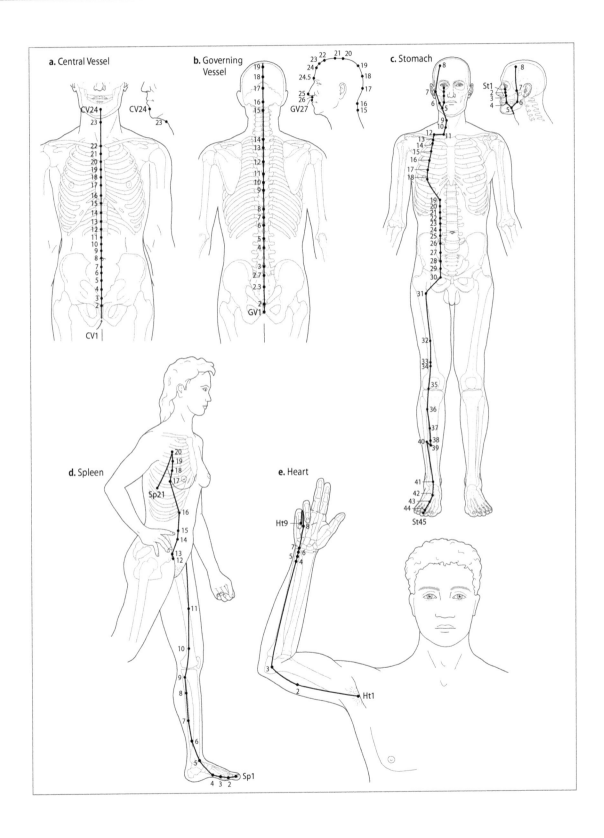

a. Central Vessel

b. Governing Vessel

c. Stomach

d. Spleen

e. Heart

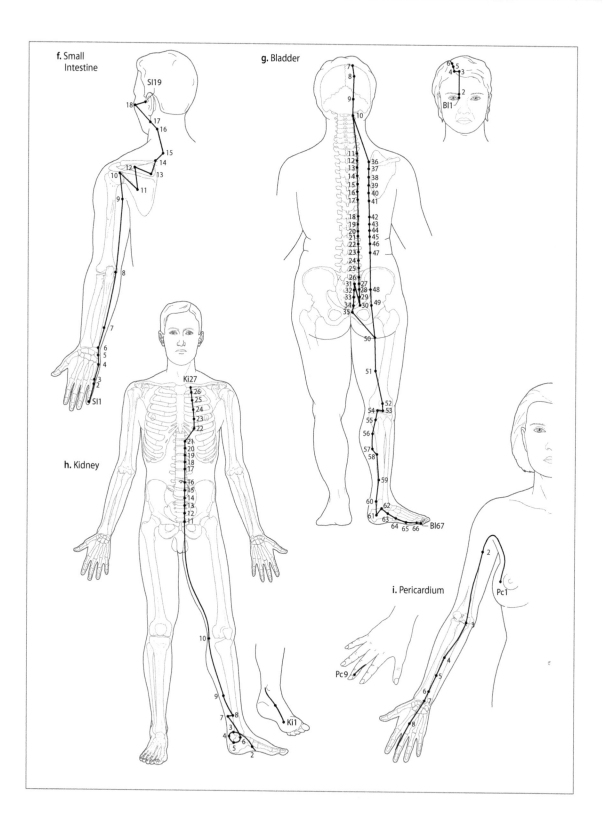

f. Small Intestine

g. Bladder

h. Kidney

i. Pericardium

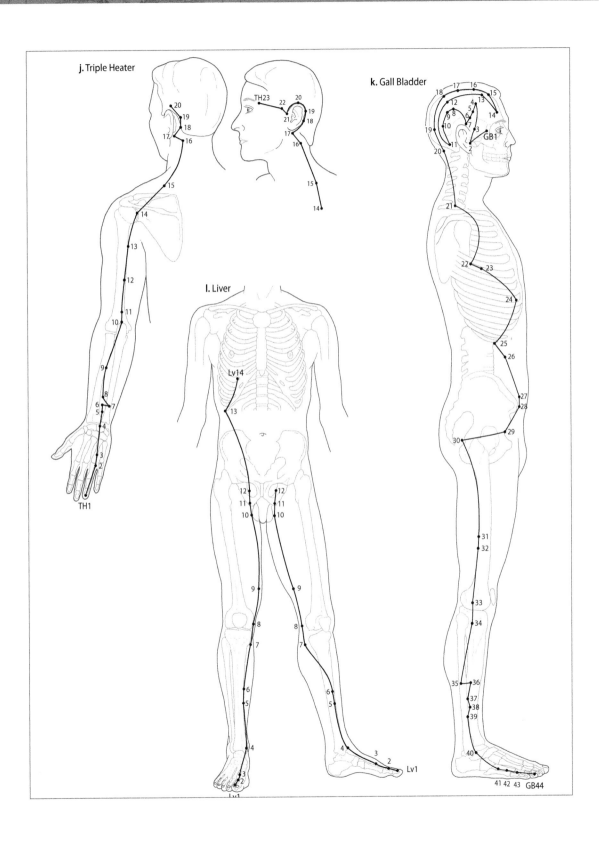

j. Triple Heater

TH23

TH1

l. Liver

Lv14

Lv1

k. Gall Bladder

GB1

GB44

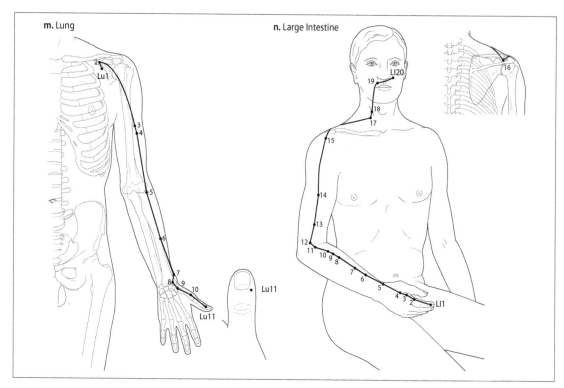

m. Lung

n. Large Intestine

Figure 6.8 continued

acupoint in the fifth intercostal space directly on the midaxillary line (a line from the center of the armpit to the waist), spleen 21. The *heart meridian* has nine acupoints and runs down from heart 1 in the mid axilla (armpit) along the inner surface of the arm to the tsing point on the ring finger side of the little fingernail, heart 9. The *small intestine meridian* has 19 acupoints and runs from the tsing point, small intestine 1, on the lateral side of the little fingernail, up the outer surface of the arm and across the shoulder and then up the neck to an acupoint on the lateral side of the face just in front of the tragus of the ear (the little trian-gular flap of the ear), small intestine 19. The *bladder meridian* has 67 acupoints and runs from bladder 1 at the inner canthus of the eye (where the two eyelids come together by the nose) up over the head, and then divides into two separate pathways down the back to the sacrum, where they again join to run down the back side of the leg and along the side of the foot to the tsing point on the outer side of the little toenail, bladder 67. The *kidney meridian* has 27 acupoints and runs up from a point directly in the center of the sole of the foot, kidney 1, and after making a circle around the inner ankle bone runs up the inside the leg and up the front of the torso just on either side of the midline to end at a dent just beneath the collarbone by the sternum, kidney 27. The *pericardium meridian* has nine acupoints and runs from just lateral to the nipple, pericardium 1, up to the shoulder and down the

middle of the inside of the arm to the tsing point by the thumb side of the middle fingernail, pericardium 9. The *triple heater meridian* has 23 acupoints and runs from the tsing point on the little finger side of the ring fingernail, triple heater 1, up the middle of the back of the hand and arm, then up the neck to end at the dent at the lateral end of the eyebrow, triple heater 23. The *gall bladder meridian* has 44 acupoints and runs from gall bladder 1 at the outer canthus of the eye (where the two eyelids meet at the outside of the eyes), up to the top of the head, and then back and forth across the side of the temple before running down the side of the torso, leg and foot to end at the tsing point on the little toe side of the fourth toenail, gall bladder 44. The *liver meridian* has 14 acupoints and runs from the tsing point on the little toe side of the big toenail, liver 1, up the medial side of the foot and leg and then up the front of the torso to liver 14 in the fifth inter-costal space on the midmammillary line from the nipple directly down to the waist. The *lung meridian* has 11 acupoints and runs down the inner surface of the arm from lung 1, in the dent below the coracoid process of the scapula, to the tsing point on the lateral side of the thumb-nail, lung 11. The *large intestine meridian* has 20 acupoints and runs from the tsing point on the thumb side of the index fingernail, large intestine 1, up the lateral side of the arm across the shoulder and up the neck to end directly next to the lateral side of the external nares (the dent next to the lateral side of the nostril), large intestine 20.

the primary vessels of acupuncture and the term *vessel* for all secondary channels.

The acupoints on each primary meridian that provide the entry to or exit from these secondary vessels are called tsing points, entry or exit points, command points, horary points, luo points, source points and Yuan points, and they control and regulate not only the energy flow within a meridian but also between the meridians and between the meridians and their associated organ. So for each meridian, rather than a straight line flow of ch'i there is a web or orb of interconnecting energy pathways connecting each meridian with every other meridian in the body.

Command points

The acupoints providing access to secondary vessels generally bear the name of the secondary vessel. For instance, the luo point provides access to the luo vessel, the Fire command point to a secondary vessel connecting each meridian to the Fire element, etc. The command points are so called because they are the entry or exit points to major secondary vessels linking the primary meridian flows to each other. Stimulation of the command point directs or commands the flow of energy in one primary meridian to another primary meridian, permitting the redistribution of energy in the meridian system and balancing the energy flows in the system as a whole.

For instance, if there were a deficiency of ch'i in the spleen meridian and an excess of ch'i in the heart meridian, stimulation of spleen 2 will 'pull' the excess ch'i from heart to fill the deficiency of ch'i in spleen by opening the secondary command vessel gate or valve, spleen 2, on the spleen end of the pipe. Energy acts like water: it always flows downhill, always seeking its own level, and it always seeks the shortest pathway. So once the spleen end of the command vessel is open, the energy will flow into the spleen meridian until the energy in both meridians is equalized.

Horary points

Each of the bilateral meridians is more yang on the right side and more yin on the left side of the body, reflecting body polarity. Hence, one type of yin–yang imbalance is when one side of a meridian has more energy than the other side, even though the meridian as a whole may have a homeostatic amount of energy. The command point of the element for the meridian on which the point is located (e.g. Earth command point on spleen meridian) is called the horary point. Stimulation of the horary point on the under-energy side of the meridian will open the horary channel. This is a secondary vessel connecting the same meridian on both sides of the body, allowing the over-energy on one side to flow into the under-energy on the other side. For instance, if the spleen meridian has too much energy on the right side (a yang imbalance), then stimulating spleen 3 on the left side meridian will permit this excess yang energy to flow into the under-energy yin side, equalizing the balance of energy between the right and left spleen meridians.

Luo points

We will briefly summarize the role of several of the major command points and their related secondary vessels. While the command points connect the primary meridians directly to each other, the luo points are the entry and exit points to the secondary vessels that connect the coupled yin and yang primary meridians of each element in the Law of Five Elements to each other (see Figure 6.9). These secondary vessels are called *luo* or *transverse vessels*. So if there is too much energy in a yang

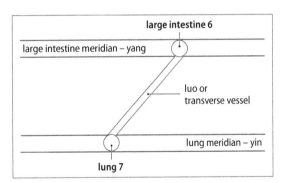

Figure 6.9 Luo or transverse vessels. Luo points are the acupoints that provide entry to and exit from the luo channel or vessel that directly connects the yin and yang primary meridian pair within each element, and are used to equalize the yin and yang energy within each element.

primary meridian of an element and too little energy in the yin primary meridian, then stimulating the luo point will open the luo vessel connecting these meridians, pulling the excess energy from the over-energy meridian into the under-energy meridian.

For example, if the large intestine meridian of the Metal element is over-energy and the lung meridian of the Metal element is under-energy, then stimulating the lung luo point, lung 7, will open the luo vessel connecting large intestine to lung meridian, pulling the excess over-energy from the large intestine meridian into the lung meridian to fill or balance its under-energy state.

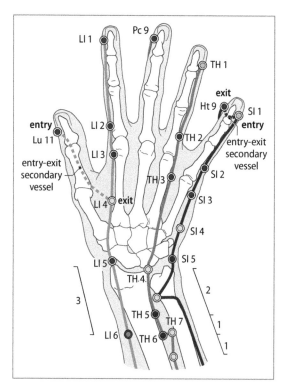

Figure 6.10 The meridian entry and exit points. Ch'i flows into a meridian via the entry point and exits that meridian via the exit point, traversing a secondary vessel called an entry–exit vessel. If the exit or entry point of one meridian is a dead end, flow is redirected to an acupoint that has direct flow to or from the previous meridian in the clock flow. Compare the flow between lung (Lu) 11 and large intestine (LI) 4, with the flow between heart (Ht) 9 and small intestine (SI) 1. Pc, pericardium; TH, triple heater.

Source points

The source point is the valve to the secondary vessel that connects each primary meridian to its associated organ. Remember that ch'i is visualized by the Chinese as the nutritive energy that sustains the energetic template needed to maintain the physical structure and function of the organ associated with that meridian. In a sense, ch'i flow is seen to maintain the energetic template of the organ or information needed to maintain the physical organ. So if the associated organ requires a greater flow of nutritive ch'i to sustain and maintain its function, stimulation of the source point will direct nutritive ch'i into the associated organ. Stimulation of the source point will also bring energy into the meridian as a whole, as they act as a transduction point for cosmic energy into subtle energy. Source points affect the entire meridian energy flow and are four times more active than any other point on the meridian.

Entry and exit points

The entry and exit points on each meridian are the ends of the secondary vessels connecting the flow of ch'i in one meridian with another meridian so that the ch'i may flow continuously through the whole meridian system. Thus the entry point is the acupoint on the meridian where energy enters the meridian, while the exit point is the acupoint, where it exits the meridian to flow on to the next meridian in the superficial cycle of ch'i flow through the body. The point of entry and the point of exit are usually the first and last points, respectively, of the meridian (see Figure 6.10).

There is an integrative pattern of flow of the ch'i through the meridian system via connection of the entry and exit points. Traditionally, this begins with the stomach meridian, then flows to spleen, heart, small intestine, bladder, kidney, pericardium, triple heater, gall bladder, liver, lung and large intestine, only to return to stomach once more. In this pattern of flow, it begins with the flow from the head to the feet, then feet to the trunk, trunk to the hand, hand to the head, and head to the feet, and this cycle repeats (see Figure 6.11).

In some cases, the points of entry and exit are not the first and last points of the meridian, and the secondary vessel uniting the consecutive meridians in the ch'i cycle do not connect at the end points, although these points are usually close to the beginning and ends of the primary meridian. Nevertheless, the remaining distal portion of the meridian before or beyond the entry or exit points is not a cul-de-sac, for there is still another secondary vessel uniting the end points of consecutive meridians, but this performs a secondary function to the secondary vessel connecting the meridian points of entry and exit. Stimulation of these acupoints helps to transmit energy from one meridian to the next if there is a blockage in ch'i flow.

Tsing points

The tsing point is the name given to the point on each meridian, either the first or last, that occurs at the extremities (e.g. beside the bed of the fingernails or toenails), sometimes called the *nail points* or *akabane points* in Japanese acupuncture (see Figure 6.12). The energy tends to pool at the beginning and end points, and these points are usually the origin of another important secondary vessel: the musculotendinous meridians.

These musculotendinous meridians are the

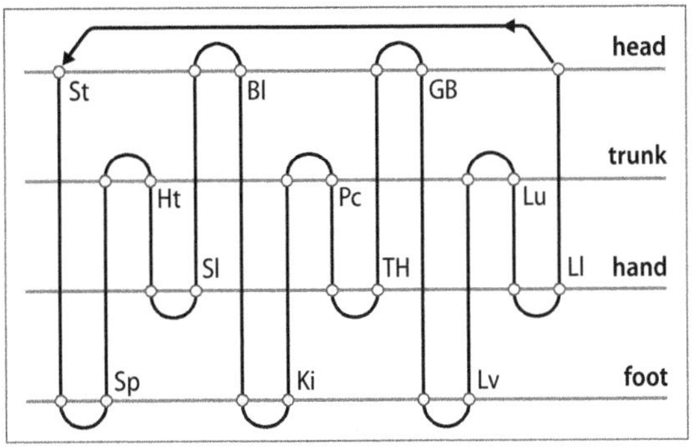

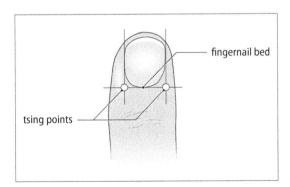

Figure 6.11 The meridian wheel or clock flows through the 12 primary meridians. Meridian ch'i flows are continuous from one meridian to the other in a specific order, but one that does not follow the deeper flows of the Law of Five Elements. Called *clock flows* or *wheel flows*, there is an orderly progression of a 2-hour peak of energy in each meridian that then flows to the next meridian in the repeated sequence, head to foot, foot to trunk, trunk to hand and hand to head, creating a 24-hour cycle. Bl, bladder; GB, gall bladder; Ht, heart; Ki, kidney; Ll, large intestine; Lv, liver; Lu, lung; Pc, pericardium; Sl, small intestine; Sp, spleen; St, stomach; TH, triple heater.

Figure 6.12 Tsing points or akabane points. The beginning or end of each meridian is what the Chinese called the *tsing point* and the Japanese call the *akabane point*. These points are located on either side of the nail bed of each finger or toe. Tsing points are located at the intersection of a line drawn from the corner of the tip of the fingernail or toenail directly up the finger or toe with a line drawn across the nail bed.

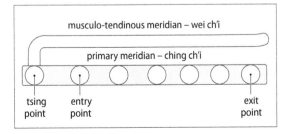

Figure 6.13 The musculotendinous meridians. Musculotendinous meridians originate at a tsing point and then flow into the superficial tissues of an adjacent body region and carry a derivative of meridian ching ch'i, called wei ch'i, that in the Chinese system ward off perverse energy.

secondary vessels that connect the primary meridian with an associated superficial region of the body, including the muscle(s) associated with the primary meridian in kinesiology. The musculotendinous meridians carry a protective form of ch'i called wei ch'i, derived from meridian ch'i, which acts as a first line of defence against invasion of perverse energy. Stimulation of the tsing point can balance the energy flow in the musculotendinous meridians (see Figure 6.13).

Association (back shu) points

Association points are acupoints on the back along the medial course of the bladder meridian on each side of the vertebral column. Excess energy from each meridian is stored in the associated point. These are also known as the *master point* for the meridian. Kidney 27 is considered the associated point for all association points, hence the more generalized effects of kidney 27 acupoints on polarity, for example switching, and even integrative neural flows across the corpus callosum underlying brain integration. The association points are all bladder meridian acupoints on the back. They act like capacitors by taking up momentary excesses of energy in the meridian flow and releasing this excess as the surge of energy passes. Acupressure on these points will often cause immediate relief of pain in the associated organ or in muscles of the back on which the point is located. Indeed one of the reasons they were painful in the first place was because the build-up of energy in the association point had spilled over into the surrounding muscle tissue, creating an over-energy state, which in the Chinese system equals pain.

These points are all paravertebral along the course of the bladder meridian one and a half cun (body inches) from the midline from bladder 13 on either side of the third thoracic vertebrae down to bladder 27 on the sacrum.

Alarm (front mu) points

Alarm points are specific indicator points that indicate over- and under-energy in the related meridian. Only the alarm points for Central, Governing, lung, liver and gall bladder meridians are on their respective meridians; the other alarm points, although not on their meridians, are basically located over the organ with which they are associated. For example, heart alarm point is over the heart area and large intestine alarm point is over the large intestine. For the 12 meridians, 6 alarm points are located on the Central meridian: 2 on the gall bladder meridian, 2 on the liver meridian and 1 each on the lung and stomach meridians. Central and Governing Vessel alarm points, Central Vessel 24 and Governing Vessel 26, are also on their respective meridians.

The alarm points are points on the secondary vessels connecting the primary meridian to its associated organ, and hence indicate disturbances in the nutritive flow of ch'i carrying organizing information to the organ that sustains its structure and function and maintains homeostasis in that organ system. It is indeed because the alarm points are located on these secondary vessels that their location often does not coincide with acupoints on the meridian for which they indicate imbalance.

Finer meridian system structure

While the primary and secondary vessels of the acupuncture meridian system have by far the greatest overall effect on the distribution of ch'i in the body, there are a number of other levels of reticulation of these ch'i channels in the body. There are tertiary vessels, quaternary vessels and so on, each connecting to various acupoints, with ch'i flow in these finer vessels being associated with more specific aspects of the body's structure and function. It is said that there are 64 levels of reticulation within the acupuncture meridian system, ending in individual cells, making this a very complex system indeed! For a thorough discussion of the acupuncture meridian system and its historical and philosophical origins, you are referred to Manfred Porkert's excellent book, *The Theoretical Foundations of Chinese Medicine*.[43]

The origin of meridian ch'i

Meridian or ching ch'i is composed of several types of ch'i derived from different sources. When you eat food, the Chinese were aware that you derive gross nutrients and energy from the food, but they also said that you derive a type of ch'i from the food, Ku Ch'i. Today, we would call this the subtle energy or vital energy of the food. The Ku Ch'i is the subtle nutritive energy from the food that sustains organ structure and function according to their theory.

Likewise, when we breathe we inhale air with all its chemical components, such as nitrogen, oxygen and carbon dioxide, but from the perspective of eastern people, we also take in a subtle form of cosmic energy called *prana* by the yogis and Ta Ch'i by the Chinese. Together, Ku Ch'i and Ta Ch'i combine to form another type of ch'i, Tsung Ch'i, which must combine with a third type of ch'i, Yuan Ch'i, to become active Chen Ch'i that flows into the yin organs, which then releases ching ch'i, which flows along the meridians, or meridian ch'i (see Figure 6.14).

This third component of meridian ch'i, Yuan Ch'i, is derived from the most fundamental ancestral energy or Hsien T'ien Ch'i stored in the kidney *energy structure*, not the kidney *organ*. This ancestral ch'i is not an active energy but only a potential to become manifest at birth with the first breath. The first breath activates the triple heater meridian

and the potential in the Hsien T'ien Ch'i manifests itself as active energy or Yuan Ch'i. Indeed, Yuan Ch'i is also necessary to separate Ku Ch'i from food. It is only when Yuan Ch'i activates the Tsung Ch'I, created by the combination of the Ta Ch'i from the air and Ku Ch'i from our food, that Chen Ch'i is created.

Chen Ch'i is then passed from the lungs directly to the yin organs of the Five Elements, with each organ retaining some of this nutritive ch'i for itself and transforming the remainder into ching ch'i and wei ch'i. Ching ch'i circulates through the primary vessels of the meridian system, while wei ch'i circulates through the more superficial tendinomuscular meridians and is the first line of defence against the invasion of perverse energy, and so is usually called *protective* or *defensive* ch'i. In the western use, the wei ch'i is regarded as part of the function of ching ch'i, and both together are referred to simply as *meridian ch'i*. It is by the active flow of meridian ch'i circulating through our meridian system that the organizing energy is distributed to the physical body, providing an energy template to maintain our physical and physiological being.

This is why in the Chinese system it is important

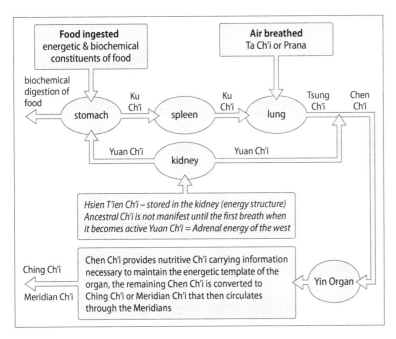

Figure 6.14 Formation of meridian of meridian ch'i. For the Chinese, food has two distinct constituents: the biochemical physical matter and an energetic constituent they called Ku Ch'i. In their view, the air we breathe also contains a more subtle energy, Ta Ch'i. When the Ku Ch'i from food combines with Ta Ch'i from breathing, this forms the precursor of Ching Ch'i or meridian ch'i called Tsung Ch'i. For both Ku Ch'i to be released from food and for Tsung Ch'i to be converted to active Chen Ch'i, Ching Ch'i requires activation by Yuan Ch'i or Ancestral Ch'i stored in the kidney energy structure.

to eat good food to maximize the quality of your Ku Ch'i, and to breathe deeply of pure air to maximize the quality and quantity of your Ta Ch'I, so you do not have to draw very strongly on your Yuan Ch'i derived from your ancestral energy. According to Chinese theory, each person is born with a certain amount of ancestral Hsien T'ien Ch'i, the source of the Yuan Ch'i essential to activate the Ta Ch'i and Ku Ch'i into active functional meridian ch'i. Therefore when the Yuan Ch'i is used up, you no longer can make meridian ch'i, and therefore there is no longer nutritive ch'i to sustain and maintain the etheric template of the organs and the energetic template disintegrates. Once the etheric template has gone, your physical body follows the second law of thermodynamics, the law of entropy, and your body begins to degenerate, leading to sickness and eventually to death.

If the quality of your food and/or air is poor, then you are deficient in Ku Ch'i and Ta Ch'i and need to draw more strongly on your ancestral derived Yuan Ch'i just to survive. From a western perspective, you can think of your Yuan Ch'i as the energy behind your ability to adapt to stressful circumstances, the equivalent of adaptation energy, as described by Hans Selye.[44] From a western physiological perspective, physiological adaptation to stress relies heavily on our adrenal energy, which in some ways plays a role analogous to Yuan Ch'i in the Chinese system.

Therefore for the Chinese it has always been clear that people will have lives of different lengths and react to stress differently. The people who come in with lots of ancestral ch'i in their 'bank account' have the potential for a long and healthy life, even if they overindulge in eating, smoking and drinking—the medical reprobates, while those people who enter this life with only a limited amount of ancestral ch'i are destined to a much shorter life no matter how well they take care of themselves! Ancestral ch'i is like a trust fund that you are born with: you can take money out but you cannot put more money back into it, and once it is empty you are bankrupt!

The Chinese found that by doing certain exercises, the basis of ch'i or qi gong and Tai Ch'i, you could build up another type of ch'i, *Ho Yuan Ch'i*, which, while it does not replace Yuan Ch'I, provides an ancillary source of energy for adapting to stress. Hence you can stretch the amount of Yuan Ch'i needed to cope with the stresses in life and hence lengthen your life. Ho Yuan Ch'i can be thought of as an ancillary bank account that you work to build up and on which you can draw for some of life's needs, thus reducing how much you need to take from the trust fund every month and therefore extending how long your trust fund will last.

Besides meridian ch'i, two other types of subtle energy flow through the meridian system: Shen and Jing. Both of these are concepts that do not directly translate into any western words, but *Shen* is usually translated as 'spirit' and *Jing* has no real translation, as it relates to the energy behind manifestation. There are also many other types of ch'i, each with its own unique contribution to your physiological and energetic function, but a discussion of these is beyond the scope of this textbook, and you are referred to the treatise by Manfred Porkert, *The Theoretical Foundations of Chinese Medicine*,[43] or Royston's Law's book *The Secondary Vessels of Acupuncture*.[41]

Meridian ch'i flow and health

According to Chinese theory, as long as the ch'i flow in every meridian is balanced with respect to yin and yang, and is neither in excess nor deficiency, the associated organ receives sufficient nutritive ch'i flow to maintain the integrity of its structure and function. Any perturbation of this flow will have immediate consequences for the function or physiology of the associated organ causing some degree of imbalance in its physiology. If the energetic imbalance is large or goes on for a period of time, the blockage of ch'i flow will then become apparent in the structure and function supported by these flows. Once the sustaining nutritive flows of ch'i are disrupted, tissues begin to degenerate following the second law of thermodynamics, the law of entropy.

The degree of structural or physiological imbalance is directly related to the degree of energetic disturbance in the meridian ch'i flow: the bigger the disturbance or blockage in energy flow, the greater will be the physiological imbalance. Hence, a minor energy blockage in a secondary or tertiary vessel may not even be noticed consciously, because at a subconscious level effective compensations have been established. However, should a primary meridian become blocked there will be an immediate overt physiological reaction easily observed by the person and others.

One approach to the perturbed physiology is to treat the symptoms arising from the disturbed physiology with a drug to counteract the physiological disturbance. The other approach would be to locate the energy blockage and the factors creating it, and then apply acupuncture or acupressure stimulation of one or more acupoints to eliminate the energy blockage, allowing the excess of energy, termed *over-energy*, to automatically flow into the area deficient in energy, termed *under energy*. Once the energy has been equalized, the physiological disturbance automatically returns to homeostasis, as the nutritive ch'i once more carries organizing information into the disturbed tissue—a process we call *healing*.

The first reaction to blocked energy flow, from the perspective of the generalized adaptation syndrome of western physiology, is the *alarm reaction* or *stage 1 stress* (see Figure 6.15). The physiology becomes overtly perturbed, with some physiological function exceeding normal homeostatic limit. If the physiologic function being observed were body temperature, this would be perceived as a fever or chills. Perceived from the perspective of Chinese medicine, this would be an energy imbalance created by an excess of yang or yin, respectively. This initiates a series of both energetic and corresponding physiological compensations to re-establish normal body temperature. If these initial rapid short-term compensations are sufficient to release the energetic blockage, and bring the body temperature back within normal homeostatic limits, stage 1 stress has been eliminated.

For instance, I become cold because I am sitting still and there is a cool breeze. This begins to lower my body temperature so I begin to shiver, a stage 1 stress response. So I then begin to walk briskly, and the heat produced from my muscular activity rapidly raises my body temperature, restoring my homeostasis, and the shivering stops. Note that sitting is passive, which is yin, and chills are also yin, so I automatically compensate by moving, increasing my yang, to increase my body temperature to counteract the heat lost to the cool breeze, which is yin.

If these initial compensations were not successful, however, and cannot bring the body temperature back within normal homeostatic limits, further more complex and ongoing compensations are implemented, leading to *stage 2 stress*, the *stage of resistance* or *compensation*. In this case, I feel the need to move more vigorously to increase the heat generated from my muscle contraction, and my body now adapts to this ongoing stressor of cold by the hypothalamus releasing thyroid stimulating hormone, causing the thyroid to release thyroxine which in turn causes all the cells of the body to increase their basal rate of metabolism, increasing body temperature in the long term.

The compensations of stage 2 stress are always energetically expensive, *but if successful, remain outside of our consciousness*. Stage 2 stress, the stage of compensation, cannot go on indefinitely, because it is dependent on putting more energy into this function than is required by homeostasis. This means that energy has to be withdrawn from other energy resources of the body to maintain these compensations. As an analogy, I need to borrow money to survive financially, so I borrow money from Peter to pay Paul. But because some compensations have compound interest on the original loan of energy, soon Peter cannot lend me enough money, so I also borrow more from Fred to pay the interest I also owe Paul, and over time I may need to even borrow more widely from Harry and James. What happens when Peter now calls in his loan as he needs the money (energy) I borrowed to survive economically? My house of cards collapses and I am suddenly bankrupt!

In many ways, this is an accurate model of what happens in the body when stage 2 stress has gone on too long. As more energetic/physiologic systems are required to support the system in stress, they reach a point where the systems lending energy suddenly have no extra energy to lend and

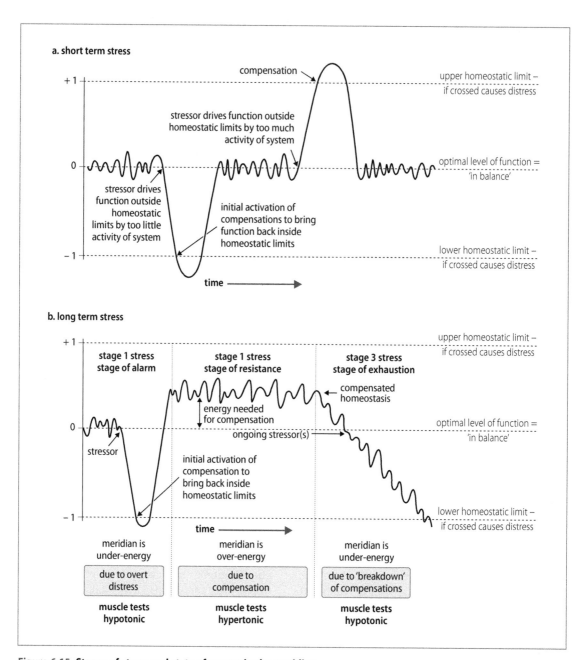

Figure 6.15 Stages of stress and state of energy in the meridian.
a, **Short-term, stage 1 stress, the stage of alarm.** A stressor has perturbed the flow of ch'i to an organ and the organ goes under-energy. With loss of organizing ch'i flows, the organ cannot sustain its normal homeostatic function and it functions less efficiently.
b, **Long-term, stage 2 stress.** In response to an ongoing stressor, the body compensates by borrowing ch'i from other organs or meridians and establishes a compensated state of balanced/imbalance, the stage of resistance. Because of the additional energy required to sustain ongoing compensations, the organ system in compensation becomes over-energy. If a stressor goes on too long, compensations begin to break down and the system enters stage 3 stress, the stage of exhaustion, and the original stress reappears as the organ or meridian goes under-energy once more.

withdraw their energetic support for the system in stress, which then results in collapse of the stressed system, leading to *stage 3 stress*, the *stage of exhaustion*. In stage 3 stress, the compensations supporting the stressed system can no longer be maintained and break down, resulting in the person becoming overtly sick or ill. At this time, they now suffer from an identifiable disease or physiological problem. If the person's physiology cannot be pushed back into the stage 2 of resistance with various types of assistance, for example drugs, surgery, good food or herbs, then the end of stage 3 stress results in death.

Stage 1 and 2 stress is reflected in the Law of Five Elements via an imbalance of meridian ch'i caused by energy blockage. The meridians upstream of the block often gain an excess of ch'i or over-energy, and at least some of the meridians downstream of the blockage become deficient in ch'i, or under-energy (see Figure 6.7). The difference between a stage 1 stress and a stage 2 stress is that the stage 1 stress represents overt uncompensated stress: one meridian is over-energy and another meridian is under-energy, and there is as yet no compensatory energy borrowing going on. If the energy blockage is resolved, for instance the person just gets more sleep, then the stage 1 stress disappears as balanced energy flow is once again re-established.

In stage 2 stress, on the other hand, the energy blockage persists, and the body compensates by redistributing the original over- and under-energies via the secondary vessels of acupuncture. Several meridians have now loaned energy to the under-energy meridian, creating a number of under-energy meridians, but each with a smaller under-energy than the original under-energy meridian. Likewise, through compensatory redistribution of the over-energy, several meridians are now over-energy, but each is less over-energy than the original over-energy meridian, so the meridian system as a whole is more balanced.

One reason an energetic imbalance may persist is that one or more of the acupoints has become blocked and can no longer maintain sufficient flow to maintain homeostasis. Using the valve analogy, a valve has become stuck or frozen, like a rusty valve, and cannot be either turned in far enough or turned out far enough to provide homeostatic ch'i flows. Therefore frozen acupoints need to develop some type of compensation to maintain function. To maintain a state of compensation, a stressed acupoint will draw on energy from another meridian to which it is connected via a secondary, tertiary or smaller vessel.

So if there is a deficiency of yin energy feeding into the point, then more yin energy will be drawn into the point from another meridian to balance the dynamics of the acupoint. Indeed, it is these compensations caused by frozen acupoints that often underlie chronic meridian-wide over- and under-energy imbalances. Therefore these frozen acupoints need to be addressed before attempting to just stimulate the acupoints according to the Law of Five Elements, or the compensated condition will just be recreated over time by the blocked flows underlying the frozen points. Frozen acupoints will be discussed in more detail in chapter 38.

References

1. Mann, F 1972, *Acupuncture: The Ancient Chinese Art of Healing and How It Works Scientifically*, Random House, New York.
   Academy of Traditional Chinese Medicine 1975, *An Outline of Chinese Acupuncture*, Foreign Language Press, Beijing, pp. 3–7.
   Xinnong, C (chief ed.) 1990 *Chinese Acupuncture and Moxibustion*, Foreign Language Press, Beijing, pp. 1–7.

2. Unschuld, PU 1989, *History of Acupuncture and Chinese Medicine*, Medical Acupuncture Publishers, Berkeley.

3. Lu, HC 1978, *The Yellow Emperor's Classic of Internal Medicine and the Difficult Cases*, Academy of Oriental Heritage, Vancouver.

4. Kaptchuk, TJ 1983, *The Web That Has No Weaver: Understanding Chinese Medicine*, Ryder, London.

Xinnong, C (chief ed.) 1990 *Chinese Acupuncture and Moxibustion*, Foreign Language Press, Beijing
Deadman, P, Al-Khafaji, M & Baker, K 1998, *A Manual of Acupuncture*, Eastland Press, Vista.

5. Xinnong, C (chief ed.) 1990 *Chinese Acupuncture and Moxibustion*, Foreign Language Press, Beijing, p. 5.

6. Grall, Y 1962, *Contribution à l'Étude de la conductibilité Électrique de la Peau*, Thesis, Algiers.

7. Niboyet, JEH 1963, *La Moindre Resistance à l'Electricite de Surfaces Punctiformes et de Trajets Catanes Concordant Avec les Points et Meridiens, Bases de l'Acupuncture*, Thesis, Marseille.
   Reichmanis, M, Marino, AA, & Becker RO 1975, Electrical

correlates of acupuncture points, *IEEE Transactions on Biomedical Engineering*, Vol. 22, pp. 533–535.

Roppel, RM & Mitchell, F, Jr 1975 Skin points of anomalously low electric resistance: current voltage characteristics and relationships to peripheral stimulation therapies, *Journal of the American Osteopathic Association*, Vol. 746, pp. 877–878.

Hyvarien, J & Karlson, M 1977, Low resistance skin points that may coincide with acupuncture locations, *Medical Biology*, Vol. 55, pp. 88–94.

Helms, JM 1995, *Acupuncture Energetics: A Clinical Approach for Physicians*, Medical Acupuncture Publishers, Berkeley, pp. 20–21.

8. Niboyet, JEH 1938, Nouvelles constalations un les proprietés électrique des points chinois, *Bulletin de la Société de'Acupuncture*, Vol. 4(30).

Bossey, J & Sambuc, P 1989, *Acupuncture et systeme nerveux: les acquis. Acupuncture et Médecine Tranditionnelle Chinois*, Paris. Encyclopedic des Médecine Naturelles, 1B-1.

Helms, JM 1995, *Acupuncture Energetics: A Clinical Approach for Physicians*, Medical Acupuncture Publishers, Berkeley, pp. 26–27.

9. Senelar, R 1979, Caractéristiques morphologiques des points chinois. In: Niboyet, JEH, ed. *Nouveau Traité d'Acupuncture*, Moulins-les-Metz, Maisonneuve, pp. 247–277.

Auziech, O 1984, *Étude Histologique des Points Cutanés de Moindre Resistance à l'Électricite et Analzse de Leurs Implications Possibles Dans la Mise en Jeu des Mécanismes Acupuncturaux*, Thesis, Montpellier.

10. Senelar, R & Auziech, O 1989, Histophysiologie du point d'acupuncture. Acupuncture et Médecine Traditionnelle Chinois, Paris. *Encyclopédie des Médecines Naturelles, 1B-2C.*

11. Bossy, J 1982 The history of acupuncture in the west: exoticism, esoterism and opposition to Cartesian rationalism, complementarity to the occidental medical system. *Nihon Ishigaku Zasshi (Journal of Japanese History of Medicine)*, Vol. 28(1) Supplement.

Souillé de Morant, G 1972, *L'Acupuncture Chinoise*. Maloine Éditeurs, Paris.

12. Porkert, M 1978, *The Theoretical Foundations of Chinese Medicine*, MIT Press, Cambridge.

Maciocia, G 1989, *The Foundations of Chinese Medicine*, Churchill Livingstone, London, pp. 15–34.

Helms, JM 1995, *Acupuncture Energetics: A Clinical Approach for Physicians*, Medical Acupuncture Publishers, Berkeley.

Deadman, P, Al-Khafaji, M & Baker, K 1998, *A Manual of Acupuncture*, Journal of Chinese Medicine Publications, East Essex, p. 671.

13. Gerber, R 1988, *Vibrational Medicine*, Bear, Santa Fe, p. 127.

Oschman, JL 2003, *Energy Medicine*, Elsevier, London.

14. Gerber, R 2000 *Vibrational Medicine for the 21st Century*, Harper Collins, New York, pp. 151–158.

15. Rose-Neil, S 1967, The work of Professor Kim Bong Han, *The Acupuncturist*, Vol. 1, p. 15.

Gerber, R 1988, *Vibrational Medicine*, Bear, Santa Fe, pp. 122–125.

16. Darras, JC, de Vernejoul, P & Albarède P 1987, Visualisation isotopique des méridiens d'acupuncture, *Cahiers de Biothérapie*, Vol. 95, pp. 13–22.

Darras, J-C, Albarède P & de Vernejoul, P 1993, Nuclear medicine investigation of transmission of acupuncture information, *Acupuncture in Medicine*, Vol. 11(1), pp. 22–28.

Darras, J-C 1989, Isotopic and cytologic assays in acupuncture.

In: *Energy Fields in Medicine*, John E. Fetzer Foundation, Kalamazoo, pp. 44–65.

17. Schlebusch, KP, Maric-Oehler, W & Popp, F-A 2005, Biophotonics in the infrared spectral range reveal acupuncture meridian structure of the body, *Journal of Alternative and Complementary Medicine*, Vol. 11(1), pp. 171–173.

18. Litscher, G 2005, Infrared thermography fails to visualize stimulation-induced meridian-like structures, *Biomedical Engineering Online*, Vol. 4(1). p. 38.

19. Popp, FA, Maric-Oehler, W, Schlebusch, KP & Klimek, W 2005, Evidence of light piping (meridian-like channels) in the human body and nonlocal EMF effects, *Electromagnetic Biology and Medicine*, Vol. 24(3), pp. 359–374.

20. Narongpunt, V, Datcu, S, Ibos, L, Adnet, F, Fontas, B, Candau, Y & Alimi, D 2004, Monitoring acupressure stimulation effects by infrared thermography, *Quantitative InfraRed Thermography Journal*, Vol. 1(2), pp. 185–204.

Yang, HQ, Xie, SS, Hu, XL, Chen, L & Li H 2002 Appearance of human meridian-like structure and acupoints and its time correlation by infrared thermal imaging, *American Journal of Chinese Medicine*, Vol. 35(2), pp. 231–240.

21. Hseuh, CC & O'Connor, J (translator) 1981, *Acupuncture: A Comprehensive Text, First Edition*, Eastland Press, Vista.

Deadman, P, Al-Khafaji, M & Baker, K 2007, *A Manual of Acupuncture*, Journal of Chinese Medicine Publications, East Sussex.

22. Brewitt B 1996, Quantitative analysis of electrical skin conductance in diagnosis: historical and current views of bioelectric medicine, *Journal of Naturopathic Medicine*, Vol. 6(1), pp. 66–75.

Ahn, AC & Martinsen, ÒG 2007, Electrical characterization of acupuncture points: technical issues and challenges, *Journal of Alternative and Complementary Medicine*, Vol. 13(8), pp. 817–824.

23. Ahn, AC, Colbert, AP, Anderson, BJ, Martinsen, OG, Hammerschlag, R, Cina, S, Wayne, PM, Langevin, HM 2008, Electrical properties of acupuncture points and meridians: a systematic review, *Bioelectromagnetics*, Vol. 29(4), pp. 245–256.

24. Litscher, G, Niemtzow, RC, Wang, L, Gao, X & Urak, CH 2011, Electrodermal mapping of an acupuncture point and a non-acupuncture point, *Journal of Alternative and Complementary Medicine*, Vol. 17(9), pp. 781–782.

25. Choi, EM, Jiang, F & Longhurst, JC 2012, Point specificity in acupuncture, *Chinese Medicine*, Vol. 7, p. 4.

26. Melzack, R & Wall, P 1965, Pain mechanisms: a new theory, *Science*, Vol. 150, pp. 971–979.

27. Hui, KK, Liu, J, Makris, N, Gollub, RL, Chen, AJ, Moore, CI, Kennedy, DN, Rosen, BR & Kwong, KK 2000, Acupuncture modulates the limbic system and subcortical gray structures of the human brain: evidence from fMRI studies in normal subjects, *Human Brain Mapping*, Vol. 9, pp. 13–25.

Yan B, Li K, Xu J, Wang, W, Li, K, Liu, H, Shan, B & Tang, X 2005, Acupoint-specific fMRI patterns in human brain, *Neuroscience Letters*, Vol. 383, pp. 236–240.

Yuanyuan Feng, Lijun Bai, Wensheng Zhang, Yanshuang Ren, Ting Xue, Hu Wang, Chongguang Zhong, Jie Tian 2011, Investigation of acupoint specificity by whole brain functional connectivity analysis from fMRI data. In: *Conference Proceedings: Annual International Conference of the IEEE Engineering in Medicine and Biology Society*, pp. 2784–2787.

28. Fang, JL, Krings, T, Weidemann, J, Meister, IG, & Thron, A 2004, Functional MRI in healthy subjects during acupuncture:

different effects of needle rotation in real and false acupoints, *Neuroradiology*, Vol. 46(5), pp. 359–362.

Zhang, W-I, Jin, Z, Luo, F, Zhang, L, Zeng, Y-W, & Han, J-S 2005, Evidence from brain imaging with fMRI supporting functional specificity of acupoints in humans, *Neuroscience Letters*, Vol. 382, pp. 1–4.

Hu KM, Wang CP, Xie HJ & Henning J 2006, Observation on activating effectiveness of acupuncture at acupoints and non-acupoints on different brain regions [in Chinese], *Zhongguo Zhen Jiu*, Vol. 26, pp. 205–207.

29. Low, RH 1984, *The Secondary Vessels of Acupuncture: A Detailed Account of Their Energies, Meridians, and Control Points*, HarperCollins, New York.

30. Maciocia, G 1989, *The Foundations of Chinese Medicine*, Churchill Livingstone, London, pp. 15–34.
Xinnong, C (chief ed.) 1987, *Chinese Acupuncture and Moxibustion*, Foreign Languages Press, Beijing, pp. 18–24.
Porkert, M 1974, *The Theoretical Foundations of Chinese Medicine*, MIT Press, Cambridge, pp. 43–76.

31. Kaptchuk, TJ 1983, *The Web That Has No Weaver: Understanding Chinese Medicine*, Ryder, London, pp. 1–33.

32. Porkert, M 1974, *The Theoretical Foundations of Chinese Medicine*, MIT Press, Cambridge, p. 46.

33. Kaptchuk, TJ 1983, *The Web That Has No Weaver: Understanding Chinese Medicine*, Ryder, London, pp. 77–114.
Gerber, R 1988, *Vibrational Medicine*, Bear, Santa Fe, pp. 176–177.
Xinnong, C (chief ed.) 1987, *Chinese Acupuncture and Moxibustion*, Foreign Languages Press, pp. 22–24.
Connelly, DM 1975, *Traditional Acupuncture: The Law of the Five Elements*, Centre for Traditional Acupuncture, Columbia, p. 15.

34. Needham, J 1974, *Science and Civilisation in China, Volume 5, Part 2*, Cambridge University Press, Cambridge, p. 92.

35. Kaptchuk, TJ 1983, *The Web That Has No Weaver: Understanding Chinese Medicine*, Ryder, London, pp. 34–49.
Gerber, R 1988, *Vibrational Medicine*, Bear, Santa Fe, pp. 188–189.

36. Rogers, C 1986, *An Introduction to the Study of Acupuncture. The Five Keys*, Acupuncture Colleges Publishing, Sydney, p. 6.

37. Kaptchuk, TJ 1983, *The Web That Has No Weaver: Understanding Chinese Medicine*, Ryder, London, pp. 7–15.

38. Rogers, C 1986, *An Introduction to the Study of Acupuncture*, Acupuncture Colleges Publishing, Sydney, pp. 7–8.
Gerber, R 1988, *Vibrational Medicine*, Bear, Santa Fe, p. 176.

39. Xinnong, C (chief ed.) 1987, *Chinese Acupuncture and Moxibustion*, Foreign Languages Press, pp. 15–18.
Maciocia, G 1989, *The Foundations of Chinese Medicine*, Churchill Livingstone, Edinburgh, p. 7.

40. Xinnong, C (chief ed.) 1987, *Chinese Acupuncture and Moxibustion*, Foreign Languages Press, pp. 108–244.

41. Low, RH 1984, *The Secondary Vessels of Acupuncture: A Detailed Account of Their Energies, Meridians, and Control Points*, HarperCollins, New York.

42. Kaptchuk, TJ 1983, *The Web That Has No Weaver: Understanding Chinese Medicine*, Ryder, London.

43. Porkert, M 1978 *The Theoretical Foundations of Chinese Medicine*, MIT Press, Cambridge

44. Selye, H 1976, *Stress in Health and Disease*, Butterworth-Heinemann, Oxford.

Chapter 7

TIBETAN FIGURE 8 ENERGIES

The aura-body interface

The aura or energy shell that surrounds the human body is connected to the physical body via three major energy systems: the acupuncture meridian system, the chakra system and the Tibetan figure 8 energy flows. Of these three energy flows, the one most intimately in contact with the physical body is the acupuncture meridian system. The ch'i (energy) flowing through the meridians is primarily etheric energy and therefore has the most direct effect on the physiology of the body, as each meridian provides essential ch'i energy to a specific organ system and muscles within the body (the basis of muscle balancing in kinesiology).

The chakras penetrate all levels of the aura, from the spiritual to the physical, and provide a conduit for cosmic energy in the form of prana to be transduced or stepped down to physiological levels via their relationship to the endocrine system and the autonomic nerve plexuses. Each of the seven major chakras is also supported in function by two of the 14 major meridians of acupuncture. In the yogic system, the energies of the body are balanced via the pranic flows of the chakras and nadis, with their concomitant effects on the endocrine and autonomic nervous systems. This, in turn, helps to balance the meridians associated with each chakra, as well as assisting in the regulation of the organ systems directly supported by each meridian. Conversely, the chakras may be balanced using acupoints related to the associated meridians, the basis of the Seven Ch'i Keys chakra balancing of Applied Physiology, which will be discussed later in this textbook.

The origins of the figure 8 energy system

The third major energy system of the body is the figure 8 energy system. While the origin of the figure 8 energy systems remains hidden in myth and speculation, recognition of these off-the-body energy flows is most often attributed to Tibetan medicine, and hence these flows are often called Tibetan figure 8 energies. One story of the figure 8 origins attributes the recognition of these energy flows to the Five Tibetan Rites, a system of exercises to revitalize the body and maintain youth and health. The Rites were first publicized by Peter Kelder in a 1939 booklet,[1] which is said to be based on the experiences of a retired British army colonel he met in California. While stationed in India, the colonel heard stories from Tibetan lamas about exercises to rejuvenate your body which were taught at a Tibetan monastery.

After retiring, the colonel discovered the monastery the lamas had spoken of and found that these Five Tibetan Rites rejuvenated him even though he was an old man at the time. In the story, the colonel mentions five energy vortices (the traditional Tibetan chakra system) and another set of energy flows that occur in a figure 8 pattern. These energy systems were the apparent mechanisms that are accessed by the Five Tibetan Rites and to which he ascribed his remarkable changes in health and vitality. Most of his story emphasized the five vortices and little is said of the figure 8 flows. However, it is undeniable that the figure 8 as a symbol has an ancient Tibetan origin; this is proven by the Tibetan rock art (dating from 600 BC to 600 AD).[2] Although the figure 8s may not be exclusively of Tibetan origin, it is an ancient Himalayan symbol that may well have inspired a modern energetic technique.

Although the origins of the figure 8s are clouded in mystery, balancing figure 8 flows has been shown in clinical practice to produce powerful anecdotal effects on physiological systems, such as reducing or even eliminating pain from tendon and muscle strains or sunburn and eliminating the symptoms of the flu.

Unlike both the chakra and the acupuncture meridian systems, the figure 8 energy system does not directly interface with the physical body but rather interfaces primarily with the acupuncture meridian system largely below it and the chakra-nadi system extending from the body to the highest spiritual layers of the aura. However, because of its position and direct interaction with the other two primary energy systems, imbalances in the figure 8 energy system may have a major impact on the balance of these energy systems. Therefore directly balancing the figure 8 energy system can rapidly rebalance either one or both of these other two major energy systems, and through their direct contact with the denser physical body can then directly affect physiological function.

Structure of the figure 8 energy system

On the trunk, the figure 8 energy flows from one hip toward the opposite shoulder; crosses in an arc to the opposite shoulder; then flows diagonally down, crossing the body to the opposite hip; and again crosses in an arc back to the side where it began, completing the figure 8. These figure 8 flows crisscross at a midpoint exactly in the middle of each body segment. The figure 8 flows are repeated over each surface of the head, trunk and legs, giving 12 major figure 8 flows over the body surfaces. There are two additional figure 8 flows: one above the head and one below the soles of the feet. This gives 14 major figure 8 energy flows in all (see Figure 7.1a).

There are also minor figure 8 energy flows associated with every joint of the body, including those in the fingers and toes. Thus, there are literally hundreds of figure 8 flows surrounding the body. Like the chakra system, however, the major flows of the figure 8 energy system dominate this system and produce the largest effects when out of balance, and they also have the greatest impact when they are brought back into balance.

When in balance, the figure 8 energy flows are not actually flowing in the normal sense of the word but rather oscillating, flowing first clockwise then counterclockwise, creating a figure 8 pattern in a slow oscillation in the top and bottom halves of the 8 flow. The point at which the figure 8 flows

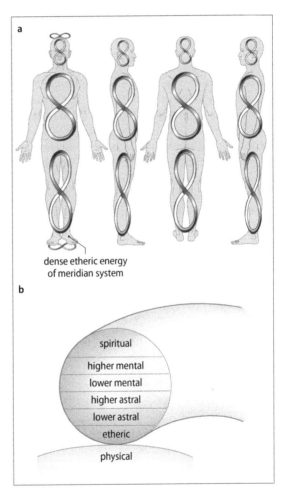

dense etheric energy of meridian system

Figure 7.1 Figure 8 energy system of the body.
a, The 14 major figure 8 energy flows. Figure 8 energy flows occur above the surface of every region of the body: the head, the trunk and legs, and above the head and below the feet. The center point where the figure 8 flows cross is called a *nodal point* and is toroid, which permits flows coming from opposite directions to cross unimpeded. **b, Auric layers of figure 8 energy flows.** Figure 8 energy flows actually extend from the etheric layer through all layers of the subtle body. Restriction of flow can be predominantly in one frequency domain, with a restriction of etheric flow having a different expression from restriction of flow in the mental layer.

cross in the middle we have termed the *nodal point*. Nodal points appear to be a toroid, a self-sustaining involuting flow that can support two flows crossing from different directions. Probably one of the most familiar (fortunately less so today) examples of a toroidal flow is a smoke ring, which smokers often created to amuse themselves or others. Another more recently discovered example is the bubble rings that dolphins can blow and then play with. These bubble rings can travel for many meters before slowly degrading, such is the self-sustaining nature of these toroidal flows, and this is in water, a medium 800 times as dense as air![3]

The figure 8 flow occurs in all levels of the aura, and thus there are flows at the etheric, astral, mental and spiritual levels (see Figure 7.1b). Therefore every layer of the figure 8 flow may be affected independently of the other layers. Normally, the factor or factors causing imbalance affect predominately one layer of the aura. Nevertheless, a disruption of homeostatic flow at one level of the aura will have an impact on the figure 8 flow as a whole.

Imbalanced figure 8 energy flows

The basis of oscillation imbalances in figure 8 flows appears to be disturbances within the auric layer that constrict flow along the pathway, as shown in Figure 7.2. These imbalances usually originate at one level of the aura, for instance an acupuncture meridian flow has been disturbed by blocked flow and thus the etheric flow of the corresponding figure 8 will be perturbed. However, at times the figure 8 flow imbalance may have a more complex origin, such as a psychoemotional issue that disturbs flow in two interacting layers: the astral and the mental. With very traumatic events, all

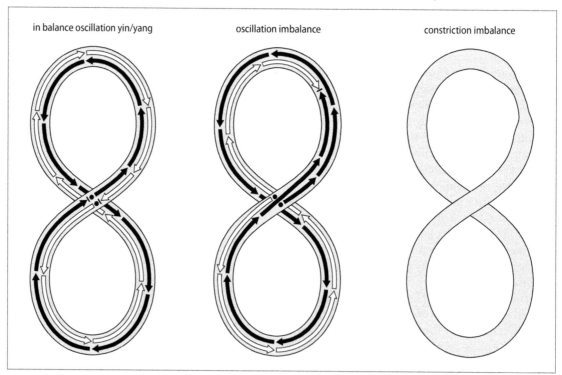

Figure 7.2 Figure 8 energy flows in balance and imbalance. Figure 8 energy flows in balance oscillate first clockwise then counterclockwise, like chakra cones (left). Loss of this even oscillation as a result of constrictions of flow disrupts these even oscillations (middle), which often results in excess oscillation in either a clockwise or a counterclockwise direction, creating an overt figure 8 energy flow imbalance. Another form of figure 8 energy imbalance is constriction in a section of the flow (right).

layers of the aura may be affected simultaneously, disturbing flow in the figure 8 as a whole.

One of the most common ways that figure 8 energy flows go out of balance is losing this even oscillation, which creates flow further in one direction than in the other, clockwise or counterclockwise. The more out of balance they become, the more rapid and further the flow of energy moves in one direction. Therefore these perturbed flows represent an excess of clockwise (yang) or counterclockwise (yin) energy flow.

Figure 8 flows can be seen as consisting of a number of segments. If the figure 8 is oriented vertically, then there is a segment from the nodal point upright to where it begins to arch to the left, a second segment arching over to the end of the arch on the opposite side and a third segment straight back to the nodal point. This same pattern of segments is repeated in the lower half of the figure 8.

These constrictions, once created, tend to remain in one area of a segment of flow, because the underlying stressor disturbing the flow is usually associated with a specific acupoint, organ or gland, chakra, etc. imbalance that is localized in, on or over specific areas of the body. Thus, these figure 8 flow imbalances can persist over time. A disturbance created by an acupoint imbalance may continuously perturb a specific chakra, organ or gland because of this ongoing disturbance of figure 8 flows.

Physiological effects of figure 8 energy flow imbalances

Although the figure 8 energy flows do not contact the physical body directly, they are in intimate contact with the acupuncture and chakra energies that do interact with the physiology of the body. Imbalances in figure 8 energy flows can therefore create imbalances within both the acupuncture meridian and the chakra systems that may then manifest as physiological disturbance within the physical body.

Because the figure 8 flows occur in the less dense etheric densities (higher vibrational energies) away from the surface of the physical body, they are the first energies to be unbalanced by physiological stresses developing within the body. They can therefore be thought of as the early warning system of the body's energy systems, because imbalances in the figure 8 flows will occur before major disturbances have yet to appear in the chakra and acupuncture systems, and well before any physiological disturbance can be perceived. For instance, when you start to come down with the flu, you often feel out of sorts, perhaps a bit spacey, but with no specific symptoms. If your figure 8 energy flows were checked at this time, they would almost always be out of balance. Even more impressive, if your figure 8 energy flows were rebalanced at this point, you would very likely never develop the flu.

An example of the power of the figure 8s to balance physiology is demonstrated by the following anecdote. When Krebs was the chief analytical chemist for the Victorian Water Quality Laboratory of the Environmental Protection Authority, he would occasionally have to go to court for prosecutions of toxic spills. Because of the legal precedent of line of evidence, the inspector who took a sample in the field must hand it directly to the chemist, who would analyze that sample. Otherwise, if another chemist should then analyze the sample they would not have direct line of evidence with the origin of the sample, and therefore this evidence would be considered hearsay in court. Krebs was coming up to a large prosecution and his chief technician Lisa was beginning to come down the flu, with runny nose, achy body and spacey feeling, the classic pre-flu symptoms. So she came to Krebs and said she would need to leave early. However, if she left early she would not finish analyzing the samples that Krebs had to present in court the next day.

So Krebs asked her to come into his office and he checked her for figure 8 energy imbalances, which are almost always out of balance in the early stages of flu. Amazingly, in the next 20 minutes, as he corrected each figure 8 imbalance one by one, Lisa went through all the flu symptoms. Her muscles began to ache more, she got a fever, then the fever broke and she began to sweat profusely, and finally she began to feel totally normal! At which point Krebs told her to 'get back out there and analyze that sample!' Significantly, she never did come down with the flu.

Correcting or activating figure 8 flows can be equally effective for treating musculoskeletal pain such as a strained tendon or ligament. Many times, Krebs has applied these figure 8 techniques over a strained joint or painful muscle to have the pain disappear after a few minutes of figure 8 treatment, especially if this was done immediately after injury!

Another amazing use of figure 8 energy flows is to reduce or eliminate the pain of sunburn. Krebs's stepson was a fair-haired and blue-eyed German, and the Australian sun is much more intense than the European sun in summer. So he was not aware how quickly he could get sunburned. After an afternoon of fun on the beach, his back was bright pink to red, and within an hour it began to burn intensely to the point that he was almost in tears. Krebs just had him lie down on his stomach and used muscle monitoring to find out which direction to sweep his hand over his stepson's back and shoulders, and then just kept sweeping his hand through the figure 8 flow in the indicated direction for approximately 45 minutes. When Krebs stopped sweeping his hand, his stepson's back was only lightly pink and he experienced no pain. Most incredibly, the next morning his back was pain-free and just slightly tanned, and he never developed blisters or peeled!

Reference

1. Kelder, P 1939, *The Eye of Revelation*.
2. Baker, I 1997, *The Tibetan Art of Healing*, Thames & Hudson, Singapore, p.53.
   Beer, R 1999, *The Encyclopedia of Tibetan Symbols and Motifs*, Shambhala Press, Boston, pp.15 & 30.
3. Dolphin Bubble Rings: http://www.youtube.com/watch?v=TMCf7SNUb-Q&feature=player_detailpage, or http://www.youtube.com/watch?feature=player_detailpage&v=wuVgXJ55G6Y (accessed August 13, 2013)

SECTION III

Understanding and applying muscle monitoring

The defining technique of Energetic Kinesiology is the use of muscle monitoring as a biofeedback tool. Muscle monitoring has proved itself to be an incredibly useful form of biofeedback because of its direct linkage to the subconscious, which largely controls muscle function. This subconscious control of muscle function interfaces with all levels of our being. Therefore muscle monitoring provides access to not only the physical realm of muscles but also the physiological, emotional, mental and psychospiritual realms of our being.

We have dedicated a whole section to understanding the mechanisms and ways of applying muscle monitoring in clinical practice because of its central role in Energetic Kinesiology. This section will explore the in-depth physiology of muscle monitoring, including the control of muscle proprioception. It will also cover the different types of states of muscle imbalance, some of which are not yet recognized in western physiology. The understanding of these 'hidden' states of muscle imbalance explain why various physical and muscular conditions often persist even after apparently effective treatment, as evidenced by the lack of any currently recognized muscle imbalance remaining.

It is also important to understand how it is possible that insubstantial inputs from our emotions and thinking might be able to impact on our physical muscle function and create states of imbalance within our skeletal and muscular systems. Likewise, these imbalances within our muscular system can reflect the unknown states of imbalance within the other systems of our body, including our physiology, feelings and state of mind. It is indeed this reciprocal linkage between the observable states of muscle imbalance and the not observable state of our feelings and emotions that make muscle monitoring such a powerful biofeedback tool, and it may produce concomitant effects on our thinking and sense of well-being.

For completeness, we have included a description of all the types of muscle monitoring that have been developed in different forms of kinesiology. While Energetic Kinesiology uses predominantly one type of muscle monitoring, isometric concentric muscle monitoring, it is important for people utilizing kinesiology to understand that there are a number of other valid types of muscle monitoring. These other types may be useful in specific circumstances or in combination with this isometric concentric muscle monitoring.

This section concludes with a discussion of the evidence supporting the ability of muscle monitoring to provide valid and reliable information about the state of imbalances within our being at many levels. We have also included a discussion of what muscle monitoring can and cannot actually tell you. This is important, because many people have a misperception of the kind of information, and the mechanisms of obtaining that information, that muscle monitoring can provide.

Chapter 8

THE PHYSIOLOGY OF MUSCLE MONITORING

What is muscle monitoring?

The basis of all Energetic Kinesiology was initially the single-position muscle testing developed by Kendall and Kendall and modified by Dr Goodheart.[1] In single-position muscle testing, the prime mover (PM) was placed in the fully contracted position and a moderately increasing pressure was applied in the direction of extension. If the muscle held against the pressure applied, it was said to be *strong*. If, on the other hand, the muscle could not hold and gave way in the direction the pressure was applied, it was said to be *weak*. While a strong muscle is easy to feel, it is difficult to describe in quantitative terms. A weak muscle may be even more difficult to feel until you have practiced enough to get a feel for the range of possible responses. This is why you often hear people describe it as the 'art of muscle testing'. Nevertheless, once you have developed the feel of a weak muscle, anyone can accurately test for the integrity of muscle response using manual muscle testing.

Muscle strength: strong and weak

To understand the concepts of muscle strength and weakness, we must first briefly present the neurology underlying muscle testing and dispel a few commonly held myths about what it is and what it is not. The first thing muscle testing is *not* is an evaluation of muscle strength. When a muscle holds, it is not strong. Likewise when a muscle gives during muscle testing, it is not weak. Even though in kinesiology today many people continue to use the terms *weak* and *strong* to describe muscle response during their muscle testing,[2] neurologically this is simply not an accurate description of what is happening.

When a muscle holds during muscle testing, the muscle has 'locked', because the level of neurological information flow between the muscle and the central nervous system is sufficient to maintain muscle contraction in opposition to the dynamic pressure applied. If the muscle gives during muscle testing, the muscle 'unlocks' or just cannot maintain the locked state, because of insufficient neurological flow between the muscle and the central nervous system or overt inhibition from another component of that muscle circuit or another part of the nervous system.

Muscle strength, on the other hand, is based on the number and size of muscle fibers in a muscle. This is usually measured by the weight that can be lifted by that muscle or force that can be exerted by the muscle (e.g. as measured on a dynamometer). A strong muscle is one that when locked can hold against a large weight, while a weaker muscle is overpowered by the same weight even when all muscle fibers are locked. Thus, the weaker muscle can still lock, that is, maintain sufficient neurological flow to hold against all pressures up to that which overpowers it. An unlocked muscle, however, cannot maintain sufficient neurological flow to hold its position, even at pressures far below that which are needed to overpower it. This is because it is not weak but rather being inhibited by inputs from some other part of the nervous system. Therefore use of the terms *strong* and *weak* with respect to muscle testing are totally misleading conceptually and incorrect in terms of neurophysiology.

To the person being tested, it does indeed feel like more pressure is being applied to the muscle when it unlocks than when it locks. However, this sense of increased force is only a subjective illusion. In reality, less pressure has actually been applied, but because of subconscious muscle inhibition it feels like more. When pressure is applied to a muscle, it initiates a load reflex that automatically matches the muscle contraction to the pressure applied outside your consciousness. All your consciousness says is 'Hold and equal the pressure', at which point the subconscious load reflex cuts in to ensure that the muscle increases its contraction to maintain its position.

When the muscle is inhibited, too few muscle fibers can contract to equal the pressure applied, and therefore the arm begins to move in the direction of pressure. Because the client is trying to resist the pressure, they now have to consciously offer resistance, which gives them the sense that the monitor is pushing harder. However, because of muscle inhibition they are now unable to do so. Even with additional conscious effort the muscle still unlocks, and it is this additional conscious effort that makes it seem like the monitor is pushing harder.

Muscle monitoring versus muscle testing

When performing a muscle test, you are not really *testing* the muscle. Testing denotes a measurement against some standard (e.g. strength as measured by weight lifted). Rather, you are monitoring the feedback to and from the muscle to check the integrity of the neurological flow between the muscle sensors (spindle cells and Golgi tendon organs) and the central nervous system.

Muscle monitoring therefore more accurately reflects the biofeedback aspect of the muscle response. In recognition of the muscle as a biofeedback device as it is used in Energetic Kinesiology, this term will be used throughout this textbook rather than the previously more commonly used term *muscle testing*.

Reciprocal facilitation or inhibition: locking and unlocking

Before further discussion of the nature of muscle monitoring, it is important to briefly discuss muscle function in general and the neurology of muscle locking and unlocking in greater detail. The fact that muscles turn on, or lock, and turn off, or unlock, is the basis of all movement and happens

millions of times a day as you move about. All muscles in the body, with only a few exceptions (the diaphragm being one), are arranged in *antagonistic pairs* of muscles that oppose each other's action. This arrangement of muscles is called *reciprocal facilitation and inhibition*, because whenever one of the pair is facilitated or turned on, its antagonist (or antagonists, as there may be several) is automatically inhibited or turned off.[3,4] Hence the turning on, or locking, and turning off, or unlocking, are both normal states of muscle function that happen all the time.

But what happens when a muscle locks during muscle monitoring? Neurologically, signals are sent to the PM to hold the position of the body part by consciously facilitating (turning on) the PM. Then, as the pressure on the body part (e.g. an arm held horizontal) is increased during muscle monitoring, the muscle sensors (spindle cells) in the PM respond by a spinal reflex arc called the *load reflex*. The load reflex increases the degree of PM contraction, while at the same time inhibiting its antagonists and facilitating their synergists.[4] Synergists are muscles that help the PM in holding the arm up, but they are not in their position of optimal mechanical advantage, so they contribute much less than the PM to establishing and maintaining this position. A muscle circuit, then, is the PM and all other muscles, both synergists and antagonists, to which it is 'wired' both at the level of the brain and the spinal reflex arcs (see Figure 8.1). The concept of muscle circuits is discussed more fully below.

Information on this response is also sent to subconscious parts of the brain, for example the cerebellum, basal ganglia and thalamus, that run prerecorded muscle programs, with the cerebellum continually making comparisons of the intended action with the actual action.[4] If the intended action was to keep the arm horizontal, but it is now actually moving downward because of the increasing pressure of the test, these subconscious brain centers will augment the automatic spinal load reflex and order additional contraction of the PM to offset movement, and the arm will remain horizontal. As long as this flow of information from muscle sensors to and from the brain remains clear

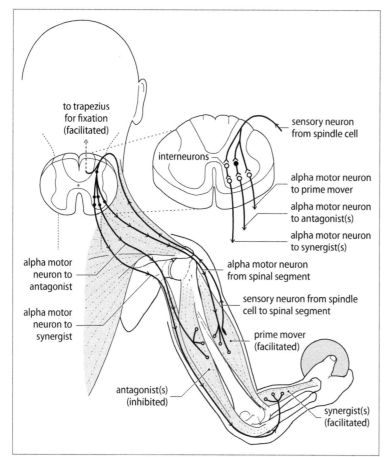

Figure 8.1 A simplified muscle circuit. A muscle circuit consists of an agonist or prime mover (the biceps), an antagonist (the triceps) or antagonist(s) and one or more synergist(s) (the brachioradialis). Spindle cells of the prime mover are wired to both its antagonist, which it inhibits, and its synergist, which it facilitates. Not shown is the reciprocal spindle cell circuitry for the antagonist (the triceps). After Walther DS, 1988, *Applied Kinesiology: Synopsis, Second Edition*, Systems DC, Pueblo.

Labels within figure:
to trapezius for fixation (facilitated)
interneurons
sensory neuron from spindle cell
alpha motor neuron to prime mover
alpha motor neuron to antagonist(s)
alpha motor neuron to synergist(s)
alpha motor neuron to antagonist
alpha motor neuron from spinal segment
sensory neuron from spindle cell to spinal segment
alpha motor neuron to synergist
prime mover (facilitated)
antagonist(s) (inhibited)
synergist(s) (facilitated)

with no interruptions, the muscle will lock and maintain its lock under continued loading until it reaches its full power of contraction. If loading continues above this point, the arm will now move down as the PM is overpowered by the downward pressure.

Recruitment

It should be noted that until approximately 80% of full contraction of the PM, it is the only muscle facilitated (turned on) to any degree. As the load on the PM approaches its limit of contraction, its synergists are then increasingly facilitated, a process call *recruitment*. However, in properly conducted muscle monitoring, the load on the PM should never exceed about one-third of the power of the muscle, and thus recruitment of synergists is minimal. This also explains why it is easier to

recruit muscles in addition to the PM when muscle monitoring is done too vigorously, which may invalidate the assessment of the actual muscle function.

When a person being monitored begins to recruit synergists, the monitor need only lighten the pressure applied, as the lighter the pressure, the more difficult it will be for the muscle to recruit synergists in addition to the PM. Because the PM has the optimal mechanical advantage in the correct monitoring position, and the pressure applied is far less force than needed to overpower the PM, a muscle with full neurological integrity will lock during muscle monitoring. That is, unless something interferes with the neurological flow of information between the muscle and the central nervous system, the muscle will be facilitated sufficiently to maintain its physical position even under increasing load. *This locking indicates a muscle in balance with its neurological circuitry.*

Under-facilitated, not weak

However, should any factor disrupt or interfere with this free flow of information between the muscle and the central nervous system, the muscle will not be able to coordinate and match its degree of facilitation to the increasing loading taking place during muscle monitoring. The arm will then move downward, appearing to give under the monitoring pressure, resulting in an unlocked muscle. Thus, a muscle that is monitored and found to unlock is *under-facilitated* relative to the pressure being applied. Note that, while the muscle may appear weak (e.g. giving under the monitoring pressure), it is not weak but just inhibited, and it is therefore not being facilitated sufficiently to resist the monitoring pressure, that is, it is under-facilitated.

Weak, as it refers to muscle strength, has nothing whatsoever to do with an unlocking muscle as found in Energetic Kinesiology, but rather only with the amount of force required to overpower the fully facilitated muscle, as discussed above. Because properly conducted muscle monitoring never *fully* facilitates the muscle (and certainly should *never, never overpower the muscle*), an unlocking muscle is not weak, it is just under-facilitated! In fact, the muscle that is unlocking is overtly inhibited by feedback from the muscle spindle cells, tendon and joint sensors or inhibitory feedback from subconscious emotional brain centers.

Proper muscle-monitoring technique

In properly conducted muscle monitoring, the degree of facilitation (turning on of contraction) of the muscle is matched by the central nervous system against increasing load, not exceeding about one-third of the muscle power. If the muscle is able to maintain sufficient coherent facilitation to hold the arm in the desired position under *slowly* increasing pressure, the muscle will lock and maintain the position against this increasing pressure.

On the other hand, should the information flow between the muscle and the central nervous system not be able to maintain facilitation equal to the rate of increase in pressure applied during monitoring, the muscle will passively move in the direction of pressure or will unlock. However, if a muscle is monitored improperly and rapid forceful pressure is applied to the unlocking muscle, it will now lock because of recruitment of its synergists and thus appear to be in homeostasis.

Muscle circuits

When using single-position muscle monitoring, it can only tell you two things: 1, the muscle was facilitated, or locked, or 2, the muscle was under-facilitated, or unlocked. As useful as this information may be, it is only a part of the story the muscle has to tell. The rest of the story is told only when the rest of the muscle circuit has been investigated.[5]

Each muscle in the body has antagonists (usually more than one) that oppose its action. The agonist or PM and its antagonist(s) are neurologically wired together via the spindle cells in the belly of these muscles. This neurological wiring is such that when a PM is facilitated (turned on), it sends signals to automatically inhibit (turn off) its antagonist(s) to the same degree to which it has been facilitated. At the same time, if the load is sufficiently large it facilitates its synergists. In this way, the limb moves in the direction of contraction, unopposed by its antagonist(s), permitting smooth and rapid movement of the limb. Likewise, facilitation of an antagonist will inhibit the PM, as the spindle cells of the antagonist(s) need to inhibit the PM in order to move the limb in the opposite direction from the action of the PM. Therefore, a complete muscle circuit includes the PM, its synergists, and its antagonists on both sides of the body (see Figure 8.1).

Why on both sides of the body? This is because the muscles of the arms and legs are reciprocally linked by a number of spinal reflexes, such as the gait mechanism. That is, when a PM on one side of the body is being facilitated, its mate on the opposite is being inhibited. Just think of walking! If the right anterior deltoid is facilitated moving the right arm forward, the left anterior deltoid is inhibited, allowing the left arm to be pulled backward by its antagonist(s).

Therefore, because of these reciprocal bilateral components of a muscle circuit, to fully investigate a muscle circuit it is important to assess the integrity of the same muscle on both sides of the body.

Contraction and extension monitoring

To learn more of the story that muscle has to tell us, the PM should be monitored not only in contraction but also in extension. That is, the muscle should be monitored first in its position of optimal contraction (pressure from contraction toward extension) and then again from its most extended position toward its contracted position (pressure from extension toward contraction).[5] This concept was first introduced to kinesiology by Richard Utt and presented at the International College of Applied Kinesiology conference in 1986.

Contraction monitoring evaluates the balance of the neurological flow to and from the sensors in the PM, while the extension monitoring evaluates the balance of neurological flow to the antagonist(s) as controlled by the sensors in the PM. Because flows to and from the PM itself and to its antagonist(s) are both part of the same muscle circuit, the state of balance within the PM and the PM's relationship to its antagonists need to be evaluated to know if the complete muscle circuit is in balance.

In extension monitoring, the antagonist(s) may either lock or unlock. However, an unlock here does not mean that the antagonist(s) are under-facilitated but rather that the PM is over-inhibiting its antagonist(s). When the PM is actively contracting, it should strongly inhibit its antagonist(s), as discussed above. However, even when the PM is in its fully extended position, the PM maintains a slight level of contraction to maintain its tone. This tonal contraction of the PM in extension creates a small level of inhibitory output to its antagonist(s), but it should not be sufficient to prevent the antagonist(s) from becoming fully facilitated and thus locking when the muscle is monitored in extension. The antagonist(s) are not being monitored in their optimal position(s) of

contraction, but rather, relative to the extended position of the PM, the antagonist(s) should be able to develop a full lock as long as the inhibitory output of the PM is within normal limits.

Should the level of contraction in the PM in its extended position exceed normal homeostatic levels, then the PM will begin to over-inhibit its antagonist(s). The antagonist(s) will then unlock when monitored with the PM in extension. While the PM may monitor in balance in contraction, it may nevertheless be over-inhibiting its antagonist(s), creating a significant imbalance in the muscle circuit as a whole. Extension monitoring is therefore really a 'readout' of stressors hidden in a part of the PM's circuitry that is *not* monitored by normal contraction monitoring alone. Nevertheless, these hidden stressors can affect the function of the PM and the integrity of the muscle circuit.

What is happening inside a muscle during contraction and extension?

A muscle fiber is made up of a fibrous sac that contains two types of fibers: thin actin fibers and thicker myosin fibers. Each muscle fiber is a long tube divided into many segments by fibrous walls called *endplates*. Each segment is called a *sarcomere*, which means 'muscle segment' in Latin. The actin fibers are embedded in the endplates and extend toward the middle of the sarcomere. In contrast, the myosin fibers lie between the actin fibers and are held only loosely in place between the endplates by fine elastic filaments.

Each myosin molecule has a rod-like tail terminating in two globular heads, and these globular heads can attach to the thin actin filaments forming crossbridges during contraction. When a nerve impulse causes the release of calcium ions into the sarcomere, the myosin heads on each end of the fiber actively grab the actin fibers and pull them toward each other, thereby shortening the sarcomere. The activation of the myosin heads and their grabbing and pulling the actin fibers is powered by energy in the form of ATP, the energy currency of the cell. When this occurs along the length of a muscle fiber, the tiny shortening of each sarcomere can cause a considerable shortening of each muscle fiber, which results in a muscle contraction.

The tendons on each end of the muscle that attach the muscle to the bones are actually just the ends of the muscle fiber without the actin and myosin fibers. Hence the tendons are continuous all the way through the muscle, and when the muscle shortens it pulls the tendons and the bones to which they are attached together, resulting in movement.

What is happening to these muscle fibers during muscle contraction and extension? And how does this relate to the position of the body part, for example the arm? The chest muscle that moves the arm toward the midline of the body, called the *pectoralis major clavicular*, is shown in various states of contraction and extension diagrammatically in Figure 8.2.

a. **PMC is in a hyper contracted state:** the actin fibres are collapsing on each other, and the myosin fibres are jammed up against the endplate. Muscle power is lost and 'pain' may cause reflex inhibition of the PMC.

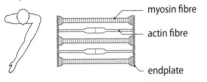

b. **In optimum contraction of the PMC:** actin fibres are touching each other and myosin fibres are almost touching the endplates. This provides maximum power of contraction and a definite 'lock'.

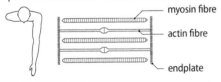

c. **PMC being monitored in full extension:** actin and myosin fibres are overlapping, but near the end of their 'travel' because it is not the fibres of the PMC that are being monitored, but rather the fibres of the antagonists in their position of optimal overlap e.g. like B above.

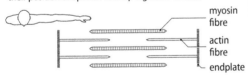

d. **PMC is hyper extended:** actin and myosin fibres just overlap at the tips and further extension will cause the muscle fibres to tear. Which is why hyperextension of a muscle 'hurts' and causes reflex inhibition of the antagonists to prevent further extension of the muscle.

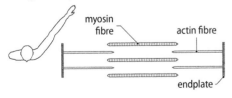

Figure 8.2 **What is happening inside a muscle during contraction: a, hypercontracted pectoralis major clavicular muscle (PMC); b, optimum contraction; c, monitored in full extension; and d, hyperextended.** The contractile unit of muscle is called a *sarcomere* and consists of two sarcomere endplates from which thin actin fibers project toward each other, with larger myosin fibers in the middle of the sarcomere that overlap the thin fixed actin fibers. A nerve impulse causes the myosin crossbridges to grab fixed actin fibers on each end and pull them together, shortening the sarcomere by pulling the endplates toward each other. This is the basis of muscle contraction.

References

1. Goodheart, GJ 1964, *Applied Kinesiology*, privately published, Detroit.
2. Walther, DS 1988, *Applied Kinesiology: Synopsis, Second Edition*, Systems DC, Pueblo.
3. Tortora, GJ & Grabowski, SR 1993, *Principles of Anatomy and Physiology, Seventh Edition*, Harper & Row, New York.
4. Guyton, AC 1986, *Textbook of Medical Physiology, Seventh Edition*, WB Saunders, Philadelphia.
5. Utt, RD 1986, *Applied Physiology I—Workshop Manual*, Applied Physiology Publishing, Tucson.

Chapter 9

PROPRIOCEPTION: THE CONTROL OF MUSCLE FUNCTION

In order to understand how muscle monitoring works at the neurophysiological level, we need to understand the control of muscle function. Muscle function is controlled by a number of different sensors in the muscles themselves, their tendons and the ligaments of the joints, among others. Together, these sensors that sense the position, length and tension of muscles are called *proprioceptors*.

There are several types of proprioceptors that provide the central nervous system (CNS) with feedback with regard to what is happening in the muscles, body position and equilibrium. The feedback from these sensors, which are actually specialized nerve endings, goes entirely to the spinal column and subconscious parts of the brain, for example the spinal segments, brainstem, basal ganglia, thalamus and cerebellum. This provides the body with information on the state of muscle contraction, the muscle and tendon tension, the position and activity of joints, and equilibrium. When stimulated, many of these proprioceptors adapt quickly and provide information on instantaneous change and rate of change in muscle activity and body position. Others adapt only slowly to stimulation and therefore provide steady state information about muscle and body position. Working together, they provide the information necessary for coordinated muscle action and movement and the maintenance of posture.

Muscle activity and states of stress in muscles are monitored primarily by two types of proprioceptors: neuromuscular spindle cells (or simply spindle cells) and Golgi tendon organs (GTOs). Information on the position of joints and stress in joints is provided by three additional types of proprioceptors: Ruffini end organs (REOs), Pacinian corpuscles and Golgi ligament organs (Golgi organs in joint ligaments). Free unmyelinated nerve fibers provide a register of pain. The structure and function of the proprioceptors of the joints will be described and briefly discussed, followed by a more comprehensive description and discussion of spindle cells and GTOs. Figure 9.1 shows the types of joint and muscle proprioceptors and their typical locations.

Joint proprioception

Ruffini end organs

Ruffini end organs, shown in Figure 9.1d, are encapsulated spray-type sensors located in the superficial layers of the fibrous connective tissue of capsular joints.[1] They are particularly common in capsular articulations such as the hip joints, where a static sense of position is important to the control of posture. REOs are usually distributed around joints in overlapping patterns such that various degrees of rotation will initiate firing of some but not other REOs.[2] Hence, which REOs have fired provides feedback on the degree of joint rotation or movement. Although REOs are found in all capsular joints, they are most numerous in the hip joints and numerous in other major joints such as the shoulder joint and temporomandibular joint of the jaw.

Ruffini end organs are unusual receptors with a biphasic (two-stage) response. Initial joint movement stimulates the REOs in the joint to fire rapidly, informing the CNS about the speed and direction of movement, but this output rapidly adapts to the new position. However, REOs also have a slowly adapting, steady state output to the CNS about the extent of that movement.[2] Because the area of activation of each REO overlaps that of its neighbor, successive firing of each REO as the joint is moved indicates the arc or direction of movement that is relayed to the CNS. This is followed by the

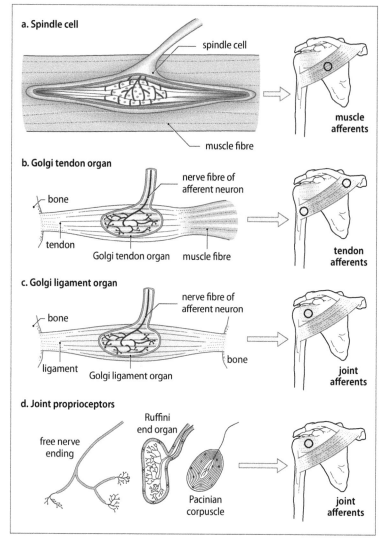

Figure 9.1 Types of joint and muscle proprioceptors and their typical locations: a, spindle cell; b, Golgi tendon organ; c, Golgi ligament organ; and d, joint proprioceptors. The primary muscle proprioceptors are the muscle spindle cells and the Golgi tendon organs, with the spindle cells located in the belly of the muscle and the tendon organs adjacent to the muscle–tendon junction. The primary proprioceptors of the joints are Ruffini end organs, Pacinian corpuscles, Golgi ligament organs and free nerve endings located in the fibrous connective tissue of the articular capsule and ligaments of the joint.

continuous steady state output from successive REOs after cessation of movement and provides feedback on the extent of movement.

Pacinian corpuscles

Pacinian corpuscles, shown in Figure 9.1d, are multilayered encapsulated proprioceptors that are highly sensitive to movement and pressure changes.[1] Structurally, there is a central nerve ending surrounded by many layers of membrane, much like the layers of an onion. They are few in number and only found in small groups in the connective tissue layers of the joint.

Pacinian corpuscles are rapidly adapting, low-threshold sensors that provide a record of transient stresses in the ligaments and capsular connective tissues.[2] When the joint moves, these sensors fire rapidly, but they cease firing as soon as movement stops. This feedback provides part of the input on which subconscious awareness of sensations of movement and pressure in joints is based.

Golgi organs

Golgi organs of the joint capsules, shown in Figure 9.1c, are almost identical in structure and function to the GTOs of the muscles. They are present only in specialized ligaments of the joints, not in the articular capsules themselves.[1]

Joint Golgi organs are high-threshold, slowly adapting receptors that along with REOs provide information about the speed and direction of joint movement. Unlike REOs, however, joint Golgi organs fire only when the speed or extent of movement is very rapid and may threaten excessive stresses on joints. When their rate of firing reaches a certain threshold, they cause reflex inhibition of muscles surrounding the joint to prevent damage to the joint ligaments and articular capsule.[2]

Free myelinated and unmyelinated nerve endings

These proprioceptors, shown in Figure 9.1d, ramify throughout the joint capsule, fat pads and synovial membranes. These are high-threshold, slowly adapting receptors that sense excessive joint movement that may cause joint damage. When activated, they cause conscious awareness of joint pain, which limits further movement to protect the joint.

Muscle proprioception
Golgi tendon organs

Although muscles have only two types of proprioceptors, these receptors account for a large percentage of the subconscious feedback to the CNS. GTOs, shown in Figure 9.1b, are located at the muscular–tendinous junction and consist of a fluid-filled capsule invested with small numbers of tendon fibers interwoven with high-speed myelinated nerve endings that ramify throughout the tendon fibers (see Figure 9.2).[1] As muscle tension increases, the tendon fibers are pulled tightly together. This squeezes the fluid-filled capsules and increases pressure on the nerve endings, which increases the output from the GTOs to the CNS. As the muscle contracts, the GTOs read the instantaneous level of tension within the tendon. When the output reaches a specific threshold, the GTOs strongly inhibit the muscle in which they are located, while at the same time turning on the antagonist(s) to this muscle to prevent overload of the tendon and possible tendon damage.[2,3] GTOs monitor and react only to muscle tension. This

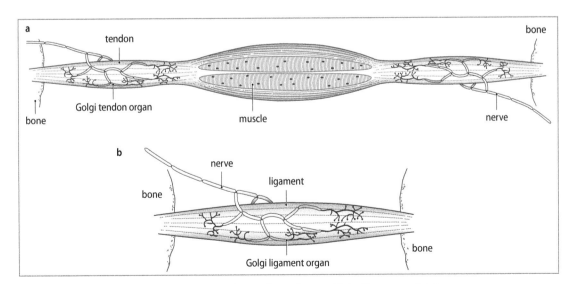

Figure 9.2 Golgi tendon and ligament organs in muscle tendons and joint ligaments. Golgi organ receptors are identical in structure with their nerve terminals, which ramify between the collagen fibers of the tendon or ligament. Both provide an instantaneous readout of tension and at threshold values initiate reflex inhibition of muscles. **a, Golgi tendon organs.** These are located at the musculotendinous junction of individual muscles. **b, Golgi ligament organs.** These are located only in specialized ligaments of the joints. After Walther DS, 1988, *Applied Kinesiology: Synopsis, Second Edition*, Systems DC, Pueblo.

information is of two types: instantaneous readout of tension, and tendon reflex inhibition of the agonist and its synergists.

1. Instantaneous readout of tension involves continuous output to the CNS, monitoring how much tension is on the muscle at any one moment, and changes in that tension over time via the rate of impulses emitted to the CNS per second. The greater the tension, the greater the number of impulses per second sent to the CNS.
2. Tendon reflex inhibition of the agonist and its synergists means that once the set point or threshold for the inhibition reflex is reached, the GTOs send inhibitory impulses to the agonist or prime mover and to its synergists that are generating the tension on the tendon to turn them off, and at the same time, facilitating impulses are sent to antagonists telling them to contract and quickly relieve tension on the

tendons of the agonist (see Figure 9.3).

The steady state tensional feedback is very important in control of muscle function for activities that involve applying various levels of force, for instance playing a piano. The instantaneous tension and the memory of that tension are what allow the pianist to play *fortissimo* (with vigor or strength) or *dolcemente* (sweet and gentle). A fine degree of tensional adjustment and virtually instantaneous local control provided by the GTOs is absolutely essential to accomplish these types of fine motor movements, which vary only in the degree of force applied.[3]

The critical feature of GTO activation, from the point of view of muscle monitoring, is the *set* point or threshold for inhibition. When this threshold or set point becomes set too low, reflex inhibition is activated long before actual damage to the tendon or muscles is likely to occur, but it limits the range of motion of the muscle. When this

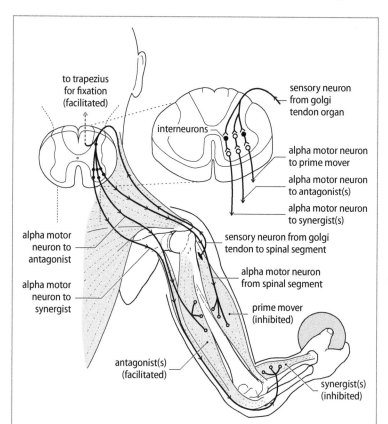

to trapezius for fixation (facilitated)

interneurons

sensory neuron from golgi tendon organ

alpha motor neuron to prime mover

alpha motor neuron to antagonist(s)

alpha motor neuron to synergist(s)

sensory neuron from golgi tendon to spinal segment

alpha motor neuron from spinal segment

alpha motor neuron to antagonist

alpha motor neuron to synergist

prime mover (inhibited)

antagonist(s) (facilitated)

synergist(s) (inhibited)

Figure 9.3 Golgi tendon organ pathways for inhibition and facilitation. Golgi tendon organs cause reflex inhibition of the prime mover and its synergist(s) and facilitation of its antagonist(s) once threshold tension has been reached. The threshold for tension is set by neurons from the brainstem either facilitating or inhibiting the interneurons separating the afferent sensory input from the efferent motor output of the spinal segment. Facilitation of these interneurons lowers the threshold of reflex inhibition, while inhibition of these interneurons increases the threshold of tendon inhibition. After Walther DS, 1988, *Applied Kinesiology: Synopsis, Second Edition*, Systems DC, Pueblo.

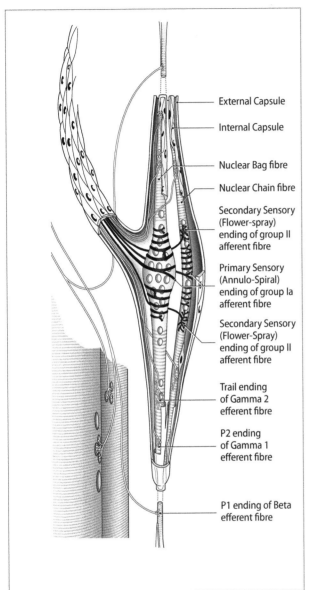

External Capsule

Internal Capsule

Nuclear Bag fibre

Nuclear Chain fibre

Secondary Sensory
(Flower-spray)
ending of group II
afferent fibre

Primary Sensory
(Annulo-Spiral)
ending of group Ia
afferent fibre

Secondary Sensory
(Flower-Spray)
ending of group II
afferent fibre

Trail ending
of Gamma 2
efferent fibre

P2 ending
of Gamma 1
efferent fibre

P1 ending of Beta
efferent fibre

Figure 9.4 Neuromuscular spindle cell. A three-dimensional reconstruction of a neuromuscular spindle, showing the spindle capsule and the nuclear bag and nuclear chain fibers. Spindle cells have two types of afferent sensory endings (black): primary and secondary. The *primary sensory endings*, called *annulospiral endings* because of the way they wrap around the non-contractile mid region of both bag and chain fibers, monitor changes in length and changes in the rate of change of length. The *secondary sensory endings*, called *flower spray endings* because they spread out across several sarcomeres, are located only on the nuclear chain fibers at the junction between the non-contractile and contractile regions. The secondary endings monitor muscle length. Both primary and secondary sensory endings send impulses into the spinal segment innervating the muscle containing the spindle cell. *Spindle cells* are also innervated by three types of motor fibers (gray). Gamma 1 efferent fibers terminate at P2 *en plaque* endings on the end of the nuclear bag fibers, just before they exit the capsule. Extrapyramidal subconscious corticospinal innervation of the gamma 1, P2 endings sets the threshold of the nuclear bag fibers for the muscle stretch or *load reflex*. *Gamma 2 efferent fibers* terminate at *en grappe* trail endings in the middle of the contractile regions on both ends of the nuclear bag and chain fibers. Pyramidal conscious corticospinal innervation of trail endings controls the length of the spindle fibers. *Beta efferent fibers* arise as a collateral branch of an alpha motor neuron innervating a slow twitch postural muscle in the neighborhood of the spindle cell and terminate at *en plaque* P1 endings outside the spindle capsule at the end of the contractile region on either end of the bag fiber at its tendinous attachment. Beta efferent fibers are the basis of reflex recruitment of surrounding extrafusal muscles. After Williams, PL & Warwick, R 1980, *Gray's Anatomy, Thirty-sixth Edition*, WB Saunders, Philadelphia

threshold is set too high, inhibition occurs too late to prevent damage to the tendon, the muscle or even the bone.

Spindle cells

Spindle cells, on the other hand, are the real 'brains' of the muscles, and are shown in Figure 9.1a. They have two types of sensory output to the CNS (annulospiral and flower spray endings) and

three types of motor input from the CNS (gamma 1, gamma 2, and beta efferent input (see Figure 9.4).[1] The sensory endings inform the CNS about muscle length, change in length and rate of change in length. The efferent motor input controls the actual rate and degree of contraction and coordinates muscle action with intended action. Hence, while the GTOs monitor tension and act as circuit breakers to prevent excessive tension from damaging the muscle and may provide feedback to assist muscle coordination, the spindle cells actively control the actual work of the muscle, that is, contraction or shortening to produce movement.

Structurally, spindle cells are highly modified muscle fibers consisting of a fluid-filled capsule containing 3–12 intrafusal or spindle fibers of two distinct types: nuclear bag and nuclear chain fibers.[1] Spindle fibers run parallel to the main or extrafusal muscle fibers and are often attached to these fibers (see Figures 9.4 and 9.5). Both types of spindle cell fibers have a mid region that is non-contractile and elastic, with two contractile regions on either end. The structure and function of the contractile ends is identical to the typical skeletal muscle fibers surrounding the spindle cells.

Muscle fibers are unusual in that they are multinucleate, that is, they contain many nuclei. The nuclear bag fibers are so named because most of the nuclei are gathered into the expanded, fluid-filled bag in the non-contractile, elastic middle of the fiber. The contractile ends of the bag fibers extend out of the spindle capsule to attach to the tendons of the main muscle fibers. The nuclear chain fibers, on the other hand, have most of the nuclei end to end in a chain in the middle of the fiber, and they attach directly to the ends of the spindle capsule. Chain fibers are contained entirely within the spindle capsule and do not extend beyond the capsule as do the longer bag fibers.[1]

Annulospiral primary endings: measuring changes in length and rate of change of changes in length

The annulospiral endings wrap around the non-contractile mid region of both bag and chain fibers, while the flower spray endings are almost entirely restricted to the chain fibers (see Figure 9.4).[1] When there is a sudden change in the length of the muscle, the annulospiral endings on the bag of the bag fibers respond very powerfully, dominating the sudden stretch reflex and causing reflex contraction of the surrounding muscle. When the muscle is stretched slowly, however, the annulospiral endings of both bag and chain fibers respond by increasing

output to the CNS, which is proportional to the degree of stretch.[2] The greater the degree of stretch, the higher the output to the CNS.

Thus, the bag fibers are primarily concerned with muscle stretch and monitor rate of change (velocity) and changes in the rate of change (changes in velocity). The bag-dominated muscle stretch reflex controls the load reflex, which initiates reflex tonification (contraction) of the surrounding extrafusal muscle fibers to automatically maintain limb position with increased load. Conversely, when the muscle is suddenly shortened, the nuclear bag output rapidly decreases or is lost altogether, and the CNS responds to this loss of information by reflex inhibition of the surrounding extrafusal fibers to stop contraction and permit muscle lengthening to regain nuclear bag output once more.

Flower spray secondary afferent endings: the measurement of muscle length

In contrast, when the contractile regions of the muscle contract or relax, the flower spray endings of the chain fibers 'fire' and send output about the change in muscle length that just occurred to the CNS and the subconscious areas of the brain. Because the flower spray endings spread out over several sarcomeres (contractile units), any contraction or relaxation of the muscle will alter the level of output from these receptors, informing the brain of changes in length. Thus, the flower spray endings of the chain fibers primarily monitor muscle length.

Together, the annulospiral and flower spray endings provide the CNS with information about what the muscle is doing and how fast it is doing it.

Motor input to the muscle from the CNS

The bag fibers receive three types of efferent (motor) nerve fibers, while the chain fibers receive only one type.[1] Both bag and chain fibers receive gamma 2 input at the trail endings. The trail endings innervate the contractile region of the spindle fibers on either side of the non-contractile mid region (see Figures 9.5 and 9.6). Gamma 2 input sets the spindle cell length. The CNS is kept informed of the length of the muscle by the output of the flower spray endings, which

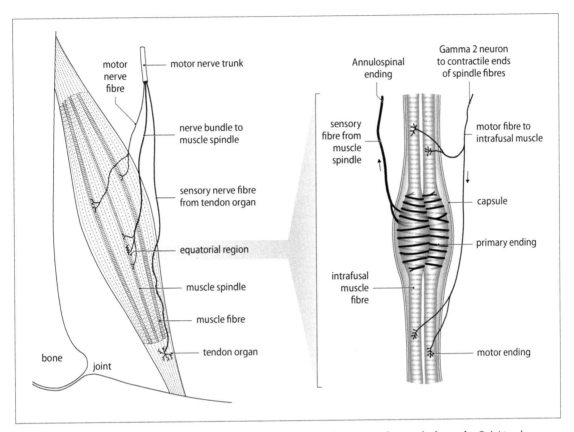

Figure 9.5 Location and arrangement of spindle cells and Golgi tendon organs in a typical muscle. Golgi tendon organs are situated in the tendons near the musculotendinous junction, while the spindle cells are small-diameter, highly modified muscle fibers that extend the length of the muscle from tendon to tendon (left). An enlarged view of the equatorial spindle capsule (right), which contains two nuclear bag fibers with the annulospiral endings wrapped around the expanded non-contractile mid region. In this schematic, only two nuclear bag spindle fibers are shown: a real spindle cell often has a dozen or more. (Nuclear chain fibers and the motor nerves to the spindle cells have been omitted for clarity.)

are compressed or stretched whenever the muscle fibers surrounding these endings change length. The degree of contraction of the spindle fibers is directly related to the degree of gamma 2 stimulation.[2] The greater the degree of contraction ordered by the gamma 2 efferents, the more the flower spray endings are stimulated to send output to the CNS, informing the CNS that the muscle is changing length.

The gamma 2 efferent–nuclear bag fibers interaction: misalignment detectors and the automatic load reflex

The spindle cells also act as alignment sensors between actual muscle response and the response intended by the brain. When the brain intends the muscle to be a specific length, for instance the forearm held horizontal to the ground, it sends impulses to the alpha motor neurons of the main extrafusal muscle fibers surrounding the spindle cells of the biceps to contract by this >−< much. At the same time, via coactivation it sends an identical signal to the spindle cell fibers via the gamma 2 fibers so that they also contract by this >−< much. As long as both the main muscle and the spindle cell fibers contract equally, the intended action *is* the actual action.[2]

If the main extrafusal fibers are lifting a load, however, they may only contract by this >−< much because of the load, while the spindle fibers *do* contract by this >—< much, as ordered by the CNS. The difference between the two lengths is made up by stretching the elastic, non-contractile central region of the spindle cell. It is this sudden stretching that initiates the myotactic or muscle stretch reflex that underlies the muscle load reflex.

Because the bag fibers are more sensitive to stretch, their stretching sends strong signals to the alpha motor neurons of the surrounding extrafusal fibers to *contract*, which causes more motor units to be recruited to cause the degree of contraction asked for by the brain, that is, this >—< much. Thus whenever the spindle fibers have contracted more than the surrounding main muscle fibers, the elastic non-contractile mid region of the bag fibers are stretched to make up the difference in the length between the main muscle fibers and the spindle cell fibers. This initiates the load reflex, which tells the main muscle fibers to pick up their game and catch up with the intended response,

that is, to equal the spindle cell length, as ordered by the CNS. Indeed, it is the gamma 2 input about intended length and the output from the stretched annulospiral endings that act as misalignment detectors between the intended and the actual muscle response. When these two do not match, it initiates contraction of the main muscle fibers to automatically compensate for varying loads (see Figures 9.4 and 9.5).[2,3]

The other two motor inputs to the spindle cells, gamma 1 and beta efferent fibers, innervate only the nuclear bag fibers. Beta efferent fibers terminate at P1 plates on the contractile region of the bag fibers that extend outside the spindle capsules just before the junction with the bag fiber tendons. The beta efferents originate as axonal collaterals (branches) from the alpha motor neurons of adjacent muscles, particularly postural muscles (see Figure 9.6).[1] When these adjacent muscles require additional muscular support to do their job, the

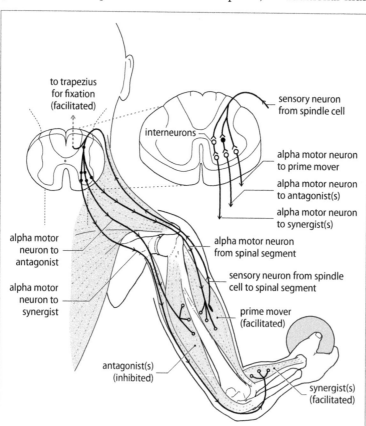

to trapezius
for fixation
(facilitated)

interneurons

sensory neuron
from spindle cell

alpha motor neuron
to prime mover

alpha motor neuron
to antagonist(s)

alpha motor neuron
to synergist(s)

alpha motor
neuron to
antagonist

alpha motor
neuron to
synergist

alpha motor neuron
from spinal segment

sensory neuron from spindle
cell to spinal segment

prime mover
(facilitated)

antagonist(s)
(inhibited)

synergist(s)
(facilitated)

Figure 9.6 Spindle cell pathways for inhibition and facilitation. Spindle cells have both afferent input to and efferent output from the central nervous system and are thus the 'brains' of the muscles, as they integrate sensory input and motor output. Note that there is a monosynaptic connection between the afferent spindle cell fibers' input and the alpha motor neurons' output innervating the main, extrafusal muscle fibers. Thus, whenever the nuclear bag fibers are suddenly stretched, they activate the surrounding muscle fibers to contract harder, which is called the *positive muscle stretch* or *load reflex*. After Walther DS, 1988, *Applied Kinesiology: Synopsis, Second Edition*, Systems DC, Pueblo.

rate of the beta efferent input to the bag fibers is increased. This beta efferent input to the bag fibers results in the shortening of these fibers, which stretches the bag fibers and initiates the muscle stretch reflex, recruiting the surrounding extrafusal main muscle fibers to help maintain posture or perform the intended action.

Recruitment: why you do not push too hard or too fast while muscle monitoring

Beta efferent input is the basis of the recruitment of surrounding muscles and why you get inaccurate results if you push too hard or too fast on a muscle when monitoring. Beta efferent fibres arise as a collateral branch of an Alpha Motor Neuron innervating a slow twitch postural muscle in the neighbourhood of the spindle cell (Figure 9.4). High level stimulation of the neighbouring postural muscle increases Beta efferent output shortening the nuclear bag fibre, which in turn stretches the 'bag' causing reflex 'recruitment' of surrounding extrafusal muscle fibres by initiating the positive muscle stretch or 'load reflex'.

Therefore, if you apply force on the muscle too rapidly and too hard, all it does is to cause the beta efferents of that muscle to recruit the surrounding muscles to turn on and help it out. This recruitment of surrounding muscles then allows even an under-facilitated muscle to appear locked. However, as long as you do not apply rapid or excessive pressure, the beta efferent output to surrounding muscles is minimal and the muscle being monitored cannot recruit its synergists to help it out. You therefore observe the correct response: an under-facilitated muscle!

The role of the gamma 1 efferents: setting the bag threshold for the muscle stretch reflex

The gamma 1 efferents terminate near the ends of the contractile region inside the spindle capsule at the P2 plates (see Figure 9.4). When P2 endings are stimulated by the brain, they set the threshold tension of the bag fibers, the threshold at which

the muscle stretch reflex is activated.[2,3] If gamma 1 input is high, then the bag is tight and the annulospiral endings are pre-stressed, such that even small changes in length will initiate the stretch reflex. However, if the gamma 1 input is low, the bag is relatively slack, and it will take a far greater degree and more rapid stretch to initiate the same response. Hence, the gamma 1 efferents control the nature of the dynamic stretch reflex and the speed and degree of the load reflex.

From a muscle monitoring perspective, when the gamma 1 input is high and the bag is tight, almost any pressure will automatically initiate muscle contraction via activating the muscle stretch reflex, which is of course *subconscious*. In this state, the muscle is over-facilitated relative to homeostasis, and even manual sedation of the spindle cells will be overridden by the overactive muscle stretch reflex, causing the muscle to lock and hold strong. In contrast, if the gamma 1 input is low, the bag may be so slack that a considerable amount of stretch will be required to initiate the muscle stretch reflex. When the muscle is monitored properly, with slow, even application of pressure to only approximately 2 kilograms, there is just not sufficient pressure to initiate the muscle stretch reflex, and the muscle will be under-facilitated and unlock or give passively under pressure.

Thus, spindle cells through their complex sensory output to and efferent motor input from the CNS control the activation and coordination of muscle function and activity throughout the body.

Use of muscle proprioception in kinesiology
Muscle sedation and tonification using proprioception

Muscles are routinely sedated and tonified using muscle proprioception in Energetic Kinesiology to check for two states of muscle imbalance: over-facilitation and under-inhibition. These sedation and tonification procedures take advantage of the reflex inhibition and tonification briefly discussed above. The pressure needs to be applied in line

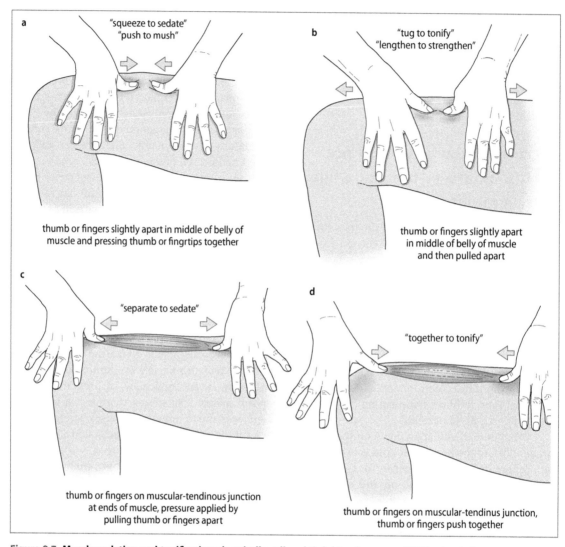

a "squeeze to sedate"
"push to mush"

thumb or fingers slightly apart in middle of belly of muscle and pressing thumb or fingrtips together

b "tug to tonify"
"lengthen to strengthen"

thumb or fingers slightly apart in middle of belly of muscle and then pulled apart

c "separate to sedate"

thumb or fingers on muscular-tendinous junction at ends of muscle, pressure applied by pulling thumb or fingers apart

d "together to tonify"

thumb or fingers on muscular-tendinus junction, thumb or fingers push together

Figure 9.7 Muscle sedation and tonification via spindle cell and Golgi tendon organ (GTO) stimulation.
a, Sedation by spindle cell stimulation. Shortening the belly of the muscle by the monitor pushing the thumbs rapidly together causes a sudden loss of feedback from the spindle cells. This would occur only if the extrafusal fibers had over-contracted, slackening the bag fibers, and thus initiates a negative muscle stretch reflex causing momentary inhibition of the extrafusal main muscle fibers.
b, Tonification by spindle cell stimulation. Lengthening the belly of the muscle by the monitor rapidly pulling the thumbs apart stretches the bag fibers, initiating a load reflex momentarily tonifying or turning on the muscle.
c, Sedation by GTO stimulation. The monitor places their thumbs at the musculotendinous junction on either end of the muscle, then rapidly pulls their thumbs apart. This initiates a positive tendon reflex, as the rapid rise in tension signals the need to inhibit muscle contraction to protect the tendon from damage.
d, Tonification by GTO stimulation. The monitor places their thumbs near the end of the tendons and rapidly pushes them together. This initiates a negative tendon reflex caused by loss of GTO output, which initiates reflex tonification of the muscle to re-establish GTO output, as continuous GTO output is needed to know what the muscle is doing.

with the muscle fibers, rather than across the muscle fibers, because the spindle cells are arranged parallel to the muscles fibers.

A way to sedate a muscle is to rapidly squeeze together the belly of the muscle (see Figure 9.7a). This reduces the tension on the non-contractile regions of the nuclear bag and chain fibers and suddenly decreases all output from the annulo-spiral endings. This in effect tells the CNS that the muscle has overshot its intended degree of contraction, resulting in reflex inhibition of the surrounding extrafusal fibers, turning off the muscle contraction and resulting in a momentary under-facilitation of the muscle so that it lengthens to once again provide output to the CNS.

Conversely, to tonify a muscle the belly of the muscle is rapidly stretched (see Figure 9.7b). This stretches the nuclear bag fibers initiating the positive muscle stretch reflex, in effect turning on contraction of the surrounding extrafusal fibers facilitating the muscle.

Shortly after physical sedation or tonification of the muscle fibers, the sensory output of the spindle cells returns to normal and a muscle in homeostasis will lock when remonitored within a few seconds. In both sedation and tonification, therefore, spindle cell response will last only for a few seconds, as the CNS constantly monitors spindle cell sensory output and makes adjustments in function based on this new output.

Therefore to sedate a muscle with spindle cells, one holds their thumbs about an inch (2–3 centimeters) apart on the belly of the muscle and then rapidly pushes them together. This will cause reflex inhibition, sedating the muscle and causing the muscle to unlock if the muscle is monitored within a few seconds of sedation. Likewise, if the thumbs tips are held together on the belly of the muscle, and then pushed rapidly apart, the resulting stretch reflex will tonify the muscle for a short time.

Therefore, whenever the nuclear bag fibres of the spindle cells are suddenly stretched by being pulled apart, they activate the "load reflex", or "positive stretch reflex", stimulating the surrounding extrafusal, main muscle fibres to contract "harder". This is the basis of "tonifying" the muscle with spindle cell stimulation. On the other hand, if the main muscle fibres surrounding the spindle cells are suddenly pushed together, releasing the tension on the nuclear bag and chain fibres, the sudden decrease in sensory output to the spinal segment results in reflex inhibition of the surrounding main muscle fibres called the "negative stretch reflex". This is the basis of "sedating" a muscle by spindle cell stimulation.

As discussed above, the GTOs can also reflexively inhibit or tonify the muscle to which they are attached. If the thumbs are placed on the muscular–tendinous junctions at each end of the muscle, and they are rapidly pulled apart, this movement will momentarily cause a rapid increase in tendon tension, resulting in sedation of the muscle (Figure 9.7c). In a sense, you have tricked the CNS into thinking the tendon might be damaged, and if the muscle is in homeostasis it will respond to protect the tendon by turning off the muscle. The muscle will be sedated and monitor under-facilitated for a short time.

Conversely, if the thumbs are placed on the muscular–tendinous junctions at each end of the muscle, and they are rapidly pushed together, the tension on the tendons is suddenly decreased, causing a large decrease in GTO output to the CNS (Figure 9.7d). In a sense, the CNS has lost contact with tendon tension, which results in reflex tonification of the surrounding muscle fibers to reestablish tendon tension. This will, in effect, facilitate or turn on the muscle, causing the muscle to lock when remonitored within a short time after manual tonification.

Sedation and tonification of inaccessible muscles

Several muscles in the body have either origins or insertions that are not physically accessible without considerable discomfort to the client. In these cases, it is necessary to use an alternative technique to activate sedation and tonification via the spindle cells and GTOs.

Two examples are the subscapularis muscle, which is underneath the surface of the scapula and whose belly is therefore inaccessible to spindle cell sedation, and the psoas muscle, whose origin is on the ventral surface of the spinal column and hence below all the viscera. In these cases, it is possible to sedate and tonify them via the spindle jam technique.

In order to sedate the muscle with the spindle jam technique, you take the muscle into the position of full contraction, then rapidly move the muscle a few centimeters further into contraction and quickly back to the original position. The muscle is then remonitored in that position. The rapid movement into further contraction causes reflex inhibition of the prime mover, because of loss of spindle cell output, allowing us to assess over-facilitation of the prime mover.

In order to tonify the prime mover, the muscle is taken into the position of full extension. Then rapidly move the muscle a few centimeters further into extension and quickly back to the original position. The muscle is then remonitored in that position. This will initiate tonification of the prime mover and reflex inhibition of its antagonist(s), assessing under-inhibition of the antagonist(s).

References

1. Williams, PL & Warwick, R 1980, *Gray's Anatomy, Thirty-sixth Edition*, WB Saunders, Philadelphia.
2. Guyton, AC 1986, *Textbook of Medical Physiology, Seventh Edition*, WB Saunders, Philadelphia.
3. Juhan, D 1987, *Job's Body, A Handbook for Bodywork*. Station Hill Press, New York.

Chapter 10

STATES OF MUSCLE IMBALANCE

The seven states of muscle response

The concept of a muscle circuit that includes monitoring in both contraction and extension was first developed in Applied Physiology, as Richard Utt recognized that there are really seven states of muscle response that can be evaluated by muscle monitoring, not just 'locked' and 'unlocked'. The seven states of muscle imbalance are summarized in Table 10.1.

Table 10.1 The seven states of muscle response
Note: PM = prime mover

CONTRACTION MONITORING (Facilitation of PM)	EXTENSION MONITORING (Inhibition of antagonist(s) by PM)
State 1: PM in homeostasis • Agonist and antagonist(s) can lock and be unlocked by sedation • North pole on PM unlocks PM • South pole on PM unlocks antagonist(s) of PM	
State 2: Under-facilitated PM • PM cannot lock	**State 3: Over-inhibiting PM** • Antagonist(s) of PM cannot lock
State 4: Over-facilitated PM • PM locks cannot be unlocked by PM sedation • North pole on PM does *not* unlock	**State 5: Under-inhibiting PM** • Antagonist(s) of PM cannot be unlocked by PM tonification • South pole on PM does *not* unlock
State 6: Flaccid paralysis • PM cannot move the muscle and thus cannot be monitored	**State 7: Spastic paralysis** • PM is highly facilitated and cannot be monitored

Homeostasis, under-facilitated and over-inhibited
State 1: homeostasis

The first state is the *balanced* or *homeostatic* (H) state of muscle function, in which the muscle has clear neurological flow with the central nervous system and can lock when monitored in contraction and lock when monitored in extension. In addition, a muscle in homeostasis can also be unlocked or sedated by either spindle cell or Golgi tendon activation. It can then be 'relocked' or tonified using the same proprioceptors.

State 2: under-facilitated

The second type of muscle response is the *under-facilitated* (UF) state, in which a stressor has interrupted the neurological flow between the prime mover and the central nervous system. In this state, when the muscle is monitored in the fully contracted position it will passively give or unlock when normal monitoring pressure is applied.

State 3: over-inhibited

The third type of muscle response is the *over-inhibited* (OI) state, in which a stressor has caused an excess of inhibitory flow from the prime mover to its antagonist(s). In this state, if the muscle is monitored in the fully extended position the antagonist (or antagonists) is (or are) inhibited and will unlock when normal monitoring pressure is applied. Remember that this is a reciprocal response, and it is the spindle cells of the prime mover that control the antagonist(s) when the prime mover is in extension and not their own proprioception. Hence, the response is a result of over-inhibition of the prime mover rather than under-facilitation of the antagonist.

Other states of muscle response

The remaining two types of muscle response, the *over-facilitated* (OF, and *under-inhibited* (UI) states of muscle balance, are the most subtle and difficult to evaluate, and they are not overtly recognized in western physiology. Both of these muscle states appear to be in balance, as indicated by a locked muscle when monitored in contraction or extension. However, both represent highly compensated states of response usually resulting from chronic imbalances.

State 4: over-facilitated

In the over-facilitated state, spindle cell or Golgi tendon sedation of the prime mover does *not* cause the prime mover to unlock. Therefore the muscle appears to be locked and apparently in homeostasis when in fact it is in a compensated state of balanced/imbalance. This means that a locked muscle can have two very different meanings: homeostasis or over-facilitation.

State 5: under-inhibited

In the under-inhibited state, spindle cell or Golgi tendon tonification of the prime mover does *not* inhibit the antagonist(s) of the prime mover, and the antagonist(s) remains locked in extension. Again, this is a compensated state of balanced/imbalance with regard to prime mover inhibition of its antagonist. This means that a locked muscle in extension has been under-inhibited by the prime mover.

Paralysis

Two other types of muscle response result from actual damage to the nervous system causing the state of *flaccid paralysis* or *spastic paralysis* in the prime mover or its antagonist(s). In both flaccid and spastic paralysis muscle monitoring is not possible.

State 6: flaccid paralysis

In the case of flaccid paralysis, either the prime mover or its antagonist(s) cannot be facilitated to move the limb or other body part even into the monitoring position. Indeed, states of flaccid paralysis, whether in contraction or extension, are evaluated by the inability to establish the monitoring position.

State 7: spastic paralysis

Spastic paralysis also results from damage to the nervous system but results in the spastic state in which the muscle maintains a high state of tone. This again prevents overt muscle monitoring, as the muscle cannot be moved, or moved only with great difficulty, from the spastic position.

Terminology

While initially only recognized in Applied Physiology, the over-facilitated and under-inhibited states of muscle imbalance are now more widely recognized in many types of Energetic Kinesiology. However, they have been referred to by a wide variety of terms, such as *frozen muscles*, *blocked muscles*, *jammed muscles* and *hypertonic muscles*. Physiologically, however, they are over-facilitated and represent a compensated state of muscle imbalance.

Muscle–organ/gland–meridian relationships

While we have been discussing only the physiology of muscle states, you must remember that the muscle is an access point for the muscle–organ/gland–meridian matrix discovered by Dr George Goodheart. Hence, a muscle imbalance does not only represent a state of muscle physiology but also an imbalance in the related organ/gland or meridian.

Applied Kinesiology developed the relationship between certain muscles in the body and corresponding organs and glands and the meridian energies affecting and affected by these organs and glands. The Chinese labeled the meridians by organ names (e.g. heart meridian), because they recognized that the meridian energies represent qualities that support the function of the related physical organs in the body.[1] The Chinese did not recognize the endocrine system, as neither did we in western physiology until the 1950s, although they did treat what western physiology considers to be endocrine conditions. They related to endocrine functions conceptually and metaphorically, although no less accurately.

For instance, the triple heater meridian in the Chinese system was related to a concept of three burners that control the energy available to the body. Through Goodheart's function–structure correlation, he discovered that the triple heater meridian is associated with the function of the thyroid and adrenal glands, the glands that control the energy available to the body. Hence, when we say the 'meridian–organ/gland relationship', it must be realized that the gland part of this relationship was added to the traditional Chinese concepts via muscle biofeedback in Applied Kinesiology.

Goodheart added specific muscles to this relationship, such that the state of balance in this network of relationships and functions (including the function of western organs) is reflected by the state of balance in specific muscle circuits. Thus, the balance in the stomach meridian not only affects and reflects the balance of energy flows but also the physiological functions of the stomach organ and the balance of several muscles in the body, for example the pectoralis major clavicular (PMC) division, biceps, neck flexors and neck extensors. Goodheart noted these relationships early on in Applied Kinesiology; for instance, when the PMC monitored unlocked or under-facilitated, he found that there was often stomach dysfunction (e.g. gastritis). Likewise, when the tensor fasciae latae monitored under-facilitated, there was often large intestine (colon) dysfunction (e.g. diarrhoea). Therefore a muscle circuit evaluated by muscle monitoring may give us a readout of stressors affecting the associated organ/gland or meridian as well as imbalances within the muscle circuit itself.

If a muscle is demonstrating an unlock caused by a physiological stress in a component of the muscle–organ/gland–meridian complex, and this stress persists over time, the body will compensate for this stress to try to re-establish the best balance

it can. Energetically, this unlocking muscle represents an under energy condition that is compensated for by the meridian system under stress, borrowing energy from one or more of the other meridians to make up the difference, so to speak. This borrowed energy needed for compensation will indeed relock the muscle by putting it into an over-energy state, resulting in an over-facilitated muscle response. The end result is a state of compensation in which the muscle is now in a balanced/imbalance state that is more functional than the overtly imbalanced state represented by under-facilitation, but that uses more energy to maintain this compensation.

Homeostasis and stress
Homeostasis: the balanced state

To understand the meaning and significance of the over-facilitated or under-inhibited states of muscle imbalance, a brief discussion is necessary of homeostasis and the nature of the compensations the body makes to maintain homeostasis in the face of chronic stress. Homeostasis is an integrated response of the body to maintain all bodily functions within narrow limits around the optimum levels of function (Figure 10.1a).[2] When a stressor drives a response toward these limits (either + or –), the body responds by changing some physiological function to bring the response back toward the optimum level. Because all systems in the body are in a state of dynamic equilibrium, the actual level of each physiological response in the body varies about this optimum level over time (see Figure 10.1b).

As long as the level of response remains within these narrow limits, the system is said to be in a true state of homeostatic balance and the body functions normally. Occasionally, a strong stressor will push the level of response outside homeostatic limits, creating a state of distress in that system (see Figure 10.1c). Immediately, the body responds by altering physiological function(s) to bring that response back within normal homeostatic limits. If it is successful, the distress is relieved and the body re-establishes normal function and homeostasis.

For instance, normally the secretion of acid in the

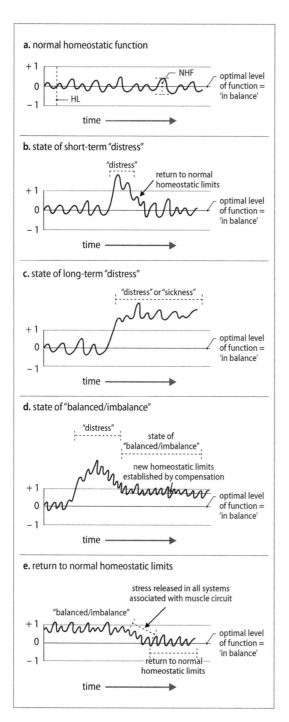

a. normal homeostatic function

+1
0
−1

NHF

optimal level
of function =
'in balance'

HL

time

b. state of short-term "distress"

"distress"

return to normal
homeostatic limits

+1
0
−1

optimal level
of function =
'in balance'

time

c. state of long-term "distress"

"distress" or "sickness"

+1
0
−1

optimal level
of function =
'in balance'

time

d. state of "balanced/imbalance"

"distress"

state of
"balanced/imbalance"

new homeostatic limits
established by compensation

+1
0
−1

optimal level
of function =
'in balance'

time

e. return to normal homeostatic limits

stress released in all systems
associated with muscle circuit

"balanced/imbalance"

+1
0
−1

optimal level
of function =
'in balance'

return to normal
homeostatic limits

time

Figure 10.1 Homeostasis and stress.

a, Normal homeostatic function (NHF). All physiological functions of the body vary around a 'normal' value because of the dynamic interactions of the many negative feedback systems involved in maintaining life. There are homeostatic limits (HLs), the range of fluctuation around this normal value that can be tolerated without disruption of homeostasis, usually denoted by +1 and −1. Each time any function moves away from the normal value for this particular function, it automatically activates compensations to return the perturbed function to optimum values of homeostasis. This results in a normal degree of variation: NHF.

b, Short-term stress: distress. When a point-in-time short-term stressor has pushed a function across the upper or lower HLs, the system goes into distress, which institutes immediate compensations to bring this function back inside HLs, ending the distress and re-establishing homeostasis.

c, Ongoing distress: sickness or disease. When a stressor has pushed some function outside the HLs, and because this stressor is both ongoing and strong enough to resist the various compensations, the body automatically activates to bring the function back inside the HLs. Sickness, such as a flu infection, usually occurs quickly, while disease (e.g. heart disease) usually develops over time and results from the breaking down of compensations.

d, State of balanced/imbalance or compensation. Following a period of ongoing distress, the body develops a series of compensations that bring the perturbed function back within homeostasis but now establishes a new level of homeostasis further from optimum values, either closer to the upper or lower HL because of the presence of an ongoing stressor. This compensated homeostatic state is often called the state of balanced/imbalance and represents ongoing compensation that although functional is energetically expensive.

e, Healing: resolution of the balanced/imbalanced state and return to normal homeostasis. When the factors creating the underlying stressor have been addressed and resolved, the function can return once more to the more energetically efficient state of normal homeostasis close to the optimum level of function.

stomach is kept within narrow limits, such that there is sufficient acid for digestion but not enough to harm the mucosa lining the stomach. However, on occasion, many people may experience the distress of an acid stomach, in which case the level of acid secretion has exceeded normal homeostatic limits. The stressor causing this over secretion of acid (the distress) may have been a bout of worry and anxiety over a financial or relationship problem (emotionally based), or perhaps it was the choice of inappropriate levels and/or kinds of food and drink.

We now know that the proximal cause is actually an infection of the stomach with *Helicobacter pylori*. This bacterium then secretes enzymes destroying the mucopolysaccharide lining of the stomach, allowing the stomach acids to now bathe the underlying stomach muscles, which burns and hurts! However, the underlying factors that permitted *H. pylori* to grow in the stomach was a condition called *hypochloria* or too little stomach acid, as the normal stomach acid of 1.5 pH will kill *H. pylori*. Indeed, it is very likely that the psycho-emotional and food choice factors identified many decades before are probably the cause of the hypochloria and ultimately the stomach ulcers.

If the stressors creating the distress are resolved (e.g. you win the lottery or else find your true love or divorce), normal acid secretion will be re-established, eliminating the *H. pylori* and allowing the stomach lining to heal, then your pain will be just a memory. If someone had been repeatedly monitoring your PMC (the muscle related to stomach function and energy) over time, they would probably have found it to monitor in homeostasis when your acid levels were within homeostatic limits. As soon as the stressors have created a state of distress, the PMC would most initially monitor unlocked or under-facilitated. The PMC would continue to monitor this way until the stressors are resolved, at which time the PMC would again lock as the levels of stomach acid are once more within homeostatic limits.

If the distress is too far outside the homeostatic limits, or if it continues for too long at high levels, the body cannot successfully compensate and a *conscious* high level of distress called *sickness* or *disease* results (see Figure 10.1c). Sickness usually

results from distress that rapidly exceeds the homeostatic limits and persists at a high level. Disease, on the other hand, usually denotes a breaking down of compensations from prolonged levels of distress. Therefore a raging viral or bacterial infection makes us sick, while we may take years to develop heart disease.

Resetting homeostatic limits: state of balanced/imbalanced

If you are *not* successful at resolving the stressors in the short term, and the stressors are ongoing, the body often compensates for this long-term stress by resetting the homeostatic limits using a series of physiological compensations that bring the stressed function back within homeostatic limits, even if this is above or below the optimal level of function (see Figure 10.1d). Hence, what was an acute distress in the short term has now been compensated for by altering the homeostatic limits to less optimum levels but with lower levels of stress in the long term. The net result of the compensation of resetting homeostatic limits to less optimum levels is less efficient physiological function and more stress on related systems that are supplying the energy to compensate for the stressed system.

To continue the example of imbalance in the secretion of stomach acid, as long as the levels of acid secretion remain outside normal homeostatic limits, permitting the growth of *H. pylori*, the related systems in the stomach would also have to be altered to reduce the damage. For instance, more stomach mucosal cells (the cells lining the stomach) may need to be produced, and the levels of protective mucopolysaccarides they produce would have to be significantly increased. This is not to mention the additional stress of the ongoing *H. pylori* infection and the effects of low acid on digestion. The increased workload to compensate for the *H. pylori* infection and disturbed digestion would, therefore, require additional energy output from a number of related systems throughout the body.

Basically, the body has created a state of balanced/imbalance as a compensation for long-term unresolved stress. If the homeostatic limits were not reset too far from the optimum level, this state of balanced/imbalance may persist for years. The person still functions well enough that all symptoms remain subclinical (e.g. you may be aware of them but not enough to make you sick). Once the body had established a state of balanced/imbalance with respect to the low-level acid secretion and the *H. pylori* secretion of enzymes eroding the stomach lining, the PMC once again monitors locked even though the symptoms of ulcers persist.

This lock would not be reflecting true homeostatic balance but rather the compensated state of balanced/imbalance. You would also find that it is not a true lock but an over-facilitation. That is, if the PMC was sedated, it would continue to lock. You may also find that while the PMC would lock in extension, tonification of the PMC would not unlock its antagonist(s). Thus, over-facilitated and under-inhibited states represent the body's way of notifying the monitor that it is doing its best to compensate for a long-term imbalance created by as yet unresolved stressors.

When you investigate the complete PMC muscle circuit on someone with a peptic ulcer, you will usually find that the PMC is both over-facilitated and under-inhibited, suggesting that these long-term chronic stresses in the stomach have created additional compensations in other related systems. This is the reason that when only single-position contraction monitoring is used, you cannot distinguish between a lock that indicates homeostasis and a lock caused by over-facilitation, the state of balanced/imbalance.

Return to homeostatic balance: resolution of stress

Without monitoring the whole PMC circuit, valuable information on the state of balance of the stomach muscle–organ/gland–meridian system will be missed. More importantly, you can only correct imbalances that you have found! Once you have located and corrected all imbalances within the PMC muscle circuit, for example rebalancing all under-facilitated, over-facilitated, over-inhibited and under-inhibited states of imbalance, you will often observe a concomitant improvement in stomach ulcers. As balanced/imbalance states of

function are eliminated from the body, the body appears to respond by resetting the homeostatic limits back toward optimum levels of function. This is perfectly reasonable if you realize that it was only unresolved stress that pushed the homeostatic limits away from optimal levels in the first place, and that prevented them from returning to these optimal levels long ago! (See Figure 10.1e.)

Significance of the state of balanced/imbalance

Hans Selye was nominated for a Nobel Prize for his discovery of the generalized adaptation syndrome (GAS). Selye found that the body responds to a wide variety of stressors (e.g. temperature, acid, mental stress and infection) with a generalized response not dependent on the nature of the specific stressor. He observed that the time course of the generalized adaptation syndrome had three distinct stages: stage 1, the stage of alarm; stage 2, the stage of resistance; and stage 3, the stage of exhaustion.[3] In stage 1 (alarm), the body is in distress as various parameters are driven outside normal homeostatic limits. If the distress persists over time, the body undergoes adaptations to develop resistance to the stressor, but at the cost of additional energy expenditure and efficiency. However, the body cannot maintain this extra energy expenditure indefinitely, and it will eventually enter the stage of exhaustion as the compensations creating the resistance begin to breakdown. The end of the stage of exhaustion is death! These stages of stress and their associated muscle states are represented graphically in Figure 10.2.

These stages of stress are indicated by specific types of muscle imbalances. Stage 1 stress of the alarm reaction is registered by under-facilitated and over-inhibited states of muscle imbalance. Even though the stage of resistance represents a successful adaptation to the on-going presence of the stressor, indicated by the balanced/imbalance state of the indicator muscle, it must be recognized that this is a compensated state, not a state of true balance. All compensations take energy to sustain and are less efficient physiologically than normal homeostatic balance.

It is like borrowing from Peter to pay Paul,

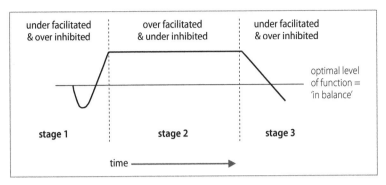

Figure 10.2 Stages of stress of the generalized adaptation syndrome and states of muscle imbalance indicating each stage of stress. a, Stage 1 stress: the stage of alarm. The body shows the changes characteristic of the first exposure to a stressor, with normal homeostatic function perturbed. At the same time, its resistance to this stressor is initially diminished and the state of distress may appear. The stage of alarm is indicated by under-facilitated and over-inhibited muscle states. **b, Stage 2 stress: the stage of resistance.** If continued exposure to the stressor is compatible with adaptation, then resistance creates various compensations in physiological function. The bodily signs characteristic of the alarm reaction have virtually disappeared, but it now requires energy to maintain the new compensated homeostasis: the state of balanced/imbalance. The stage of resistance is indicated by over-facilitated and under-inhibited muscle states. **c, Stage 3 stress: the stage of exhaustion.** Long-term exposure to a stressor to which the body has adapted by various levels of compensation, and for which eventually even more compensations were employed, eventually exhaust the energy needed for adaptation. The signs of the alarm reaction reappear, but now they rapidly become irreversible, and if prolonged the individual will die. The stage of exhaustion is also indicated by under-facilitated and over-inhibited muscle states.

because at some point Peter has to be paid back, and if the borrowing has gone on for too long or at too high a level, you may be bankrupted trying to pay Peter back. Likewise, in the body if stage 2 stress goes on for too long, the systems supporting the compensations needed for resistance begin to break down leading to the stage of exhaustion.

Stage 3 stress of exhaustion is once again uncompensated and registered by under-facilitated and over-inhibited states of muscle imbalance. However, although stage of alarm and stage of exhaustion are both represented by under-facilitated and over-inhibited muscle states, they are clearly not the same thing. In the stage of alarm, the muscles are under-facilitated and over-inhibited and the person displays distress, which may be only short term. In the stage of exhaustion, these under-facilitated and over-inhibited states represent a system that is collapsing and the person looks ill or sick.

Therefore by being able to directly monitor for stage of resistance by identifying the over-facilitated and under-inhibited states of muscle imbalance, we are able to balance for these compensated states within the body. This allows us to move the body closer to normal homeostatic limits, reducing the energy needs of the associated system, and hopefully further from the stage of exhaustion. *This clearly has tremendous significance in helping people to return to more optimal levels of health!*

Accurate indicator muscle monitoring

There are two different ways in which a muscle can indicate stress. First, a muscle can be a direct indicator of stress within the muscle–organ/gland–meridian related circuit. In this case, the muscle imbalances directly reflect imbalances within the associated organ/gland–meridian. Second, the muscle can be an independent indicator muscle for generalized stress in any part of the body.

When the muscle is used as an indicator specifically for its associated organ/gland–meridian matrix, any overt states of muscle imbalance (under-facilitation, over-inhibition, over-facilitation or under-inhibition) mean there is an imbalance within some component of this energetic matrix. It may also indicate an overt imbalance within the associated physiological systems.

The muscle can also be used as a generalized biofeedback tool indicating stress or a stressor affecting any component of the whole body–mind system. However, a muscle used as a general indicator of stress must have no overt muscle imbalances (under-facilitation, over-inhibition, over-facilitation or under-inhibition), otherwise it would not be known whether the imbalance was in the indicator muscle's circuit itself or within the system you are investigating or assessing. Therefore a muscle must be cleared of all its muscle circuit imbalances before it can be used as a generalized indicator.

The significance of clear circuit muscle monitoring

A clear balanced muscle circuit is one in which: 1, a lock is observed in both contraction and extension monitoring; 2, the locked muscle can be unlocked by sedation of the prime mover in contraction monitoring; and 3, the locked antagonists can be unlocked by tonification of the prime mover in extension monitoring. A muscle demonstrating any imbalanced state, (e.g. under-facilitation, over-facilitation, under-inhibition or over-inhibition) *cannot* be reliably used as a generalized indicator muscle.

Perhaps even more important, a muscle will *not* be able to indicate many imbalances hidden in these over-facilitated, under-inhibited or over-inhibited states of muscle response, unless those states are directly investigated. Therefore if only single position contraction muscle monitoring is used, the presence of any or all these states of imbalance may well obscure significant information. For instance, your PMC indicator may be in a balanced state in the clear when not thinking of anything in particular. But the minute you are asked to think of your mother, it may very well (and often does) go into an *over-facilitated* state, rather than the more observable *under-facilitated* state. Using only single position contraction monitoring, this important response would be missed, and the monitor would incorrectly assume that thinking of

your mother was not stressful because your muscle stayed locked!

For instance, only single-position contraction monitoring was initially used in Applied Kinesiology. In Walther's *Applied Kinesiology: Synopsis*, he states that 'the muscle–organ/gland association should not be considered absolute. An individual may have a gastric ulcer confirmed by radiology but the PMC may not test weak'.[4] However, because the person's PMC was not monitored for over-facilitation, the strong muscle test may not be indicating balance but rather compensated imbalance. We have *never* found a person with a confirmed peptic ulcer whose PMC did not show at least one, and usually several, of the following imbalances: under-facilitation, over-facilitation, under-inhibition or over-inhibition. Most often, it will monitor over-facilitated or under-inhibited, and not uncommonly both, while it will very often not monitor under-facilitated or over-inhibited, the more overtly observable states. Why? Because peptic ulcers are chronic long-term problems for which the body has ample time to compensate by creating the stage 2 stress of resistance!

From the above example, it is clear that a locked indicator muscle can indicate two quite different states of muscle response. The first is the homeostatic state, in which the muscle is locked, indicating that there is homeostasis within its energetic and physiological systems. In this state, the prime mover can be sedated and hence unlock. The other possibility is that the muscle is over-facilitated, in which case it locks but cannot be sedated and thus it is in a compensated state of over-facilitation, indicating an ongoing stressor.

Because the purpose of muscle monitoring is to evaluate and correct stressors in the muscle–organ/gland–meridian system, much of the information muscle monitoring can provide may be lost unless an indicator muscle is cleared of all imbalances in all four monitoring positions: contraction and extension on both sides of the body.

You may ask, 'But why on both sides of the body?' This is because of the fact that there are a number of bilateral neurological circuits that link each muscle on one side of the body with the same muscle on the other side of the body. Via these bilateral circuits, an imbalance in a muscle on one side of the body can produce interfering input to the balanced circuit on the other side of the body. Therefore, to be sure to have established a clear muscle circuit, the indicator muscle of choice must be in homeostasis on both sides of the body.

References

1. Black, D 1989, *Chinese Healing Principles—Can They Work for Us?* Issue in the Healing Current Series, Spectrum Marketing Services, Toorak.
2. Tortora, GJ & Grabowski, SR 1993, *Principles of Anatomy and Physiology, Seventh Edition*, Harper & Row, New York.
3. Selye, H 1936, A syndrome produced by diverse nocuous agents, *Nature*, Vol. 138, p. 32.
4. Walther, DS 1988, *Applied Kinesiology: Synopsis, Second Edition*, Systems DC, Pueblo. p. 14.

Chapter 11

EMOTIONAL CONTROL OF MUSCULAR RESPONSE

Subconscious rules

Through the muscle monitoring techniques of kinesiology, the body can be asked direct questions. By *body*, we mean that integrated unit of the physiological, emotional, mental and spiritual realms of your being: you. We underline that this access is possible because muscle response is predominantly controlled from the subconscious and can thus interface with the other domains of your being.

Most of us think that we run our body consciously, yet if you consider it from a physiological point of view, even when you are standing still there are hundreds of muscles in various states of contraction operating to keep you upright. Consciously, you are not involved, but every second millions of bits of information are being processed in your subconscious.

The reason you are not aware of these 5-10 million impulses per second is because most of the information goes directly into the totally subconscious brainstem and cerebellum, the subconscious components of the basal ganglia and subconscious components of your limbic system. Only a small amount of that sensory data is passed into your conscious limbic and cortical areas for you to perceive. In a sense, what you perceive consciously is only a summary statement of everything that is happening subconsciously.

You tell your body to stand up. That simple instruction constitutes conscious input into the subconscious areas of your brain that run the motor system; they then issue instructions for your muscles to contract and synchronize in a way that allows you to stand up. To perform this action requires millions of pieces of sensory data, yet all your conscious brain needs to know is the fact that you are standing up.

When you walk, the decision to move is conscious. Once you start walking, however, you can begin thinking about something else entirely. The body can go into autopilot, a subsystem of subconscious programs that interact with the consciousness to some degree but that largely leave your consciousness free to think about other things. This subconscious programming is extremely powerful, because at times it can and must supersede conscious instructions. When we examine muscle responses, we see that the mechanism is set up in such a way that ultimately these subconscious control circuits cannot be overridden by the conscious. When it comes to the more important program of survival, or of protecting the body from harm, the subconscious rules.

If, for instance, you consciously wish to be stupid and try to pick up a weight that would violate your physical integrity by loading so much tension onto the body that muscles and tendons would tear and bones would break, the subconscious sensors measuring the increasing rate of tension would tell the subconscious control centers that damage is likely to occur. These subconscious centers would then send inhibitory signals to turn the muscles off, overriding your conscious instructions. You can see this happen in any weight-lifting competition. Just as a finalist is pushing the barbell above their head, they begin to tremble and then drop the barbell. To protect their physical integrity, their subconscious control centers and sensors simply overrode their conscious desire to break the world record. It would not allow them to damage their structural integrity even to fulfil a consciously desired goal.

So while we think we are in charge of our

physical activity, we are actually aware of very little of it. The vast majority is subconsciously driven, and the subconscious has its own agenda: survival.

Survival first

Scientific experiments have established that neuropathways are activated by the simple act of remembering an event, and not surprising, they are the same neuropathways that fired when you actually experienced the event.[1] While this aspect of recalling from memory powerfully loaded survival experiences is useful for our physical well-being, it can become an equally powerful impediment to our personal growth.

These mechanisms have their roots in our evolutionary origins. The traditional lifestyles of indigenous peoples allude to the idea that mankind basically grew up as a social species who lived in small kinship groups and who spent most of their lives eking out a living from their environment, an environment that contained considerable physical risk. In prehistoric times, there was much more danger in the immediate surroundings. Real physical threat occurred on a daily basis, and because of these conditions the brain evolved in a way that ensured survival.

It also evolved in a way that helped maintain emotional harmony, interaction and cooperation in small, dependent social groups, because an individual had a much better chance of survival by being a member of a group. This has left us with an emotional structure that is built around both physical and social survival. Taboos and rituals developed to facilitate our social survival as much as reactions to threat developed for our physical survival. While physical threat alone was necessary to initiate physical survival programs, mechanisms to survive emotional threat evolved to ensure cultural survival. Primary among the mechanisms that aid social survival is guilt, shame and blame.

The emotion of guilt is programmed into us in a social context before we are capable of rational thought, and hence it becomes one of our basic survival programs. When you do something that is considered outside the norms of your group, you are told or made to feel that you are bad. Children learn very early that when they are bad they are not liked, and love is often withheld. Therefore children quickly realize that when they do something bad, they feel bad. This is the essence of the guilt program. How many adults, including yourself, do you know who are often run by their guilt programming?

You can see that there are powerful subconscious emotional programs that drive our behavior. Guilt is only one, but an important one. While the sight of a charging bull will trigger your physical survival program ('Run!'), unspoken disapproval can just as powerfully trigger your emotional survival program (guilt!).

This is particularly true of children, who operate on a much more intuitive, feeling level. Unspoken gestures and vocal tone have much more power and meaning than spoken words, which children largely do not comprehend. The power of these signals is that they activate or trigger strong emotions that are linked to similar negative emotional experiences that have occurred in the past. When this happens, the child is now reacting not to the current circumstance but rather to their emotional experience of a similar circumstance in the past. The past becomes now for them, and the emotion of the past dominates their current state.

To the brain, remembering an event happening is no different from experiencing the event in real time. A memory that you are currently experiencing is, to your brain, your current reality. A situation that you are thinking about, even one that may not occur until the future, can also have the same impact or emotional charge to the brain. The brain responds to both real, remembered or imagined impulses in the same way, as if they are occurring right now. Brain time is now time.

This now-time programming triggered by past experiences is the basis of a muscle 'unlocking' or being inhibited when we merely think about a past experience or event. When a muscle is monitored and the person accesses a negative memory, the guilt or other associated negative emotions activate brainstem nuclei that send inhibitory signals to the spinal segments inhibiting the load reflex, and the muscle unlocks.

Muscle–emotion interface

How can something that I only thought or felt, particularly something from the past or that may happen in the future, affect my muscle now?

The subconscious areas of the brain that control or elicit our emotions is located in the limbic cortex and brainstem, the ancient brain centers developed in our evolutionary past. There are direct neurological connections between these brain centers and the pathways that control our muscle tone and tension.[2] Why do you think your neck gets tight when you are anxious and worried? Why does your stomach churn? Why do purely mental events have such a telling physical effect?

It is because the parts of the brain that control our emotional and physical survival programs also subconsciously set the tone of our muscular system. Therefore the emotional tone of a person is directly reflected in their muscular tone. If you see someone walking down the street with their head down and shoulders slumped, and with drooping mouth and downcast eyes—all states of muscle tone—you would probably correctly surmise that this person is depressed or unhappy. It is interesting to note that somehow western medical science has been largely blind to an observation of the effect of emotions on muscular tone that even young children make: 'Mummy, are you unhappy?' Our emotional states are very graphically echoed in our physical postures.

Clearly, because kinesiology monitors subconscious muscle tone, it is directly linked to the emotional centers that are setting that tone. When monitoring a muscle, you are interacting directly with the interface between the neurological physical body and the emotions and thoughts that affect that body. Furthermore, the muscle also monitors the interface between the physical body and the energetic systems of Chinese acupuncture. If you recall, the Chinese recognized that each energy flow was affected by specific emotional states. What kinesiology adds is the physical response linking energy flows and emotions. Figure 11.1 illustrates this relationship.

The initial step is the transduction of the emotional and mental fields generating our feelings and thoughts into neural impulses representing the states of these feelings and thoughts as patterns of neurons firing in different limbic areas, or by these emotional and mental fields generating distortions in or disrupting the flows of ch'i or prana in the energy systems, which are then transduced into patterns of neurons firing in different limbic areas or other neurological interfaces of the brainstem and autonomic nervous system.

Recent research has indeed demonstrated that small magnetic vortices or *Strudels* (German for 'vortex') appear spontaneously above the parts of the brain that are associated with specific types of mental processing that the person was asked to do while being scanned. These Strudels appear just before activation of these areas, as seen in

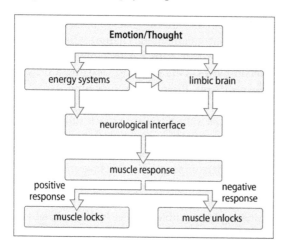

Figure 11.1 The emotion–muscle interface. Emotions and thoughts may affect muscle function through two pathways. One is via the limbic brain and the effects of the reticulospinal pathways on muscle tone. The other is via the energy systems, as each meridian, chakra and figure 8 energy flow has an association via frequency resonance with a specific emotion. These associations then have effects on the balance of these energy systems, which are in turn transduced into effects on the physiology of muscle response.

functional magnetic resonance imaging scans, suggesting that it may indeed be the transduction of these magnetic vortices that are represented.

Limbic and brainstem control of gamma 1 output

One of the most common and remarkable observations in kinesiology is when a person is asked to think of a negative emotion or emotional circumstance as they are monitored and suddenly their arm unlocks. But why should this happen? Clearly, a muscle response is a neurophysiological event, while emotion is a psychoemotional event. How are the two connected?

Because the ultimate event is physical, the arm giving or unlocking, then there must be neurological circuitry that underlies this event, but a search of the traditional anatomy and physiological literature appears to offer few clues. However, after studying the in-depth neurological circuitry of muscle spindle cells and Golgi tendon organs and their connection to the brainstem and brain, we have pieced together at least a reasonable explanation that is consistent with current neurological knowledge. We then go further afield and suggest the interface between the mental event of thinking and emotions and the physiological response to these psychoemotional events: an unlocking muscle.

Current anatomy and physiology textbooks are fuzzy on the details of exactly what part of the brain controls gamma 1 output to the spindle cells. Piecing together the apparent and possible connections between the upper motor neurons descending from the brain and the gamma 1 lower motor neurons setting the muscle stretch reflex threshold, the following scenario arises.

The gamma 1 motor neurons are not directly connected to descending motor tracts but rather by interneurons receiving input from several sources. The most probable sources are the medial (pontine) reticulospinal tracts and lateral (medullary) reticulospinal tracts (see Figure 11.2).[1] Both of these tracts terminate at all levels within the spine in the medial parts of the ventral gray horns adjacent to the gamma 1 motor neurons and are linked to gamma 1 motor neurons via interneurons

from both of these tracts, as well as direct spinal tracts projecting from the brainstem nuclei of the reticular formation. We believe these multiple connections to these subconscious reticular nuclei to be the neurological interface of the emotion–muscle response.

The medial (pontine) and lateral (medullary) reticulospinal tracts arise from several major reticular nuclei that receive direct input from the areas of the brain known to be involved with the origin and expression of our survival emotions: the amygdala, the hypothalamus, and the periaqueductal gray matter (PAG), as well as limbic centers such as the anterior cingulate gyrus, the guilt–shame–blame center of the brain. The amygdala appears to be one of the primary subconscious emotional centers in the brain, in charge of the survival-oriented fight-or-flight responses, and gives rise to our primary emotions of fear, punishment, escape, rage and pleasure. Fibers project directly from the amygdala to the hypothalamus, which then creates our physical and physiological reaction to these powerful emotions, for example the dry mouth, tightness in the stomach, the clenched jaw and sweaty palms. Fibers also project directly from the central nucleus of the amygdala to the PAG, which initiates our behavioral reactions to fear: the dilated pupils, gasp and withdrawal reflex.

The autonomic nervous system centers in the hypothalamus and PAG do this by projecting their influences directly to spinal levels via the lateral (medullary) reticulospinal tracts. The emotional content of these messages is then relayed via interneurons directly to the gamma 1 motor neurons. Likewise, fibers also project directly from the amygdala, hypothalamus and PAG to other reticular nuclei including the pontine and medullary nuclei, which via the medial (pontine) reticulospinal, lateral (medullary) and other reticulospinal tracts transmit the emotional content to the gamma 1 motor neurons via the interconnecting interneurons (see Figure 11.2). Depending on the nature of this emotional content, the gamma 1 motor neurons will either be facilitated, potentially leading to over-facilitation, or inhibited, potentially leading to under-facilitation of the associated muscles.[1]

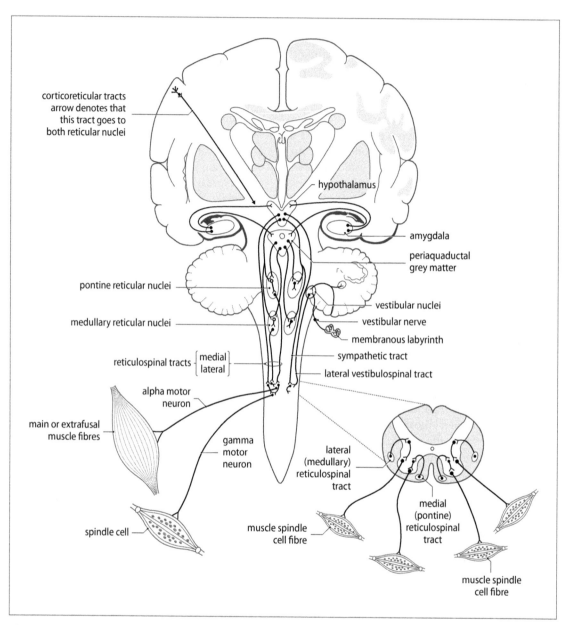

Figure 11.2 The emotional control of muscle function: the descending motor pathways. Subconscious emotional centers of the limbic and brainstem survival emotional centers project fibers directly to the pontine and medullary reticular nuclei. These directly alter muscle tone via interneurons to the gamma 1 motor neurons corresponding to the type of survival emotions that were activated. Thus, these extrapyramidal tracts control basal muscle tone and set the load reflex controlling muscle function.

Emotion–brain interface[3]

While it is fine to suggest that output from the emotional areas of the brain (the amygdala, hypothalamus, PAG, etc.) initiates the neurological response to emotional stress, with the rest just being a neurological cascade down through the brain from these limbic and reticular areas to the gamma 1 motor neurons, and their effect on the nuclear bag fiber control of the muscle stretch reflex, it begs the question, 'How does the subtle energy of the astral and mental bodies in which emotions and thought forms are created interface with the physiological emotional areas of the brain?'

What follows is totally speculative, but it at least provides a cognitive model through which to understand the muscular response to emotional states. Thought forms (mental body phenomena) and vibrational patterns associated with emotions (astral body phenomenon) are both generated in the subtle vibrational bodies of Man, but they are then stepped down into etheric energy patterns, which are in turn transduced into physiological patterns of nerves firing within the emotional centers of the brain, such as the amygdala and the PAG. Neural output from these emotional centers then follows the neurological cascade described above to the gamma 1 motor neurons that ultimately results in either over-facilitation or under-facilitation of the muscle being monitored.

Perhaps an example will clarify the rather detailed description above. You have cleared an indicator muscle and performed all pre-checks. You then ask the person, 'Think of your mother [or father]!' and monitor the indicator muscle. There are three possible responses: 1, the muscle locks, and when sedated unlocks, demonstrating homeostasis and hence no stress to whatever thought forms were accessed; 2, the muscle locks but will not unlock when sedated, demonstrating over-facilitation, a state of compensated stress; or 3, the muscle unlocks, registering overt uncompensated stress.

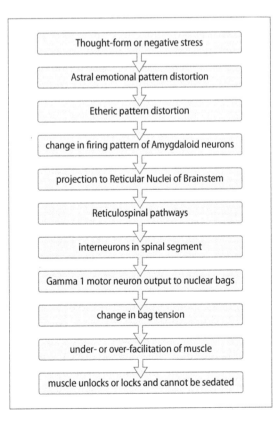

Figure 11.3 Flowchart of the emotion–brain interface. In the energetic model presented here, negative emotions and thoughts are first represented as astral and mental field vibrational patterns that are stepped down into etheric field distortions. These distortions are then transduced into changes in the firing pattern of neurons in the amygdala or other limbic or brainstem emotional centers. The output of these centers is projected to reticular brainstem nuclei and their descending reticulospinal pathways to spinal segments. Via interneurons, this input to reticular brainstem nuclei alters gamma 1 pathway output to the nuclear bag fibers, changing bag tension and altering the load reflex. It also creates either under-facilitation if the bag fibers were inhibited or over-facilitation if the bag fibers were facilitated.

In this case, the muscle unlocks. According to the above model, the thought form generated an astral body reaction to the associated stimulus, that is, Mother (or Father). This astral emotional pattern distorted the denser etheric body of the acupuncture system, and this distortion was in turn transduced into an electromagnetic pattern that altered the neural firing patterns within the amygdala. This pattern of neural activity in the amygdala was then projected to the hypothalamus, the PAG, other brainstem nuclei, etc., as well as directly to reticular nuclei in the brainstem.

These reticular nuclei in turn relayed this pattern via the medial and lateral reticulospinal and other reticular fibers to the interneurons in the spinal segment containing the gamma 1 motor neurons innervating the nuclear bag fibers of spindle cells within the indicator muscle. This change in gamma 1 input to the bag fibers suddenly inhibits or turns down the tension of the bag fibers. The sudden slackening of the bag fibers caused the threshold for the muscle stretch reflex to dip below the stretching caused by the muscle being monitored, and therefore the muscle just gave way under the monitoring pressure; the indicator muscle unlocked. See Figure 11.3.

The unlocked indicator thus indicated some type of emotional stress for this person around their mother or father. The person may even state, 'I get along very well with my Mother [or Father], and we love each other!' This may well be their conscious understanding of their relationship with this person, but the indicator muscle just demonstrated a stress reaction informing the person and the monitor that somewhere in this person's subconscious there lurk some unresolved issues. This is not surprising when you note that the muscle response was controlled not by the conscious part of the brain saying 'Hold your arm up', but rather by the subconscious emotional centers beyond our conscious knowledge or understanding that actually set the tone of the spindle cells controlling the muscle response.

While the nature of the subtle body interface with the amygdala and PAG are as yet unknown, the etheric effects of acupuncture point stimulation on the neuronal firing rates and patterns in the amygdala have been demonstrated.[4] Stimulation of specific acupoints has been shown to alter the discharge rate and pattern of firing in specific neurons in a rabbit amygdala. Stimulation of another acupoint caused a different pattern of neural activity in the same amygdaloid neurons, while the exact same stimulation of non-acupoint (or sham) points had no effect on the rates of neural discharge in these amygdaloid neurons.

The emotion–muscle interface for Golgi tendon organs

In Figure 9.3, it can be seen that the GTOs also have interneurons between the input from the sensory fibers of the GTO capsule and the motor neurons controlling muscle response. The same reticulospinal pathways carrying the emotional content of the amygdala reaction to a thought form could also change the set point for the GTO threshold for muscle inhibition. Should the amygdala reaction relayed by the reticulospinal pathways strongly inhibit the GTO circuit interneurons, then GTO output would need to be very high to cause any degree of reflex inhibition, hence the muscle would monitor over-facilitated with respect to GTO sedation. Tendon sedation would not inhibit the muscle. If, on the other hand, the emotional content strongly facilitated the GTO circuit interneurons, only slight GTO activation would cause strong reflex inhibition of the muscle, hence the muscle would monitor under-facilitated and unlock.

In the model presented, it is hypothesized that thoughts and emotions generate subtle body disturbances that in turn are transduced into patterns of activation in the subconscious brain centers that create survival emotions and reactions. The output of these subconscious brain centers to the gamma 1 pathways via the reticulospinal tracts, then resets the threshold of the load reflex, which results in changes in the muscle response observed via muscle monitoring. If the threshold for inhibition is set too high, the muscle will monitor over-facilitated, whereas if the threshold is set too low, the muscle will monitor under-facilitated.

References

1. Guyton, AC 1991, *Textbook of Medical Physiology, Eighth Edition,* WB Saunders, Philadelphia, p. 646.

   Kosslyn, SM, Alpert, NM, Thompson, WL, Maljkovic, V, Weise, SB, Chabris, CF, Hamilton, SE, Rauch, SL & Buonanno, FS 1993, Visual mental imagery activates topographically organized visual cortex: PET investigations, *Journal of Cognitive Neuroscience,* Vol. 5, pp. 263–287.

   Damasio, H, Grabowski, T, Damasio, A, Tranel, D, Boles-Ponto, L, Watkins, GL & Hichwa, RD 1993, Visual recall with the eyes closed and covered activates early visual cortices, *Society for Neuroscience Abstracts,* Vol. 19, 1603.

2. Noback, CR, Strominger, ML & Demarest, RJ 1991, *The Human Nervous System, Fourth Edition,* Lea & Febiger, Philadelphia.

3. Williams, PL & Warwick, R 1980, *Gray's Anatomy, Thirty-sixth Edition,* WB Saunders, Philadelphia.

   Guyton, AC 1991, *Textbook of Medical Physiology, Eighth Edition,* WB Saunders, Philadelphia.

   Juhan, D 1987, *Job's Body,* Station Hill Press, New York.

4. Zhongfang, L, Qingshu, C, Shuping, C & Zhenjing, H 1989, Effect of electro-acupuncture of 'Neiguan' on spontaneous discharges of single unit in amygdaloid nucleus in rabbits, *Journal of Traditional Chinese Medicine,* Vol. 9, No. 2, pp. 144–150.

Chapter 12

DOES MUSCLE MONITORING WORK?

Is muscle monitoring a useful biofeedback tool?

Krebs has a rigorous scientific background, so when he was first introduced to manual muscle monitoring he immediately wanted to validate what he was doing, only to find out that this was much harder than he ever conceived it would be! His first attempt was using physics, by simply placing a force transducer between his hand and the arm or other body part he was monitoring. Much to his surprise, the results were 'all over the place' and made no sense. Harms-Ringdhal found that electromyographs and dynamometers often produce false positives and negative findings when compared with manual muscle testing, as these instruments appear to measure different aspects of muscular activity than those accessed by manual muscle monitoring. In addition, just slight variations in position change the dynamics of the force measured by the force transducer.[1]

As discussed earlier in this book, we distinguish between manual muscle testing and manual muscle monitoring because they use two quite different protocols when accessing muscle function. Most of the existing literature has assessed the Applied Kinesiology (AK) chiropractic and/or physiotherapist muscle assessment procedures, which are significantly different from Energetic Kinesiology muscle assessment procedures and are used in a different way. Therefore it is predictable that they may yield relatively different outcomes.

While technically AK is a form of Energetic Kinesiology as it employs various aspects of the Chinese meridian theory and has acupressure-based corrections,[2] in practice it is more structurally focused than other modalities of Energetic Kinesiology. AK also uses a variation of the more traditional form of manual muscle testing found in other physical therapies (e.g. physiotherapy, academic kinesiology and orthopedic therapies).

In contrast, the more energy-based kinesiology modalities use a different approach from that of manual muscle testing used by AK chiropractors, termed *muscle monitoring*, to access all domains of our multidimensional body, often with greater emphasis on feedback from the subtle energy domains than from the physical domain.

However, before discussing AK manual muscle testing and then Energetic Kinesiology muscle monitoring in greater depth, there are a number of factors that underlie both types of manual muscle biofeedback that may affect the application, interpretation and outcome when either of these types of manual muscle testing is employed.

Factors affecting muscle response during muscle testing or monitoring

There are a number of factors involved in the seemingly simple act of manual testing a muscle. The two primary factors are the complexity of the physics of even simple manual muscle monitoring, and the complexity of the hidden subconscious control of our muscle function. Even assuming that the muscle is placed in the correct position to accurately monitor a specific muscle, and then the pressure is applied in exactly the correct direction at exactly the right level of pressure, the actual interaction between the monitor's hand and the client's limb is quite complex! However, this complexity is hidden from our consciousness as it results largely from the interaction of various subconscious sensory–motor loops, several of which are spinal reflexes involving no consciousness at all!

Indeed, this is what separates our subjective perception of what is happening from what *is* actually happening, and why our subjective perception of what is happening is largely objectively incorrect. Our consciousness is unaware that it normally activates only subconscious servo circuits rather than actually running the show. This is because there are two totally separate pathways that control our muscles: one is largely subconscious and sets the basal muscle tone controlling basic spinal reflexes such as the load reflex (which in turn actually control our primary muscle functions), and one that is totally conscious and that allows us to tell our muscles what to do and how we want it to be done!

The subconscious extrapyramidal pathways run from sets of brainstem nuclei, primarily the reticular nuclei of the pons and medulla controlling our basal muscle tone, and the vestibular nuclei controlling our equilibrium and balance.[3] These reticulospinal and vestibulospinal tracts run down the spinal cord primarily to alpha motor neurons controlling the basal tone of the postural muscles of the body, and to the gamma 1 motor neurons controlling the muscle stretch or load reflex.[4] Being brainstem in origin, they are totally subconscious and controlled by reflexes. However, these subconscious nuclei and tracts provide the substrate on which the second set of conscious pathways operate. The pyramidal corticospinal tracts run from our motor cortex down the spinal cord to the spinal segments and synapse via interneurons with the alpha motor neurons that contract individual muscles of the body and orchestrate individual muscles to give us direct conscious control of our movements.[5]

Thus, when subconscious extrapyramidal output inhibits muscle tone, including the load reflex that in turn directly controls our muscle responses as well as other spinal reflexes, our consciousness can no longer make our muscles do what we have asked them to do! Try as you might with your consciousness, you will not be able to make muscles whose subconscious reflexes are inhibited ever 'lock'. But to you, it subjectively feels that you are trying really hard to hold your arm or leg up, because indeed you are sending streams of signals from your cortex down your pyramidal pathways, saying 'Hold', but to no avail, as it is the subconscious substrate that actually controls the ability of your muscles to lock and thus obey your conscious commands.

Perhaps an analogy will clarify why our conscious experience of muscle testing/monitoring seems so at odds with what happens. You can think of your muscles as light bulbs, with the big muscles being 100-watt bulbs; your consciousness can only turn the light switch on or off. Normally, when you decide to flip the switch on, it makes a bright light (100 watts of power). However, the catch is that your subconscious controls the dimmer switch! Therefore, no matter how many watts the bulb is, if the subconscious dimmer switch has turned down the power to your bulb, when your consciousness switches the light bulb on, you have only a dim light! It is still a 100-watt light bulb, but you are now getting only 20 watts of power.

Add to this a relatively complex set of physics phenomena and you can understand why the conscious experience of manual muscle testing/monitoring bears little resemblance to what is actually happening! To the untrained eye, the physics of manual muscle testing/monitoring appears quite straightforward: 'Push the arm in this direction!' The muscle response is either weak ('unlocks') and moves in the direction of pressure, or is strong (locks) and holds its position against the increasing pressure applied.

What is actually happening from a physics and mathematical perspective, however, is quite complex and designed to deceive your conscious perception. When I push on your arm, there are two independent phenomena happening together, one from physics and the other from mathematics. First, I am pushing on a lever system, so there are vectors of force that vary with what the arm actually does, that is, lock or unlock. And second, manual muscle monitoring is the interaction of two separate nervous systems, each with its own set of automatic reflexes and conscious inputs that generate second- and third-order differential relationships. Therefore the outcome of muscle monitoring, whether the muscle locks or unlocks, is the solution of these vectors and subvectors of force with the second- and third-order differential interactions, as the cerebellum has been doing calculus long before Newton or von Leibniz wrote down their equations.

One of the most common statements that clients make when they are being muscle tested/

monitored is, 'You're pushing differently! That's why my arm gave way!' And this is indeed how it feels, because of the physics of vectors. When I push on the lever of your arm and the shoulder muscle locks, the direction of force (called a vector in physics) is straight down the shaft of your arm into the shoulder joint. However, when the muscle unlocks, the arm now begins to transit an arc as it moves toward the table. The pressure applied is indeed straight down toward the table, but because of the mechanics of the joint, the arm cannot move straight down toward the table but rather travels through an arc. This means that the single vector of force straight down the arm into the joint of the locked muscle now begins to break down into a series of subvectors. The subvectors are rapidly changing as the arm transcribes an arc of the arm, following the movement permitted by the mechanics of the joint when the muscle unlocks!

Thus, while the practitioner pushed exactly the same way in both instances, it clearly felt to the client that the practitioner pushed differently on the locked muscle than on the unlocked muscle. Even though this is not objectively true, it is how it feels! In addition, it also felt like the practitioner pushed harder on the unlocked muscle than on the locked muscle. Again, this is not true objectively; in fact, it is exactly opposite to the objective truth!

The feeling of the practitioner pushing differently was a direct consequence of the change in vectors as the arm moved through the arc of the joint. And the feeling that the monitor was pushing harder when the muscle unlocked compared with when it locked was a direct consequence of the subconscious inhibition of the basal muscle tone required to activate the load reflex that locks the muscle. Once the load reflex has been inhibited, it is no longer possible to lock the muscle, but in an attempt to hold the arm in the test/monitoring position, the client now uses increasing conscious effort to activate the very muscle or muscles that are now being overtly inhibited by the subconscious!

Until relatively recently, scientists have generally dismissed manual muscle testing/monitoring as being subjective and therefore not a credible technique worthy of further scientific investigation. This point of view resulted from both the lack of effective instrumentation capable of accurately assessing all aspects of these complex interactions of the two nervous systems during manual muscle testing/monitoring. It was also reinforced by the false subjective perception of what is actually happening during muscle testing/monitoring.

How is the muscle testing/monitoring performed?

The procedures used in manual muscle testing in the more physical therapies, especially when used in orthopedic testing, to a fair degree match their name—the Manual Muscle Test (MMT)—as the pressure is generally applied quickly and with moderate to strong force, depending on the practitioner and the muscle being tested. Historically, physiotherapists, Structural Kinesiologists and AK chiropractors applied moderate force, as indeed it was a test of the relative muscle strength and used to detect any muscle weakness.

Over the years, many AK chiropractors began to use considerably less force and see muscle testing as an art in which the force applied to the client is increased at a constant rate until the tester feels the muscle *begin* to give way, and then just follows this movement. As Walther has stated, 'Once the muscle is in motion, the muscle test is over, as it is the amount of force required to initiate motion that is the parameter to be measured in an accurate MMT.'[2] The classic break test used by physical therapists also tests this same phenomenon but rates it on a scale of 1–5 (with 5 representing a fully locked muscle),[6] rather than the binary scale of Energetic Kinesiologists, in which the muscle is perceived to hold strong or lock or to give way and appear weak when it unlocks. This more recent AK Manual Muscle Test is an approach more in line with the type of muscle activation generally taught in the various Energetic Kinesiology systems today.

Therefore a good deal of the difference between mechanoelectrical measurements of dynamometers and manual muscle testing/monitoring results from how the testing/monitoring is performed. In the more biomechanical applications, such as orthopedic testing, the muscles are tested for their ability to hold against linearly increasing load that brings the muscle toward its maximal limits. Likewise, the force applied by a dynamometer is relatively linear and invariant, and it is increased relatively rapidly. Therefore dynamometric testing largely activates a first-order differential, the linear rate of change response from the muscle, and is thus testing different aspects of neuromuscular control than the tests against variable resistance used in Energetic Kinesiology, including AK.

Before evaluating the validity of muscle testing/monitoring in Energetic Kinesiology, we will first discuss AK manual muscle testing and the AK research literature. This is followed by a discussion of Energetic Kinesiology muscle monitoring and the Energetic Kinesiology research literature.

What is AK muscle testing accessing and why is it important?

In both AK and Energetic Kinesiology, the muscle is being used as a biofeedback tool to determine where in the body there is an active stressor. The focus in AK, however, is on the neuromuscular interactions with the musculoskeletal structural system. Therefore AK uses the muscle response, the AK MMT, to determine if there are stressors affecting muscular and skeletal function. Because the skeletal system depends on integrated muscular function to maintain its integrity, muscular imbalance will result in the loss of skeletal–structural integrity and the distortion of normal posture and function. This is especially true, as the spinal system is maintained by tensegrity, the coordinated activity of intervertebral muscles pulling the spine erect from the skull, with the intervertebral muscles of each vertebra lifting the vertebra below it upward, thus maintaining an erect spine.[7]

Therefore, muscle imbalance causes skeletal–postural imbalances by specific muscles becoming either too tight, the over-facilitated state of imbalance, or more commonly, various muscles being inhibited, often by output from another muscle or another component of the musculoskeletal system (e.g. the Golgi tendon and Golgi ligament organs, fascial stretch receptors, and nociceptors). The commonly held belief that most muscle pain and skeletal distortion results from some form of tonic muscular hyperactivity that creates and maintains the chronic pain and dysfunction is giving way to the view that the real culprit is muscle inhibition, with the inhibited muscle now having to be compensated for by other muscles, often synergist(s) of the prime mover or another muscle(s).

However, each muscle in the body is a prime mover for a specific action, and is attached to the skeleton in such a way as to give this muscle maximal mechanical advantage to do a specific action when it contracts. So if for any reason the prime mover of a specific action is inhibited, another muscle, usually a synergist of the inhibited agonist, must now take over the job of the inhibited muscle(s), as well as its own job! More importantly, the recruited or compensating muscle is now at a distinct mechanical disadvantage and has to work really hard to maintain the muscle position normally easily maintained by the inhibited prime mover. In fact, synergist–agonist substitution for inhibited muscles is common in neuromuscular dysfunction.[8]

An analogy may clarify. You are designed to carry buckets of sand directly by your side, and even heavy buckets can be carried easily this way. But just think how much heavier the same buckets of sand feels when you attempt to carry the two buckets with your arms held out horizontally; this is exactly what happens when a muscle, for example an intervertebral muscle, is inhibited and its synergist(s) has to take over. This may indeed cause the synergist(s) that is now working at a mechanical disadvantage to become over-facilitated, or over-energy from the energetic perspective. And an over-facilitated muscle always over-inhibits its antagonist, creating a reciprocal problem.

But what would cause this inhibition? Data from several studies suggest that the body's reaction to injury and pain is not primarily increased muscular tension and stiffness, but rather muscular inhibition![9] This is a protective reaction sometimes called the tendon or ligament guard reflex. If you have strained a tendon or have torn a muscle, the nervous system then activates a series of compensatory reactions to both protect the damaged structure from further damage and to permit healing to take place. Inhibition of the muscle that is torn or has a strained tendon reduces the mechanical stress on this damaged tendon or muscle, permitting the tissue to heal. However, once the muscle is actively inhibited, when further force is applied to the muscle it not only activates further tendon and ligament reflex inhibition but the loss of muscle contraction creates increased physical tension or stress on the tendons and ligaments, which in turn fire nociceptors (pain receptors), causing pain and often resulting in further muscle inhibition.

Lund and colleagues suggest that the old pain–spasm–pain model, in which muscle tension is necessarily increased when pain is present, and indeed, it is the pain that inhibits the muscle causing weakness, should be replaced with the pain-adaptation model.[10] Rather than pain causing increased tension when pain is present in various musculoskeletal disorders, there is decreased activation or overt inhibition of muscles during movements in which they act as the agonists, and increased activation during movements in which they are antagonists. This is exactly what Edgerton and coworkers found in patients suffering from chronic neck pain resulting from whiplash; there was underactivity of agonist muscles and overactivity of synergistic muscles. Indeed, this pattern of inhibited and over-facilitated muscles allowed them to discriminate people with chronic neck pain from those who had recovered, with 88% accuracy.[11]

There is now evidence that impaired strength resulting from muscle inhibition occurs in close relationship with the development of specific joint dysfunction, inflammation or injury and will produce ongoing inhibition of muscle function.[12] Also, most other parameters of dysfunction identified in low back pain and neck pain patients have been shown not to precede the pain but rather only accompany it. An important exception is muscle strength which can predict future low back pain and neck pain in asymptomatic individuals.[13]

But how is an AK chiropractor to know of muscle weakness resulting from muscle inhibition? Equally important, where does this inhibition originate, and therefore what would be the most effective treatment to apply, or what further investigation may actually prevent the onset of future pain, discomfort and dysfunction? One of the most direct and efficient approaches is the use of the AK MMT if you are a chiropractor or muscle monitoring if you are an Energetic Kinesiologist. Indeed, Schmitt and Cuthbert state, 'Where diagnostic methods have a capacity to specify the form of therapy needed or the prognosis or long-term course of a disorder or imbalance, this diagnosis has increased value.'[14]

Thus, the MMT has diagnostic value to both identify a functional disorder (muscle inhibition), and then to assist in locating the chiropractic manipulative technique to correct the observed inhibition. Equally important, the MMT can then be used once more to confirm that the initial muscle inhibition underlying the postural or structural imbalance has been resolved. The immediate improvement in muscle strength and its covariance with the client's dysfunctions after chiropractic manipulative technique that has been reported clinically supports this correlation.[15]

A brief review of Manual Muscle Testing research used in AK

A primary issue that needs to be addressed in order to determine whether manual muscle testing used in AK and muscle monitoring used in other Energetic Kinesiology modalities are valid tools to provide feedback about the various states and conditions in the body that are of diagnostic or treatment value is: 'Does it work?' To determine this, the MMT has to be assessed for its reliability and validity. The reliability of a diagnostic or treatment method is a measure of the consistency of the measurement when repeated. Depending on the type of measurement performed, different types of reliability coefficients, such as the Cohen's kappa coefficient, can be calculated, and the closer to 1, the higher the reliability.

There are two types of reliability that must be considered. First is intraexaminer (or intrarater) reliability: the ability of the same tester or monitor to consistently achieve similar values in test–re-test studies. Second is interexaminer (inter-rater) reliability: the ability of two or more testers or monitors to achieve similar values or outcomes when tested or monitored by several practitioners. Intraexaminer reliability is necessary to evaluate the reproducibility and consistency of the test, while interexaminer reliability is necessary to assess the meaning or validity of the test, as it measures the relative variability of the same test performed by different examiners.

To establish the validity of both intra- and interexaminer reliability, there must be another means of measuring the factor or issue being assessed to provide a reference or standard measurement with which to compare the observed results. This reference value may be quantitative, for example how many kilograms of force were actually applied, or qualitative, for example the use of a pain or subjective effort scale, with 0 being none, and 10 being the most pain of this type you have ever felt or the most effort you can make. Traditionally, the reference value has been a mechanical testing device called a dynamometer, an instrument to directly measure mechanical force by applying pressure to a force transducer, an electrical device that converts pressure or force into an electrical signal that can be recorded and calibrated. Use of a dynamometer in manual muscle testing is sometimes called quantitative muscle testing (QMT).

Dynamometric versus manual muscle testing

While it would appear that dynamometers are the logical gold standard for the MMT, as they produce hard quantitative data, direct comparisons can be problematic when handheld dynamometers (HHDs) are used, because of the complexity of manual muscle tests, as discussed earlier in this chapter. There is also evidence that dynamometers do not measure the same aspects of muscle activity as manual muscle testing,[15] especially if the muscle unlocks rather than resisting the linear force applied. Also, slight variations in the position or

angle of the contact point of the dynamometer on the body can produce false negative and positive values because of the fact that, until recently, all force transducers were highly directional in design. Thus small changes of angle of application of the HHD on the body may produce aberrant values.[16]

This is exactly what Krebs found when he tried to apply a simple unidirectional force-transducer to validate his manual muscle monitoring. If the muscle can develop a strong lock and the device can be placed in such a way that linear pressure can be applied to the muscle, results are generally consistent. However, if the muscle begins to unlock as the angle of application constantly changes, the values recorded often vary considerably. Because of the constantly changing angles of contact of the force transducer with the body and the directionality of the force transducer, the force transducer may capture only a small part of the actual force applied and thus is not able to record the actual force applied.

There have been a number of studies in AK attempting to use HHDs to measure the force or pressure applied to a muscle and then compare this quantitative value with the outcome of the MMT; was the force more when the muscle locked and less when the muscle unlocked? However, the results of various studies have been highly variable, with some studies showing good agreement between HHDs and the MMT.[17] Comparison of two studies, one by Marino and colleagues[18] and one by Wadsworth and colleagues,[19] showed significant reliability between HHD and MMT scores. Scores measured with HHDs were consistent with the examiners' determination of muscle weakness ($P < 0.001$) in both studies. However, other studies demonstrated considerable differences between HHD data and MMT assessments of muscle function,[20] with the study by Kenney and coworkers finding no correlation between QMT and MMT evaluation of muscle strength with regard to an assessment of nutrient status.[21] It should be noted that they employed a research design that did not reflect the clinical practice and principles of AK, and the study does not reflect anything the International College of Applied Kinesiology supports or teaches. Another study, by Escolar and colleagues, showed that QMT was more reliable than the MMT performed by inexperienced examiners. However, with adequate training of these novice examiners, an interclass correlation coefficient > 0.75 was achieved between the QMT and MMT.[22] In yet another study using blind trials with sugar or a placebo placed in the mouth, computerized dynamometric (QMT) testing found no significant correlation, while the MMT revealed a highly statistically difference ($P = 0.006$) between the control and experimental groups.

In a more recent study by Fosang and Baker, while there was reasonably good correlation between QMT and MMT in general, dyanometric tests were not sensitive to changes in strength or strength measurements below grade 3 (on a 1–5 scale), while MMT tests revealed changes on grade 3 and even below.[23] The human examiner is still the most sensitive instrument we have to interpret the MMT, and according to Walther, 'Presently the best "instrument" to perform manual muscle testing is a well-trained examiner, using his/her perception of time and force with knowledge of anatomy and physiology of muscle function.'[24]

Intraexaminer and interexaminer reliability

Regardless of the method or equipment used, to standardize the MMT in a research setting it is most important that test protocols be highly reproducible both when the same examiner makes a series of tests (intraexaminer reliability) and when different examiners repeat the same tests as previous examiners (interexaminer reliability). We will just summarize the findings here of two recent comprehensive reviews of AK manual muscle testing research that surveyed the literature for both intraexaminer and interexaminer reliability, and you are referred to these excellent reviews for an extensive analysis of this important topic.[25]

The levels of agreement for interexaminer reliability in 10 studies, including three randomized controlled trials (RCTs), based on +/- one grade, were high, ranging from 82% to 97%, and from 96% to 98% for test–retest intraexaminer reliability. The results of these studies suggest that in order to be confident that a true change in strength has

occurred, MMT scores must change at least one full grade, the change from an inhibited or weak muscle to a facilitated or strong muscle, which is a common result of successful treatment.[26] Leisman, Zenhausern and colleagues found that there was a significant difference in strong versus weak muscle-testing outcomes, and showed using force measurements from both practitioner and patient that these changes were not attributable to decreased or increased testing force from the practitioner performing the test.[27]

Several studies have shown good intra- and interexaminer reliability with both groups of upper and lower limb muscles, as well as testing individual limb muscles.[28] Pollard and coworkers found good interexaminer reliability between two practitioners of differing skill when using repeated testing on the deltoid (k 0.62) and psoas (k 0.67),[29] while Jepson and colleagues found inter-rater reliability for two examiners (blinded as to patient-related information) who classified 14 muscles on the right and left sides of the body in terms of normal or reduced strength, and reduced strength was significantly associated with the presence of symptoms. This study also demonstrated a comparable or better reliability than that of other diagnostic tests in common use for upper limb dysfunction.[30] A recent study of interexaminer reliability for the MMT of lower limb muscles blinded the examiner for ideomotor cues yet found good reliability, with interexaminer agreement of 70–90%, depending on the specific muscle tested.[31]

Taken in total, the AK manual muscle testing research literature provides reasonable support for acceptable levels of intraexaminer and interexaminer reliability, and there is an increasing body of literature supporting the validity of MMT as a diagnostic tool for the treatment of a range of musculoskeletal dysfunctions. A review in 2007 of the AK research literature by Cuthbert and Goodheart using very carefully constructed criteria for selecting over 100 research papers in AK concluded that manual muscle testing is both a science and an art, but that *there is substantial research evidence for reliability, interexaminer consistency, and validity*.[25]

The scientific research up to this point certainly

supports the view that manual muscle testing has validity in specific types of conditions, such as lower back pain[25,32] and mechanical neck pain,[33] and for various specific conditions, such as juvenile idiopathic inflammatory myopathies,[34] but suffers from the lack of rigorous RCTs in many other areas in which it has been applied.[25] Indeed, Cuthbert and Goodheart conclude that, 'MMT as employed by chiropractors, physiotherapists and neurologists was shown to be a clinically useful tool, but its ultimate scientific validation and application requires testing that employs sophisticated research models in areas of neurophysiology, biomechanics, RCTs and statistical analysis.'[25]

What is Energetic Kinesiology muscle monitoring accessing and why is it important?

Both AK and Energetic Kinesiology use the integrity of proprioceptive feedback and relative muscle strength rather than absolute muscle strength in accessing the feedback from manual muscle monitoring; this is the *art* in the art and science of manual muscle testing or monitoring. In Energetic Kinesiology, however, the monitor is not only monitoring the physical function of the muscle, but rather is using the observable muscle responses as an interface to reference and locate stressors or imbalances within subconscious and subtle body energy systems. Therefore they are truly using muscle function to monitor for potential imbalances or stressors, rather than test the muscle for relative strength.

Perhaps the primary difference between the AK MMT and Energetic Kinesiology muscle monitoring is how the muscle to be tested or monitored will be employed. In AK, muscles are assessed via the MMT to locate muscles demonstrating inhibition and that thus appear weak. So if the muscle being tested was not inhibited, and did not give way to the monitoring pressure, the practitioner would then go to another muscle to investigate which muscles have imbalance or are overtly being directly affected by a stressor of some type. Thus in AK, the muscles tested are being assessed for

their direct relationship to the stressor causing the muscle imbalance. In contrast, in muscle monitoring an indicator muscle is selected as a generalized indicator to detect stressor(s) (see chapter 10) in any domain of physiological or energetic function.

Indeed, before a muscle can be used as an indicator muscle in Energetic Kinesiology, it first must undergo a series of pre-checks (discussed in chapter 22) to establish that it is in physiological homeostasis, and that there are no extraneous factors currently perturbing its function. Then this balanced indicator muscle is employed as a monitoring tool to access and assess imbalances or stressors affecting subconscious physical, etheric, emotional and mental processes, or imbalances within the subtle energy systems of the body. Thus, the indicator muscle will be in homeostatic function and locking when the monitor circuit locates an acupoint. If the indicator muscle remains locked, it indicates that there are currently no active stressors affecting this acupoint or the energetic circuits or systems with which it is interfaced. If the indicator muscle unlocks when the acupoint is touched, it indicates that there is currently an active stressor creating an imbalance in the acupoint or energy flow in that specific meridian, and the type of muscle response gives the monitor information about the types of stressors and likely effect of this imbalance.

Besides this difference in how muscles are used in AKMMT and muscle monitoring, the monitoring procedure is also considerably different. To monitor a muscle in Energetic Kinesiology, the monitor applies pressure slowly, increasing pressure to approximately only 2 kilograms of force, sustains this pressure for approximately two full seconds, and then slowly releases the pressure. While applying pressure for a full two seconds has long been a part of Energetic Kinesiology muscle-monitoring protocol, recent research has demonstrated exactly how important it is to maintain the pressure on the muscle or limb for at least the two seconds. Conable conducted a pilot study to investigate the difference between short (1-second) and long (3-second) muscle tests on strong or facilitated versus weak or functionally inhibited muscles.

He observed that longer test durations demonstrate muscle weakness not evident on the short 1-second tests of the same muscles.[35] Therefore it appears maintaining the monitoring pressure for a full two seconds before beginning to decrease pressure will achieve more accurate results than shorter test durations, and be more effective at detecting imbalances or stressors affecting the body's homeostasis.

Because even small muscles in the body, even those of children, cannot be overpowered by only 2 kilograms of force, you are never assessing the muscle's strength in Energetic Kinesiology, which is also why the terms *locked* and *unlocked* are used rather than the more testing-based terms *strong* and *weak* traditionally used in AK manual muscle testing. Rather than strength, you are assessing the subconscious neural circuits as an interface with all levels of your multidimensional being.

In Energetic Kinesiology, force is also applied more slowly on the muscle and limited to force well below that which would *fully* activate the load reflex, as just enough pressure is applied to *feel* the muscle lock. Once the muscle has locked, the monitor can increase the monitoring pressure considerably, but the response will remain the same until the monitoring pressure begins to overpower the muscle. However, the monitor never needs to apply very much pressure to clearly identify a locked muscle. To paraphrase Walther in AK, 'Once the muscle has clearly locked there is no need for the monitor to increase the monitoring pressure.' Rather than the AK focus on structure and postural integrity, in Energetic Kinesiology the focus is on the muscle responses to reveal subconscious and subtle energy body integrity and balance.

However, the source of many physical issues result from deeper subconscious origins that normally remain unknown but that are now suddenly observable, or at least the effects of their presence becomes both observable and felt when the muscle is monitored. The client does not need the monitor to tell them that some stressor has been activated when their formerly locked muscle suddenly unlocks. Likewise, when a formerly unlocking muscle suddenly returns to normal function and locks, the client immediately has a conscious experience of positive change in a function or state.

Research supporting muscle monitoring and Energetic Kinesiology methods

The very fact that muscle response can indicate energetic imbalances places Energetic Kinesiology well outside of the accepted scientific and medical model that doubts—or should we state more correctly, is ignorant of—the energy systems of the body. A scientist or doctor cannot say that ch'i or prana do not exist, for to do so you would first have to be able to measure ch'i and prana, something not yet possible with current scientific instrumentation, although the development of the measurement of biofields is progressing rapidly.[36] Something you cannot measure, and hence cannot know about, is something that you are ignorant of, and ignorance is not a particularly strong place to argue from! So kinesiology, like all other energetic systems (such as homeopathy), has had an uphill battle to prove that it is a valid and reliable method for successfully addressing physiological, nutritional and/or psychoemotional imbalances of the human body.

As Energetic Kinesiology is in the early stage of development, there have been only a few scientific studies on the use of muscle monitoring and the Energetic Kinesiology model presented above, as opposed to the numerous studies completed with AK manual muscle testing. Also, like the AK research literature, the studies that have been done tend to be small with either one or two examiners, and generally with small sample sizes that limit the statistical power of the study, and they have often had only limited statistical analysis of the data, if any was done at all.

One of the first studies to address the use of an indicator muscle and to validate its use was by Rolfes in her PhD thesis, *The Phenomenon of Indicator Muscle Change. An Explanation of its Validity and Meaning.*[37] The term *indicator change* has been used throughout this book and in the kinesiology literature in general to indicate a change in muscle response, either from a locked muscle to an unlocked muscle or from an unlocked muscle back to a locked muscle. Rolfes elucidated two aspects of what she termed the 'phenomenon' of indicator muscle change, which is the basis of the whole field of kinesiology in all of its manifestations. These two aspects are a sensory bodily experience, the transient loss of muscle strength and how this bodily experience is intellectually processed: the felt experience and the cognitive experience. The cognitive experience tries to understand the felt experience in intellectual terms, such as a cause and effect relationship between an intervention and the phenomenon of the muscle response, the indicator change, which is suited to a quantitative experimental design. In contrast, the sensory bodily experience of the indicator muscle change was explored by a qualitative design using a structured interview of the subject's felt experiences and what this had meant to them.

Rolfes examined two areas for the validity of an indicator muscle to accurately respond to specific stressors in two different domains: a response to detect imbalance or alterations in ch'i flows in meridians, and the response to negative emotional states in an experimental setting. Important contextual parameters such as the emotional and intellectual dependency in a client–therapist setting, preconceptions of the therapist and client, and expectations of the outcome of the procedure were removed, using a double-blind setting for the acupuncture system tests and a single-blind setting for the emotional tests. Two examiners, Rolfes and another Energetic Kinesiologist, did all the testing. The qualitative results of structured interviews with the subjects following the study provide insights to the client's perception of the experience, which had not previously been examined systematically.

Rolfes used the discovery by Goodheart that magnets applied to the sedation points of traditional Chinese acupuncture would also sedate or inhibit meridian-related muscles.[38] AK research had shown both the triceps muscle of the arm and the latissimus dorsi muscle of the shoulder to be spleen meridian–related muscles, and thus placing the magnet on the sedation point spleen 5 should inhibit both these muscles once applied. In a double blind, once the triceps or latissimus muscle of the arm was correctly positioned for monitoring,

an assistant applied either a 3000-gauss rare earth button magnet or a placebo shirt button of similar size, color and weight to spleen 5. Then each of these two muscles was monitored in turn and the results recorded. Application of the north pole of the magnet to spleen 5 consistently inhibited both meridian-related muscles and were statistically significant ($P < 0.001$ for the triceps and $P < 0.01$ for the latissimus dorsi), and there was good inter-examiner reliability. This result has been replicated in the more recent study of Moncayo and Moncayo using stimulation of sedation points and measuring meridian-related muscle response confirmed by surface electromyography (sEMG) and the MMT.[39]

In her study of effects of negative emotional states on muscle response, Rolfes used mental imagery of an anxiety theme, with subjects being told that they had failed an important examination (subjects were all currently students), or of a placebo theme, that the subjects were lying comfortably on a massage table and resting. Once they had been informed of their theme, they were then asked to explore the feelings this theme generated for them. The subjects were then monitored during this exploration phase. There was a significantly different occurrence of indicator muscle change during the imagery of the anxiety theme compared with the placebo theme ($P < 0.03$ for the triceps muscle and $P < 0.009$ for the latissimus dorsi). Interestingly, anxiety is the emotion found to be associated with the spleen meridian, and this association was expressed by the spleen meridian–related muscles. A study by Monti and colleagues confirmed that subconscious emotional responses control the outcome of the indicator muscle response. They investigated differences in manual muscle test outcomes after subjects were exposed to congruent and incongruent semantic stimuli. The order in which the statements were repeated was controlled by a counterbalanced design. Overall, significant differences were found in muscle test responses between congruent and incongruent self-referential semantic statements ($P < 0.001$).[40]

In her post-study structured interviews, Rolfes was able to evaluate some of the qualitative effects on their personal perception of the subjects from their observation of the indicator muscle changes that occurred during the experiments. The subjects' perception of what they personally gained by participation in this study can be summarized in several statements. First, observing their indicator muscle change, the physical event of becoming weak or the muscle remaining strong in the different contexts of the study, made them acutely aware of the mind–body connection, a connection with one's inner being, including, as some subjects stated, access to their intuition. Second, the indicator muscle change was a physical event felt and observed by the clients, to which they ascribed a quality of 'feeling the body responding' to a part of reality on which they did not normally focus— increased consciousness of their energy fields and its interweaving with their body, including problem areas or disturbances in their energy field—and which provided them with information about themselves that they could not access or retrieve with the intellect.

The only recent review of kinesiology that includes Energetic Kinesiology practitioners or manual muscle testing performed in the style of muscle monitoring was done by Hall and coworkers.[41] In fact, this type of muscle testing was one of their inclusion criteria. They reviewed the research done primarily in AK, but their review included a few Energetic Kinesiology-based studies. The review had three aims: 1, to assess whether the diagnostic accuracy, including intra- and interexaminer reliability, has been established; 2, to review whether there is evidence for therapeutic effectiveness; and 3, to critically assess the quality of the relevant studies.

The study involved an electronic search of databases for relevant studies, which were then analyzed and scored for methodological quality and quality of reporting using standard quality assessment tools. What they found was that the studies that met their inclusion criteria were generally of low quality and therefore difficult to assess for effectiveness. However, they make the following unabashed statement: 'Based on this review of the studies there is insufficient evidence to suggest that kinesiology (of any type) has any specific

therapeutic effect for any condition ... or that the validity of muscle testing has been established.'

This statement far exceeds the scope of the research study the authors had undertaken. They did a literature review, so the only scientifically true statement they could formulate is that 'the studies conducted and published to date in kinesiology do not fulfill the requirements necessary to ascertain a positive score when being measured by the QUADAS tool (Quality Assessment of Diagnostic Accuracy Studies), Jadad scale, Standards for the Reporting of Diagnostic Accuracy Studies and Consolidated Standards of Reporting Trials methods for assessing the quality of methods and reporting used in these studies.' Their conclusion at the end of the review that there is no evidence of therapeutic effectiveness is flawed and inaccurate, because if there is just no literature on the therapeutic effectiveness, this does not imply that there is no evidence that kinesiology treatments are not effective, when there is over 30 years of clinical evidence that it works!

Despite the above conclusion of Hall and colleagues, the three studies they reported for effectiveness in Table 1 of their review were all conducted by Energetic Kinesiologists and showed highly statistically significant results. One study showed significant reduction in stress and ability to cope, as measured by the Perceived Stress Scale, with a reduction in the mean score of $P < 0.0005$, and in a larger study with 88 women with mastalgia there was a significant reduction in pain after the first treatment ($P < 0.00001$). The third study was a controlled study with 26 subjects suffering from recurring disturbing dreams. The mean dream frequency was reduced in the treatment group compared with the control group (anova), with $P < 0.006$. Therefore, despite the poor methodological and reporting quality of these studies, they appear to have been quite successful by demonstrating perceptible and reproducible effect on the people receiving these treatments.

A 2010 study by Muehlboeck at the University of Salzburg studied the effect of kinesiology from the perspective of the clients and confirmed that clients perceived positive outcomes for a number of different types of conditions from a number of different kinesiology practitioners.[42] Two hundred clients each received five treatment sessions from 29 Energetic Kinesiologists practicing in Salzburg, Austria. The measurement instrument applied was a dichotomous semantic differential or polarity profile consisting of 38 word pairs describing physical, emotional, mental and social properties, for example weak–strong, tight–relaxed, ill–well, tired–awake or rested, troubled–unconcerned, nervous–calm, timid–courageous, frustrated–motivated, and unfocused–focused. The polarity profile covered physical issues, emotional states, mental states, social interactions and overall well-being. The subjects evaluated each word pair by choosing which emoticon, from a very happy face to a very sad face on a seven-face scale, best represented their current state of being with regard to that word pair.

The subjects were asked to evaluate their state of being by filling out a polarity profile before receiving the five treatments and then after completion of the five treatments. It should be noted that the subjects were seeing their practitioner for a variety of reasons, from physical pain to stress-related issues, social or personality issues, psychoemotional issues and even spiritual issues. On the seven-point polarity profile scale of well-being, a 7 for any property means that you are currently experiencing the most positive state of this property you can experience, while a 1 means that you are currently experiencing the most negative state of this property that you can experience. The 38 word pairs were chosen to represent different aspects of how you feel about your life, from physical factors affecting your life to psychoemotional states, social relationships and individual factors that increase or decrease our sense of well-being.

The pretreatment mean value for each item of polarity profile for all of the subjects varied from 2.55 for the psychoemotional pair (stressed–active) to 4.57 for the social pair (indignant–friendly), with all except seven out of 38 pretreatment values less than 4. Following the five Energetic Kinesiology treatments, the range was now 5.28 for the psychoemotional pair (worried–carefree) to 6.20 for the personal state pair (desperate–confident), with the property values for all pairs now being significantly greater than 4. The average increase in well-being scores of all property pairs was 2.4, an increase of 34.3% over the pretreatment values, and the improvement in scores ranged between 2.26 (32.2%) and 2.55 (36.4%). The subjects were also interviewed after treatment for their perception of any changes in overall well-being, and they reported improvements in pain and physical well-being and psychoemotional states but less improvement in their social states.

Two things that emerged from the post-treatment interviews that speak directly to subjects' perception of the value of these kinesiology treatments were: 1, that the great majority stated they would have further kinesiology treatments and they would recommend that others try kinesiology; and 2, the subjects felt better, not only in regard to their specific presenting issue but also in overall well-being. The other interesting observation was how the subjects found their kinesiologist. It was almost entirely word-of-mouth recommendations from friends, acquaintances, family members or work colleagues—a clear statement that these referring people have also had a positive experience with Energetic Kinesiology.

The conclusion of Hall and coworkers regarding kinesiology from their review of methodological quality was that 'There is insufficient evidence for diagnostic accuracy within kinesiology, the validity of muscle response for any condition and the effectiveness for any condition.' However, from the studies by Rolfes and Muehlboeck, people's *actual* experience with kinesiology treatments appears to support their effectiveness and the client's satisfaction with the outcomes of their treatments. In fact, their satisfaction is high enough that they are willing to put their money where their mouth is and seek further Energetic Kinesiology treatments, as well as recommend these treatments to their family, friends and work colleagues! Muehlboeck is currently beginning a follow-on study to define in more detail the relationship between Energetic Kinesiology treatments and outcomes.

One of the major problems in validating Energetic Kinesiology techniques scientifically is the types of studies that are considered the gold standard for clinical research today: the double-blind RCTs. These are designed to evaluate largely single factors, for example a drug or another limited-context factor, and require that a standardized treatment protocol be applied to each subject and that this treatment protocol is set in advance by the experimenter. For single-action or single-factor studies such as individual drugs, which work by a single enzyme or biochemical pathway, this may be appropriate. However, RCTs are an inappropriate experimental design to validate multifactor and multidomain therapies such as Energetic Kinesiology protocols and their application in practice.

A unique and significant component of the practice of Energetic Kinesiology is that it is a client-based therapy in which biofeedback from the client directs each step of the therapy. In applying the kinesiology protocol, the monitor follows the ongoing muscle biofeedback provided by the client using muscle monitoring. However, this feedback may originate in one or more of the domains comprising our multidimensional being: the physical, etheric, emotional, mental and even spiritual levels. This means that every treatment is unique as each person may have a number of different interacting factors contributing to the same presenting issue and represented in several domains. Therefore, inherent to the structure and methods of Energetic Kinesiology, it cannot not fulfill a major research criterion demanded for RCTs, which is to employ standardized treatment protocols. These treatment protocols are generally limited to one domain and often involve just one area of the body, for example neck or lower back pain.

From the perspective of Energetic Kinesiology, people are *multidimensional beings* who may express the effects of stressors on their homeostatic function primarily at one level or domain, or in two or more interacting domains. Energetic Kinesiology can detect and treat imbalances in all these domains, and many Energetic Kinesiology treatments or corrections involve multiple factors, which are often in different domains. For example, one component of the treatment may involve stimulating acupoints in the etheric domain, another

component may involve identifying trigger words in the emotional domain using alarm points in the etheric domain, while the final correction may be balancing a chakra in the auric domain.

Currently, western scientists are attempting to isolate individual components and the role of each component in order to understand the functioning of the human body. But are we really just the sum of all our parts? Are we just a biomechanical machine? One observation that has been consistently made in science is that in complex interacting systems, and the human body and mind certainly qualify, the interaction of the parts often produces higher order structures and functions that are not predictable from the mere summing of their individual parts. The rejection of Man as a multidimensional being by western science was largely because of the separation of mind and body into the res cognitans and the res extensa by Descartes,[43] and the development of rational reductionist thinking generating the biochemical–biomechanical paradigm. This separation of mind and body was supported during its development by a mechanical clockwork universe of Newtonian physics, which explained what we could see and touch and which followed logical, rational rules.

However, a primary factor behind the rejection of the energetic paradigm in western science was that unlike the physical world so well described and so easy to confirm with observation, the energetic systems of the East were unseen and not measurable by scientific instrumentation. So a mysterious unseen world in which Man is represented as a multidimensional being controlled by unknown energies such as prana and ch'i seemed hardly credible. Without a means to objectively measure these unseen fields and validate their existence, and hence their potential to heal or have an effect on our physical body, these energy systems were dismissed as myth or primitive belief systems more aligned with superstition than with science.

Indeed, the greatest challenge for any therapeutic system that represents the body at many levels and can be influenced by the interconnections between these levels is this: how do you design a study to take all these interacting factors into account and partition out which factors have which effect? An example is the connections between immune system competence, nutritional deficiency, spleen meridian energy balance and/or psychoemotional stress, with each factor individually involved in the observed dysfunction, but with the effect or impact of each factor on this dysfunction varying with each individual subject of the study. This makes it difficult to assess which type of therapy will be most appropriate for each subject. But how do you design a research protocol with this degree of variability in application without losing the ability to determine how much of the effect observed is the result of each of these multiple factors? This problem is resolved in RCTs by a priori standardizing the treatment protocol, limiting the number and types of techniques applied and the domains in which they may be applied.

Perhaps the greatest issue for proving the validity of kinesiology is the types of experimental designs that are currently used and considered valid and evidence of scientific proof. In relatively context-free systems or in limited-contextual systems such as single-reaction drug tests, double-blind studies may be a valid means of determining an effect. However, in complex context-dependent systems such as the multifactor, multidomain energy systems of the body, the double-blind model as it is is invalid, as it requires you to eliminate context to satisfy its rules of the study, when it is the context that determines effect. Clearly, in contextual healing to eliminate context is to eliminate the mechanisms via which healing occurs![44]

Indeed, the weakness of RCTs is that they *are* designed for single-factor treatments to single-factor causes, while the cause of most physiological problems is multifactorial, even for seemingly simple muscular problems. Any RCT involving a practitioner working in a multifactorial system, using multidomain therapy, which is strongly context-dependent, may well produce limited or poor outcomes because of the limitations of the experimental design, not the treatment being applied. This is a fact now being openly discussed in western medicine![45]

All double-blind studies could be challenged on the premise that no biological system or subsystem can ever be context-free. By their very nature, biological systems are complex, dynamically interacting sets of equilibria, in which it is virtually impossible to eliminate all contextual input. Hence all double-blind studies ignore a number of contextual factors that may affect the outcome, but because these factors are *believed* to have only a small effect they are ignored. However, as discussed in section 9, biological systems are self-organized chaotic systems in which a small input at a critical time during a phase transition may result in reorganization of the whole system. Indeed, this is one of the reasons why outcomes of biological studies are so variable from study to study and there is a need for sophisticated statistical analysis to determine effect!

Future directions in muscle monitoring research in Energetic Kinesiology

One of the limiting factors in kinesiology research has been instrumentation capable of accurately measuring the actual force applied by the monitor during muscle monitoring, because of the complexity of the dynamics of muscle–muscle interactions and the change in vectors depending on what the muscle did (i.e. lock or unlock). Both these factors combine to create a false subjective conscious perception of what is happening during muscle monitoring, that is, 'You're pushing harder this time!' Without this single piece of data, how hard did the monitor actually push on the muscle? Muscle testing and muscle monitoring will forever remain subjective even while sEMG can now give real-time feedback on the objective degree of muscle contraction of the client's muscles during manual muscle testing and muscle monitoring. Only in the past year have these devices been developed, such as the microFET-2 muscle tester (Hoggan Scientific, Salt Lake City, Utah) and the NeuroPro Tester (Buhler Athletic Injuries & Human Performance Clinic, Kaysville, Utah).

These new devices now provide a means of using multidirectional force transducers to record quantitatively the objective amount of force that the monitor is applying to the muscle during a manual muscle test. When actual force is coupled with sEMG, both components of the systems interacting can be objectively measured simultaneously and can be directly compared. Krebs and colleagues are currently beginning a series of experiments using sEMG and quantitative three-dimensional force transducers, as well as a subjective effort scale. Ongoing research is now being conducted using multidimensional force transducers at the Muscle Physiology Laboratory, University of Colorado, Boulder, Colorado and the Institute of Sport Science, Johannes Gutenberg University, Mainz, Germany to provide feedback on the absolute force applied to the muscles during muscle monitoring; also, sEMG power spectra are being used to assess what is happening in the muscles when they lock and unlock, and a subjective effort scale is being used to fully understand both the objective and the subjective aspects of muscle monitoring. Therefore all three components of manual muscle monitoring—the objective force applied by the monitor, the objective degree of contraction of the client's muscle, and the client's subjective conscious perception of the force applied—are being recorded at the same time. Thus both the subconscious control of muscle function (the muscle locking or unlocking) and the conscious perception of this event ('You pushed harder' when the muscle unlocked or 'You did not push as hard' when the muscle locks) have an external reference point: the actual objective force applied, which allows objective validation of the outcome of the muscle monitoring.

There are two other major factors that portend to play a major role in validating the effectiveness of muscle monitoring and testing as meaningful and accurate tools for providing biofeedback from the different domains of our multidimensional being. First is the rapid development of techniques to objectively detect and measure the biofields of the human body, the flows of ch'i and prana of the body's energy systems. The second is development of new research methods to assess techniques and therapies that are highly contextual in application and multidomain in effect. The future of research in Energetic Kinesiology is both bright and exciting!

Use of muscle monitoring in Energetic Kinesiology: factors that need to be considered

There are a number of factors that need to be addressed and discussed with regard to the use of Energetic Kinesiology in order to understand how these factors affect the application and outcome of this broadly applicable healing technique. Failure to understand these factors and the limitations of what muscle monitoring can tell and cannot tell you have led many well-meaning Energetic Kinesiologists to make statements about how it works, what it can tell you and the outcomes it can produce that are incorrect or overtly untrue.

Is muscle monitoring subjective or objective?

One of the major reasons why kinesiology has often been dismissed is that it is based on people's subjective experience when a muscle is being monitored. People universally report two subjective experiences when being monitored, as discussed in detail above: 1, when the muscle unlocks, it feels as if the monitor is pushing harder than when the muscle locks, and 2, people consistently report that the monitor pushed differently when the muscle locked than when it unlocked.

To our knowledge, the current studies of Krebs and coworkers are the first time in kinesiology research that a subjective effort scale has been used to directly evaluate the subjective experience of individuals being monitored.[46] These studies were carried out at the Institute of Sport Science at the Johannes Gutenberg University in Mainz, Germany and at the Motor Physiology Laboratory at the University of Colorado in Boulder within the past year and are now being replicated and the results prepared for publication.

Subjects were given a subjective effort scale to evaluate how much effort they were exerting to hold the muscle in its monitoring position against the monitor's pressure. The effort scale ranged from 0, being no effort, to 10, being the most effort they can make, and they were instructed to evaluate only their effort to hold the arm in its monitoring position, not what happened during the monitoring, for example whether the muscle locked or unlocked.

Surprisingly, when the muscle unlocked the subjects reported that they were making a 7–10 effort to hold the muscle in position; they were trying very hard to hold against the monitoring pressure. However, objective sEMG recordings of the number of motor units being recruited showed relatively few motor units actually recruited, with an increase in the number of motor units recruited as pressure was initially applied, but then a rapid decrease back to baseline levels as the muscle passively gave in the direction of pressure. Clearly, once the recruitment of motor units in the muscle begins to decrease, the monitor cannot push harder, as the degree of resistance has been reduced and continues to decrease until back at baseline.

When the same muscle was treated to correct the muscle imbalance, and it now locked on being monitored manually, the subjects then reported an effort of only 2–4. In direct contrast to their subjective experience, the electromyographic

results now showed a large recruitment of muscle fibers that continued until the pressure was released. Thus it appears that the only thing subjective about muscle monitoring is the person's subjective experience of the monitoring pressure, which happens to be totally incorrect.

How could the subjective effort evaluation be so inaccurate with regard to what was actually happening in the muscle? Remember that there are two primary spinal pathways that control our muscle function: the subconscious extrapyramidal spinal pathways and the conscious pyramidal corticospinal pathways, as discussed above.

The extrapyramidal spinal pathways are totally subconscious in origin and set basal muscle tone and thus the load reflex of each muscle, while the pyramidal corticospinal pathways provide direct conscious voluntary control of these same muscles. When the output of the subconscious extrapyramidal pathways have correctly set both the muscle tone and the load reflex, all the consciousness has to do is send a request to hold the muscle in the monitoring position via the conscious pyramidal pathways to move the limb or body part into a

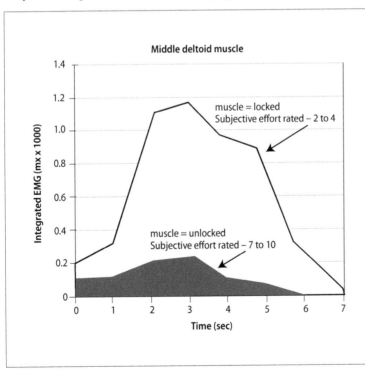

Figure 12.1 Electromyographic power spectra of a locked muscle and an unlocked muscle. A locked muscle rapidly recruits motor units and then sustains contraction until the monitoring pressure is released, while an unlocked muscle initially begins to recruit motor units but then, because of inhibition, this recruitment just drops away back to baseline. Note that the subjective effort from the perspective of the client is rated only 2–4 out of 10 when the muscle is locked, so the client feels like they are putting in relatively little effort. However, when the muscle is unlocking the subjective effort goes up to 7–10 as the client is consciously trying very hard to keep the muscle locked but unconscious inhibition of the muscle makes this impossible.

particular position, and then hold it in that position. The subconscious load reflex then automatically increases contraction to match the increase in pressure during monitoring (see Figure 12.1).

Thus the actual increase in muscle contraction to match the increasing monitoring pressure almost entirely results from the subconscious spinal reflex pathways, that is, until the load approaches the limit of power of that muscle. At this point, the person being monitored will now have to apply greater and greater conscious effort to hold against the increasing pressure until the force applied exceeds the number of motor units this muscle can recruit, at which point the muscle is overpowered and will then move in the direction of pressure.

But what part of the brain actually sets the tone of the muscle and the load reflex controlled by the extrapyramidal pathways? The subcortical survival centers such as the amygdala, brainstem nuclei and the limbic emotional areas all have pathways that project directly from these survival centers into the reticular and vestibular spinal nuclei that then set basal muscle tone and the load reflex. Therefore output from any of the subcortical survival centers can alter basal muscle tone, resetting the load reflex and altering the normal muscle response to increased load.

If the basal muscle tone is set too low, the annulospiral endings of the spindle cell bag fibers cannot be stretched strongly enough to activate a load reflex of sufficient strength to fully lock the muscle, and therefore it gives way in the direction of the pressure. To offset the loss of automatic recruitment of muscle fibers by the load reflex to resist the increasing monitoring pressure, the client now has to consciously increase muscle contraction by telling the muscle to 'HOLD!', which leads to the overt perception of increased effort on the part of the client and the recruitment of synergist muscles. However, despite this increased conscious effort, without the support of the subconscious pathways that actually control muscle function it is not possible to provide enough resistance to hold the muscle in place, and the muscle now passively gives in the direction of force.

Thus, contrary to the belief that muscle monitoring is subjective, *it is only the perception of the person being monitored that is subjective.* The muscle is objectively recruiting fewer muscle fibers when the muscle is unlocking, and far greater numbers of muscle fibers when the muscle is locking. What is subjective is the person's perception of their conscious effort needed to resist the pressure, not the actual amount of pressure applied.

What muscle monitoring can and cannot tell you

This is one of the most contentious issues in Energetic Kinesiology, both between practitioners of different modalities and from the outside point of view in the assessment of the validity of kinesiology. It is also probably one of the greatest stumbling blocks to the acceptance of Energetic Kinesiology in the mainstream. Claims for what kinesiology can tell you run from the obvious to the sublime to the ridiculous!

Unfortunately, one of the first truly 'popular' books in the mainstream on kinesiology was Dr John Diamond's *The Body Does Not Lie.*[47] The title is true in the absolute sense that the body never overtly lies. The body used in this case to mean the muscle responses from monitoring muscles to ask questions, or more accurately to assess the subconscious processing underlying muscle function, as discussed above. Indeed, the body never knows the truth, and then deliberately distorts this truth or lies, *but it does not mean that the result of every muscle test is true!*

There are a number of factors that can result in a muscle response not accurately reflecting the correct or true objective answer, or providing an accurate assessment of stress involved, when various types of muscle monitoring are employed. Lack of knowledge of how these factors may perturb the outcome of muscle monitoring means that the answers provided by way of the muscle response do not necessarily provide either accurate or meaningful answers to the questions asked.

Just pushing on a muscle after asking a question and observing what it does is not a valid or reliable mechanism to determine the objective, external truth! If adequate pre-checks for the reliability and homeostatic function of a muscle have not been assessed before pushing on the muscle, the response could merely reflect an extraneous factor causing a spurious change in muscle function. These spurious changes may include subclinical dehydration; various forms of functional and structural dysfunction, either within the muscle itself or in the many neurological circuits to which it is connected; psycho-emotional factors subconsciously altering gamma 1 pathway output, changing basal muscle tone; incorrect muscle monitoring technique; and strong mental or emotional intention on the part of the monitor or the client. Each of these factors could potentially alter the muscle response to the question being asked!

Then there is the issue of how the question was asked: 1, as a verbal question or a verbal challenge; 2, as a challenge to an acupoint, for example circuit locating an alarm point; or 3, as an acupressure format, a sequence or series of hand modes in combination with circuit locating (touching) an acupoint or acupoints. Verbal questions are by far the easiest and require the least knowledge to employ, but they are also the most difficult to use correctly, and they are limited by both the knowledge of the person asking the question and the context of the question, *as muscle response is totally contextual*. Furthermore, part of the context of the final muscle response is indeed the intention of the person asking the question, as the intention of the monitor can have a direct effect on the outcome of the muscle response when monitored. *When the person asking the question is not aware of this fact, that their intention is part of the context, then the muscle response can be very biased by this lack of awareness of the role their intention played in the muscle response observed!*

Also, when asking verbal questions, the monitor has to understand that the muscle response is an all-or-nothing response, in which it can only lock or unlock; there is no *maybe*! This means that the question asked must be extremely clear with only a 'yes' or 'no' answer possible. Because there are only two possible outcomes when a muscle is monitored, if the question asked does not have an absolute clear 'yes' or 'no' answer, what is the body to do? Whatever response it gives will be incorrect, because if it locks the monitor will incorrectly

think this means the answer is 'yes', but if it unlocks, then the monitor will incorrectly think the answer is 'no', when in fact the question they actually asked does not have a clear 'yes' or 'no' answer!

We have personally seen many poorly trained kinesiologists ask totally open-ended questions, that we could not answer with a 'yes' or a 'no'. These kinesiologists would then get a muscle response and then ask the next totally open-ended question, assuming that whatever the last response they got from muscle monitoring was true! In no time at all, the answers they are getting were total nonsense, but unfortunately they believe them to be the truth! 'The body does not lie' phenomenon is often cited by many untrained Energetic Kinesiologists to validate the 'answers' they received via muscle monitoring.

To counter this 'yes-no' or 'unlock–lock' problem, a better approach when using verbal access to gain information from manual muscle monitoring is to use a verbal challenge. A challenge is made by making a statement to the person, both heard by the conscious aspect of brain function and processed before conscious perception in the subconscious systems of the brain, for example the survival systems of the brainstem and limbic system. The survival systems monitor every sensory input to the brain and make rapid associations based on this input with sensory input from the past that was similar, and then often alter muscle response based on the survival emotions activated by these previous associations. In a challenge, it is not 'yes' or 'no' indicated by the muscle response, but rather stress associated with the challenge, the statement made, the acupoint touched, etc., in which case the muscle will unlock, indicating a stress reaction to the challenge presented. If, on the other hand, the challenge statement or acupoint has no 'stress' associated with it, the muscle will remain locked.

Therefore, when using a challenge, you offer the body three possible responses: 1, the challenge elicits a stress association or frequency match, causing an indicator change, either from locked to unlocked or from unlocked to locked; 2, the challenge does not create stress or match stress in the circuit and therefore there is no indicator change; or 3, the challenge is *totally irrelevant* to the frequency of imbalance in the circuit, and therefore again there is no indicator change.

Asking questions as verbal challenges or using hand modes are forms of frequency matching is, from the energetic perspective, like asking electro-magnetic–energetic questions of the subconscious that already speaks this electromagnetic–energetic language. The subconscious does not speak English, French or German but rather this electromagnetic-energetic language of neurological and energy flows. This subconscious interface of the energetic circuits to the neurological muscle circuits is the basis of the indicator change observed in muscle monitoring. The indicator change then indicates a frequency match, suggesting an active stress in this circuit, or a match to the stress that is already in the circuit. Likewise, if this electromagnetic–energetic question poses no stress or stress below threshold levels, then the indicator muscle will not change, indicating no frequency match or active stress associated with the challenge.

The primary advantage of challenging, especially with acupressure formatting, is that you are in a sense talking to the body in the same language it already speaks, and therefore there is no translation needed! Verbal questions that use only 'yes' and 'no' as answers unfortunately must first be translated through the subconscious before the answer can be determined. And as anyone who is involved with translation between languages is well aware, translation errors are a major source of inaccuracy and confusion in information transfer!

The discussion provided below is only our point of view from over 20 years in clinical practice and having a comprehensive understanding of both the research science and the energetic sciences underlying the field of Energetic Kinesiology. While we discussed the anatomy and physiology of muscle function and how this relates to the traditional muscle monitoring above, below we would like to present what we consider the important considerations and limitations when using this wonderful direct biofeedback tool. *If muscle monitoring is to be used as an effective and accurate means of accessing mean-ingful information from the muscle response, it is essential the monitor comprehends the following limitations.*

Muscle monitoring is contextual

How the muscle responds is totally context-dependent. This is partly because it is an all-or-nothing response and therefore must sum up all the negatives and positives, many from subconscious brain areas, and can then respond only by a lock or unlock! A lock response says only that the stressor was not of sufficient magnitude to disrupt the coherency of the feedback maintaining the muscle load reflex. Likewise, an unlock response indicates only that some factor(s) reached the threshold of interference to disrupt muscle feedback, causing a loss of coherent muscle response.

Any question you are asked verbally is always context-dependent. For example, you are sitting in a chair and a friend asks you, 'How are you today?' But you are allowed only an all-or-nothing response: 'good' or 'not good'. You must first rapidly evaluate every level of your life, physically, emotionally, mentally and spiritually, and then add them all up, all the positives and all the negatives, to give a 'good' (locked) or 'not good' (unlocked) response. So while you twisted your right ankle yesterday and it hurts when you put pressure on it, you are sitting down and it does not hurt right now, hence your answer may well be 'good'! However, if your friend changes the context and now says 'How is your right ankle today?', you will now reply with 'Not good. I twisted it yesterday and it hurts like hell when I try to stand on it!' So which are you, good or not good? It all depends on the context of the question! Therefore whenever asking a question, the monitor must be extremely aware of the context that they are providing.

Also, for better or for worse, the intention of the monitor also provides a frequency signature that becomes part of the context of the question or challenge and as such can influence the outcome of the muscle response. If a monitor is not aware of this possibility, then their intention becomes an unknown bias in the outcome of the muscle response, perhaps of sufficient magnitude to change the outcome from locked to unlocked! However, if they are overtly aware of the role that their intention may play in the outcome, they can consciously correct for this bias and be as neutral as possible in intention while they monitor the indicator muscle.

Beginning students always ask, 'What is the muscle supposed to be doing?' We always answer, 'It is not *supposed* to be doing anything; it is just locking or unlocking! Your job is to, as neutrally as possible, just observe one thing: what is the muscle doing? Once you have made this observation "Oh! It is locking", then and only then should you begin to think about "What does this mean?"'

Muscle response is a >50% phenomenon

An indicator muscle will lock up to the point at which the interference exceeds 50%. This is once again the result of the all-or-nothing aspect of muscle function, the summing up of all the excitatory (+) and inhibitory (−) inputs to the motor neurons contracting the muscle. Once the feedback interference exceeds 50%, then muscle inhibition will exceed muscle facilitation and the muscle will unlock.

This means that there may be stressors within a muscle circuit yet the muscle will lock, because it will not unlock until the stressors exceed 50% of stress. Second, when it does unlock you do not know if it represents 51% stress or 99% stress in the muscle circuit. Hence, the muscle does not indicate the degree of stress, only that the stress exceeds 50%. Likewise, if it locks it indicates only that there is less than 50% stress in the circuit. However, the qualitative change in muscle response may indicate to some extent the degree of stress in the circuit. In circuits that have extremely high levels of stress, the muscle will unlock completely offering almost no resistance, while in a less stressed circuit the muscle will unlock but still offer moderate resistance.

Muscle monitoring provides only subjective feedback with regard to internal states

Muscle monitoring cannot tell you anything about objective external reality, only the specific internal reactions of the client's subjective perspective of reality. However, this is what causes them stress; not objective reality but rather their subjective perspective of it—the glass is half full or half empty, and your subjective perspective determines your experience of which it is. Hence muscle monitoring is often very unreliable with regard to strong emotionally laden issues if these issues are related to yourself, as your emotional reactions become important components of the context of the muscle response to monitoring! This is one of the reasons beginning students so often find it difficult to monitor their family members, especially spouses, but have no difficulty monitoring classmates.

Muscle monitoring can give you feedback only about the subjective personal experience of the person being monitored. Because much of personal experience is controlled by subconscious survival reactions that color our conscious perceptions even before we can consciously think, it is not a reliable indicator of the objective truth! This is one reason why eyewitness reports are so often unreliable and do not match each other or what objectively happened as determined by a camera.

As stated above, technically the body never overtly lies, that is, knows the truth and indicates something else. However, the feedback loops and mechanisms involved in the output from the body via muscle monitoring are often affected by many factors, such as hydration, electromagnetic polarity reversals (switching), deep-seated emotions, irrational beliefs and fears. These factors may result in a muscle response that indicates exactly opposite information to the objective truth, that is, what is true in the external reality. For example, we have found that monitoring a woman for whether she is or is not pregnant has often no better than 50% chance, because being pregnant is such an emotionally charged issue for many women, yet she *is objectively* either pregnant or not pregnant!

However, muscle monitoring is an exceedingly good feedback mechanism for revealing any stressors, both conscious and subconscious, of the client's subjective experience. Indeed, it is this subjective experience that creates stress for the person, not the objective events that have happened. Krebs is disabled and lives in pain every day. These are objective facts; however, how he responds to these objective facts may or may not cause him stress, which is his subjective reaction to this objective reality! Being disabled and having constant pain signals sent to his cortex is just how it *is*, whether this creates frustration and anger and he suffers from these signals, creating an experience of stress, is totally a result of his subjective relation to this objective state of his body.

So some days he copes well with these difficult objective experiences and has pain but no suffering; pain is only an experience, a bunch of nerve impulses activating part of the brain. On these days, he experiences pain but no suffering from the stress of these objective impulses. Other days, his subjective experience is one of suffering as a result of these same impulses, and he feels stressed by them. If you monitored him about pain on the 'good' days, he would not show an indicator change as this causes no subjective stress. In contrast, if you monitored him on one of his 'bad' days, he would show an indicator change, indicating that these same objective signals were now causing him subjective stress.

Beliefs, emotions and thoughts influence muscle monitoring

Muscle monitoring can be influenced by the beliefs, emotions and thoughts of both the monitor and the client, because it is subjective and so intimately connected to the subconscious areas of the brain generating emotions and thoughts. This is not problematic as long as you understand that this is part of the context of a muscle response. A monitor can never be totally objective, as they, like everyone else, have deep-seated beliefs and subconscious emotional programs. However, by knowing this the monitor can choose to put themselves into a neutral space during monitoring using conscious intent.

Frank Mahony, the developer of Hyperton-X, would often do a demonstration for beginning students to make this point. He would hold up a matchbox and then say, 'This is full of white sugar.' Now every budding kinesiologist 'knows' that white sugar is the work of the devil! Not surprisingly, as he tested the class almost everyone would

show an unlocked muscle. Then he would take another matchbox and say, 'This contains matches', then again test all the students, and most people would now show a locked muscle. Then he would open both matchboxes to reveal only matches! Clearly, the muscle response to the white sugar was only a reaction to the person's belief about white sugar, not the objective reality of matches.

Does this invalidate muscle monitoring? No, of course not; it just shows that the person's belief is an important part of the context in terms of the muscle response. Likewise, if the monitor has a strong belief about white sugar and is not actively monitoring their own neutrality in the muscle-monitoring process, they may also perturb the outcome of the test, because they 'know' that white sugar is bad for everyone! This just points out the need for each monitor to be ever-vigilant to maintain as much as possible a neutral space from which to monitor.

Richard Utt, founder of Applied Physiology, made a statement that all muscle monitors should repeat often to themselves when assessing the outcome of muscle monitoring, 'If you are not surprised by the outcome of your muscle monitoring a reasonable percentage of the time, but are always "finding" what you knew would be the muscle response, suspect unintentional internal bias—basically self-fulfilling outcomes largely generated by your intentional biases or beliefs!'

The monitor's confidence is important

The monitor's trust in himself or herself and feel for the locked or unlocked state of the muscle may impact on the outcome of muscle monitoring. Some people have a natural sense for the muscle response and can easily feel the different muscle states, while others have difficulty knowing when the muscle has locked or is unlocked. However, this is a trainable skill, and with practice it can become extremely reliable and consistent for everyone. Hence the difference in validity and interexaminer reliability between practitioners with little muscle-monitoring experience and those with over five years' experience demonstrated in the research literature.[46]

For novice monitors, two factors often result in

the 'battle for the indicator muscle'. The first is learning the proper muscle-monitoring technique, and the second is to apply this technique with consistent increasing pressure. Often, a novice monitor begins to apply pressure to a muscle but as the pressure is applied at first the client's muscle begins move in the direction of the pressure applied, as it takes the load reflex a fraction of a second to kick in. Then instead of the monitor properly continuing to apply increasing pressure, at the point the client's muscle begins to give, the monitor decreases their pressure, just as the load reflex is beginning to react to the initial pressure by increasing contraction, which now moves the client's muscle up against their hand just as they are beginning to reduce their pressure on the muscle. This then results in the monitor increasing pressure on the muscle once more, just as the client's muscle is beginning to reduce its degree of contraction! The end result is the muscle seesawing—first down, then up, then down, then up—making it difficult for the monitor to feel whether the muscle is locking or unlocking.

We have also seen beginning students monitor another person and get a clear lock but then monitor it again and again because they do not yet know the feel of a locked muscle, or more often did not trust themselves and what they had actually clearly felt. Often, after a few of these repetitive unnecessary tests, the subconscious of the person being monitored will over-facilitate, blocking the muscle response, and the student can no longer monitor anything as the indicator muscle can no longer respond. Hence there can be no indicator change. It is as if the body's innate wisdom is saying, 'I told you three times! If you don't trust yourself enough to listen to me, I'm not letting you into my biocomputer!'

Muscle monitoring cannot reveal absolute truths

From our perspective, because muscle monitoring cannot tell you external truths, it also cannot tell you objectively about absolute truths, such as what level of spirituality you or another person has attained, what is your true life's purpose or who is your soulmate. It can suggest only what areas and issues relate to these absolute truths and whether these create stress for you subjectively. This is something important for you to know if you wish to clear these issues to assist in your personal growth!

In this regard, we cannot support books that we feel misrepresent the scope of muscle monitoring by stating that muscle monitoring can provide objective truths or future unknown events.[48] To use muscle monitoring to divulge objective truths, such as where a person is with regard to their level of personal development and spirituality, or who is your true soulmate, we would call a misuse of this valuable feedback tool. We consider these types of claims for the use of muscle monitoring to do much more harm than good to kinesiology as a whole, because of all the bad press that it gets! It also damages the credibility of serious practitioners who use muscle monitoring correctly: as an effective biofeedback tool to assist people to resolve their physical, psychoemotional and spiritual stresses and difficulties. If only muscle monitoring could tell us of future objective truths, we would both be very wealthy from winning the lottery repeatedly!

In a similar vein, many uninformed or misinformed kinesiologists with limited training may perform what we call the ouija board school of kinesiology. In this approach to kinesiology, which is all too common, a person with very little training believes that the muscle response is a mystical event controlled by a power outside themselves, infallible and all-knowing! We call it *talking to God at the end of the indicator muscle!* Because God knows everything, the monitor does not have to know anything! They even go so far as to justify their ignorance with statements like, 'Oh, knowledge would contaminate or interfere with my intuition!'

Clearly, from the previous discussion, the muscle response is very definitely of this world. In fact, it has a rigorous neurophysiological basis (discussed in detail in chapters 8 and 9), even while it may interface with our emotions, thoughts and even our spiritual nature.

The fallacies of the ouija board school is twofold: 1, God is not at the end of the indicator muscle but rather a switched, confused and belief-biased subconscious generating many unsubstantiated stressors and ungrounded fears when viewed from an external perspective; and 2, even if God were at the end of an indicator muscle, this model suffers another insurmountable problem. Muscle monitoring only answers questions or challenges generated by the monitor; it can *never* ask questions or talk back to you to tell you what to ask next or what you should do! Only knowledge provides you with the ability to ask relevant and meaningful questions, tools needed to effectively utilize the biofeedback provided by muscle monitoring.

Muscle monitoring and intuition

Muscle monitoring does *not* invalidate or block your intuition but rather provides an external guide to use your intuition more effectively! All too often we have heard again and again, 'Oh! Using muscle monitoring will decrease my intuitive abilities!' Quite to the contrary, muscle monitoring can assist you to use your intuition in a far more effective way. While intuition may correctly identify the stress that is present, what intuition often cannot tell you is the context of this stress. Sometimes, correctly identifying a stressor that is highly compensated and then dragging it onto center stage in the person's life may not only be unhelpful but may be harmful.

When we have deep-seated issues, often these are issues that we could not cope with at the time we experienced them, as they created great stress in our lives. So to cope we figuratively buried these issues often deep in our subconscious by creating effective compensations to keep them out of sight so we could function once again in our lives. What we have observed over and over again in clinical practice is that by following the kinesiology process with integrity, often an issue we may indeed know intuitively is true for the client does not come up for several sessions.

Because my intuition may be telling me that this is the central issue from the first session, why does it take five balances before it is finally revealed through the biofeedback of muscle monitoring? What intuition does *not* tell you is how this person has compensated their core issue to protect themselves, as they cannot cope with this issue upfront at this time. What is happening in these first four balances is a gentle decompensation of the central issue. As the surrounding issues are resolved (each representing a compensation for the core issue), this permits the core issue to now be directly addressed. When the stress has been reduced enough, and there are sufficient resources available to allow the person to cope effectively, the issue will then come to the surface and perhaps even provide the key to completely resolve this issue!

The discussion above is meant to provide a reasoned and cogently argued perspective on the role of muscle monitoring and its use in Energetic Kinesiology, addressing the mechanisms of muscle response, the power and limitations of muscle monitoring and the critical role of context in its application. These are our personal views and are offered from this perspective.

References

1. Harms-Ringdahl, K 1993, *Muscle Strength*, Churchill Livingstone, Edinburgh.
2. Walther, DS 1998, *Applied Kinesiology: Synopsis, Second Edition*, Systems DC, Pueblo.
3. Garcia-Rill, E, Homma, Y & Skinner, RD 2004, Arousal mechanisms related to posture and locomotion: 1. Descending modulation, *Progress in Brain Research*, Vol. 143, pp. 283–290.
4. Guyton, AC 1991, Cortical and brainstem control of motor function. In: Guyton, AC, ed. *Basic Neuroscience: Anatomy and Physiology*, WB Saunders, Philadelphia, pp. 214–217.
5. Robert, MB & Levy, MN 2000, *Principles of Physiology, Third Edition*, Mosby, London.

6. Harms-Ringdahl, K 1993, *Muscle Strength*, Churchill Livingstone, Edinburgh.
   Kendall, FP, McCreary, EK & Provance, PG 1993, *Muscles: Testing and Function, With Posture and Pain*, Williams & Wilkins, Baltimore.
   Daniels, L & Worthingham, K 2002, *Muscle Testing—Techniques of Manual Examination, Seventh Edition*, WB Saunders, Philadelphia.
7. Levin, S 2010, *The Tensegrity-Truss as a Model for Spine Mechanics: Biotensegrity* [online] Available at: http://www.biotensegrity.com/tensegrity_truss.php
8. Lund, JP, Donga, R, Widmer, CG & Stohler, CS 1991, The pain-adaptation model: a discussion of the relationship between

chronic musculoskeletal pain and motor activity. *Canadian Journal of Physiology and Pharmacology*, Vol. 69(5), pp. 683–694.

Goldberg, EJ & Neptune, RR 2007, Compensatory strategies during normal walking in response to muscle weakness and increased hip joint stiffness, *Gait and Posture*, Vol. 25(3), pp. 360–367.

9. Liebenson, C, ed. 2007, *Rehabilitation of the Spine: A Practitioner's Manual, Second Edition*, Lippincott Williams & Wilkins, Philadelphia.

Panjabi, M 2006, A hypothesis of chronic back pain: ligament subfailure injuries lead to muscle control dysfunction. *European Spine Journal*, Vol. 15(5), pp. 668–676.

Janda, V 1983, *Muscle Function Testing*, Butterworth-Heinemann, Oxford.

10. Lund, JP, Donga, R, Widmer, CG & Stohler, CS 1991, The pain-adaptation model: a discussion of the relationship between chronic musculoskeletal pain and motor activity. *Canadian Journal of Physiology and Pharmacology*, Vol. 69(5), pp. 683–694.

11. Edgerton, VR, Wolf, SL, Levendowski, DJ & Roy, RR 1996, Theoretical basis for patterning EMG amplitudes to assess muscle dysfunction. *Medicine and Science in Sports and Exercise*, Vol. 28(6), pp. 744–751.

12. DeAndrade, JR, Grant, C & Dixon, AS 1965, Joint distension and reflex muscle inhibition in the knee. *Journal of Bone and Joint Surgery*, Vol. 47, pp. 313–322.

Stokes, M & Young, A 1984, Investigations of quadriceps inhibition: implications for clinical practice, *Physiotherapy*, Vol. 70, pp. 425–428.

Spencer, JD, Hayes, KC & Alexander, IJ 1984, Knee joint effusion and quadriceps reflex inhibition in man, *Archives of Physical Medicine and Rehabilitation*, Vol. 65(4), pp. 171–177.

Hossain, M & Nokes, LDM 2005, A model of dynamic sacro-iliac joint instability from malrecruitment of gluteus maximus and biceps femoris muscles resulting in low back pain, *Medical Hypotheses*, Vol. 65(2), pp. 278–281.

Zafar, H 2000, Integrated jaw and neck function in man. Studies of mandibular and head–neck movements during jaw opening–closing tasks, *Swedish Dental Journal Supplement*, pp. 1–41.

13. Edgerton, VR, Wolf, SL, Levendowski, DJ & Roy, RR 1996, 'Theoretical basis for patterning EMG amplitudes to assess muscle dysfunction.' *Med Sci Sports Exerc*, 28(6):744-751.

Biering-Sorensen, F 1984, 'Physical measurements as risk indicators for low-back trouble over a one-year period.' *Spine*, 9(2):106-19.

Karvonen, MJ, Viitasalo, JT, Komi, PV, Nummi, J & Jarvinen, T 1980, 'Back and leg complaints in relation to muscle strength in young men.' *Scand J Rehabil Med*, 12(2):53-9.

Barton, PM & Hayes, KC 1996, 'Neck flexor muscle strength, efficiency, and relaxation times in normal subjects and subjects with unilateral neck pain and headache.' *Arch Phys Med Rehabil*, 77(7):680-687.

Cady, LD, Bischoff, DP, O'Connell, ER, Thomas, PC & Allan, JH 1979, 'Strength and fitness and subsequent back injuries in firefighters.' *J Occup Med*, 21(4):269-272.

14. Schmitt, WH Jr & Cuthbert, SC 2008, Common errors and clinical guidelines for manual muscle testing: 'the arm test' and other inaccurate procedures, *Chiropractic & Osteopathy*, Vol. 16, p. 16

15. Leisman, G, Zenhausern, R, Ferentz, A, Tefera, T & Zemcov, A 1995, Electromyographic effects of fatigue and task repetition on the validity of estimates of strong and weak muscles in applied kinesiological muscle-testing procedures, *Perceptual and Motor Skills*, Vol. 80, pp. 963–977.

Marino, M, Nicholas, JA, Gleim, GW, Rosenthal, P & Nicholas, SJ 1982, The efficacy of manual assessment of muscle strength using a new device, *American Journal of Sports Medicine*, Vol. 10(6), pp. 360–364.

Basmajian, JV 1978, *Muscles Alive: Their Functions Revealed by Electromyography, Fourth Edition*, Williams & Wilkins, Baltimore.

MacConaill, NA & Basmajian, JV 1977, *Muscles and Movements: A Basis for Human Kinesiology*, Robert E. Krieger, Huntington.

Rosenbaum, R 1999, Carpal tunnel syndrome and the myth of El Dorado, *Muscle & Nerve*, Vol. 22, pp. 1165–1167.

Pollard, HP, Bablis, P, Bonello, R 2006, Can the ileocecal valve point predict low back pain using manual muscle testing?' *Chiropractic Journal of Australia*, Vol. 36, pp. 58–62.

Pollard, H, Lakay, B, Tucker, F, Watson, B & Bablis, P 2005, Interexaminer reliability of the deltoid and psoas muscle test, *Journal of Manipulative and Physiological Therapeutics*, Vol. 28(1), pp. 52–56.

Escolar, DM, Henricson, EK, Mayhew, J, Florence, J, Leshner, R, Patel, KM & Clemens, PR 2001, Clinical evaluator reliability for quantitative and manual muscle testing measures of strength in children, *Muscle and Nerve*, Vol. 24(6), pp. 787–793.

16. Karin Harms-Ringdahl, K 1993, *Muscle Strength*, Churchill Livingstone, Edinburgh.

Kendall, FP, McCreary, EK, Provance, PG 1993, *Muscles: Testing and Function*, Williams & Wilkins, Baltimore.

Daniels, L & Worthingham, K 2002, *Muscle Testing: Techniques of Manual Examination, Seventh Edition*, WB Saunders, Philadelphia.

17. Fosang, A & Baker, R 2006, A method for comparing manual muscle strength, *Gait and Posture*, Vol. 24(4), pp. 406–411.

Bohannon, RW 1986, Manual muscle test scores and dynamometer test scores of knee extension strength, *Archives of Physical Medicine and Rehabilitation*, Vol. 67(6), pp. 390–392.

Marino, M, Nicholas, JA, Gleim, GW, Rosenthal, P & Nicholas, SJ 1982, The efficacy of manual assessment of muscle strength using a new device, *American Journal of Sports Medicine*, Vol. 10(6), pp. 360–364.

18. Marino, M, Nicholas, JA, Gleim, GW, Rosenthal, P & Nicholas, SJ 1982, The efficacy of manual assessment of muscle strength using a new device, *American Journal of Sports Medicine*, Vol. 10(6), pp. 360–364.

19. Wadsworth, CT, Krishnan, R, Sear, M, Harrold, J & Nielsen, DH 1987, Intrarater reliability of manual muscle testing and hand-held dynametric muscle testing, *Physical Therapy*, Vol. 67(9), pp. 1342–1347.

20. Daniels, L & Worthingham, K 2002, *Muscle Testing: Techniques of Manual Examination, Seventh Edition*, WB Saunders, Philadelphia.

21. Kenney, JJ, Clemens, R & Forsythe, KD 1988, Applied kinesiology unreliable for assessing nutrient status, *Journal of the American Dietetic Association*, Vol. 88(6), pp. 698–704.

22. Escolar, DM, Henricson, EK, Mayhew, J, Florence, J, Leshner, R, Patel, KM & Clemens, PR 2001, Clinical evaluator reliability for quantitative and manual muscle testing measures of strength in children, *Muscle and Nerve*, Vol. 24(6), pp. 787–793.

23. Fosang, A & Baker, R 2006, A method for comparing manual muscle strength, *Gait and Posture*, Vol. 24(4), pp. 406–411.

24. Walther, DS 2000, *Applied Kinesiology: Synopsis, Second Edition*, Systems DC, Pueblo.

25. Cuthbert, SC & Goodheart, GJ 2007, On the reliability and validity of manual muscle testing: a literature review. *Chiropractic and Osteopathy*, Vol. 15(1), p. 4.

    Schmitt, WH Jr & Cuthbert, SC 2008, Common errors and clinical guidelines for manual muscle testing: 'the arm test' and other inaccurate procedures, *Chiropractic & Osteopathy*, Vol. 16, p. 16.

26. Schmitt, WH Jr & Cuthbert, SC 2008, Common errors and clinical guidelines for manual muscle testing: 'the arm test' and other inaccurate procedures, *Chiropractic & Osteopathy*, Vol. 16, p. 16.

27. Leisman, G, Zenhausern, R, Ferentz, A, Tefera, T & Zemcov, A 1995, Electromyographic effects of fatigue and task repetition on the validity of estimates of strong and weak muscles in applied kinesiological muscle-testing procedures, *Perceptual and Motor Skills*, Vol. 80, pp. 963–977.

28. Jepsen, JR, Laursen, LH, Hagert, CG, Kreiner, S & Larsen, AI 2006, Diagnostic accuracy of the neurological upper limb examination I: inter-rater reproducibility of selected findings and patterns. *BMC Neurology*, Vol. 6, p. 8.

    Jain, M, Smith, M, Cintas, H, Koziol, D, Wesley, R, Harris-Love, M, Lovell, D, Rider, LG & Hicks, J 2006, Intra-rater and inter-rater reliability of the 10-point Manual Muscle Testing (MMT) of children with juvenile idiopathic inflammatory myopathies, *Physical and Occupational Therapy in Pediatrics*, Vol. 26(3), pp. 5–17.

    Pollard, H, Calder, D, Farrar, L, Ford, M, Melamet, A & Cuthbert, S 2011, Inter-examiner reliability of Manual Muscle Testing of lower limb muscles without ideomotor effect, *Chiropractic Journal of Australia*, Vol. 41, pp. 23–30.

29. Pollard, H, Lakay, B, Tucker, F, Watson, B & Bablis, P 2005, Interexaminer reliability of the deltoid and psoas muscle test, *Journal of Manipulative and Physiological Therapeutics*, Vol. 28(1), pp. 52–56.

30. Jepsen, JR, Laursen, LH, Hagert, CG, Kreiner, S & Larsen, AI 2006, Diagnostic accuracy of the neurological upper limb examination I: inter-rater reproducibility of selected findings and patterns, *BMC Neurology*, Vol. 6, p. 8.

31. Pollard, H, Calder, D, Farrar, L, Ford, M, Melamet, A & Cuthbert, S 2011, Inter-examiner reliability of Manual Muscle Testing of lower limb muscles without ideomotor effect, *Chiropractic Journal of Australia*, Vol. 41, pp. 23–30.

32. Pollard, HP, Bablis, P, Bonello, R 2006, Can the ileocecal valve point predict low back pain using manual muscle testing? *Chiropractic Journal of Australia*, Vol. 36, pp. 58–62.

33. Cuthbert, SC, Rosner, AL & McDowall, D 2011, Association of manual muscle tests and mechanical neck pain: results from a prospective pilot study, *Journal of Bodywork and Movement Therapies*, Vol. 15(2), pp. 192–200.

34. Jain, M, Smith, M, Cintas, H, Koziol, D, Wesley R, Harris-Love, M, Lovell, D, Rider, LG & Hicks, J 2006, Intra-rater and inter-rater reliability of the 10-point Manual Muscle Testing (MMT) of children with juvenile idiopathic inflammatory myopathies. *Physical and Occupational Therapy in Pediatrics*, Vol. 26(3), pp. 5–17.

    Rider, LG, Koziol, D, Giannini, EH, Jain, MS, Smith, MR, Whitney-Mahoney, K, Feldman, BM, Wright, SJ, Lindsley, CB, Pachman, LM, Villalba, ML, Lovell, DJ, Bowyer, SL, Plotz, PH, Miller, FW

    & Hicks, JE 2010, Validation of manual muscle testing and a subset of eight muscles for adult and juvenile idiopathic inflammatory myopathies, *Arthritis Care and Research*, Vol. 62(4), pp. 465–472.

35. Conable, KM 2010, Intraexaminer comparison of applied kinesiology manual muscle testing of varying durations: a pilot study, *Journal of Chiropractic Medicine*, Vol. 9, pp. 3–10.

36. Korotkov, K 2002, *Human Energy Field: Study With Gas-Discharge Visualization (GDV) Bioelectrography*, Backbone, Fair Lawn.

    Korotokov, K 2004, *Measuring Human Energy Fields: State of the Science*, Backbone, Fair Lawn.

    Schlebusch, KP, Maric-Oehler, W & Popp FA 2005, Biophotonics in the infrared spectrum reveal acupuncture meridian structure of the body, *Journal of Alternative and Complementary Medicine*, Vol. 11(1), pp. 171–173.

    Swanson, C 2010, *Life Force: the Scientific Basis*, Poseidia Press, Tucson.

37. Rolfes, A 1997, *The Phenomenon of Indicator Muscle Change. An Explanation of its Validity and Meaning*, privately published, Newrybar.

38. McCord, KM 1991, Applied Kinesiology: an historical overview, *Digest of Chiropractic Economics*, Vol. 34, pp. 20–27.

39. Moncayo, R & Moncayo, H 2009, Evaluation of Applied Kinesiology meridian techniques by means of surface electromyography (sEMG): demonstration of the regulatory influence of antique acupuncture points, *Chinese Medicine*, Vol. 4(1), p. 9.

40. Monti, D, Sinnott, J, Marchese, M, Kunel, E & Greeson, J 1999, Muscle test comparisons of congruent and incongruent self-referential statements. *Perceptual and Motor Skills*, Vol. 88, pp. 1019–1028.

41. Hall, S, Lewith, G, Brien, S & Little, P 2008, A review of the literature in applied and specialised kinesiology, *Forschende Komplementärmedizin*, Vol. 15, pp. 40–46.

42. Muehlboeck, A 2010, Kinesiology, as seen from the client's perspective?, unpublished study, University of Salzburg.

43. Spinoza, B 1963, *Earlier Philosophical Writings: The Cartesian Principles and Thoughts on Metaphysics*, Bobbs-Merrill, New York.

44. Black, D 1990, *Inner Wisdom: The Challenge of Contextual Healing*, Tapestry Press, Springville.

    Black, D 1991, *Fine Tuning: The Promise of Contextual Healing*, Tapestry Press, Springville.

45. Topol, E 2012, *The Creative Destruction of Medicine: How the Digital Revolution Will Create a Better Health Care*, Basic Books, New York.

    Topol, E, *Get Rid of the Randomized Trial; Here's a Better Way* [online video recording] Available at: http://www.medscape.com/viewarticle/768635

46. Caruso, B & Leisman, G 2000, A force/displacement analysis of muscle testing, *Perceptual and Motor Skills*, Vol. 91, pp. 683–692.

47. Diamond, J 1990, *Your Body Does Not Lie*, Harper & Row, Sydney.

    Diamond, J 1992, *Life Energy*, Harper & Row, Sydney.

48. Hawkins, DR 1995, *Power vs. Force (Revised Edition): The Hidden Determinants of Human Behavior*, Hay House, Carlsbad.

    Hawkins, DR 2006, *Truth vs. Falsehood: How to Tell the Difference*, Hay House, Carlsbad.

SECTION IV

Core kinesiology tools

While muscle monitoring is the technique that defines kinesiology as a therapy, there are a number of other techniques that over the past three decades have become core techniques used in every session by practitioners of modern Energetic Kinesiology. They can be thought of as the tools used in this field. These non-verbal mechanisms are used together with muscle monitoring to provide the information needed for performing an effective kinesiology balance.

This section will discuss in detail each of these techniques, including the pause lock mechanism, powers of stress, hand modes, specific indicator points and acupressure formatting. In addition, this section concludes with a discussion of the proper use and application of verbal questioning and challenges in combination with muscle monitoring. In all these cases, the information comes from muscle feedback and is often unknown to or unknowable by the client.

To our knowledge, pause lock, the ability to hold an energetic pattern of information over time so that its relationship to other aspects of the imbalance may be investigated, is a novel technique unique to Energetic Kinesiology. This ability to enter an imbalance into circuit and investigate what other information or imbalances may be related to this presenting issue, including the timeline of this issue in the person's life, often permits far deeper and long-lasting resolution of the presenting issue.

Muscle monitoring relies on the ability of a muscle to indicate states of imbalance by 'locking' and 'unlocking'. This is called an *indicator change* in Energetic Kinesiology and is basically a form of frequency matching. However, when an imbalance is entered into circuit with sufficient magnitude of stress, or the underlying issue has been well compensated, the indicator muscle may become incapable of change. Thus, it has lost its ability to indicate the presence of imbalances, much like an electrical circuit that when overloaded will automatically flip the circuit breaker, switching off all electrical flow.

In order to re-establish electrical flow, you need to flip the circuit breaker back on again. Similarly, to re-establish information flow you need to be able to switch the indicator muscle on again. This process has been termed *entering powers of stress*, the overload in the circuit represented as excess energy. This excess energy is then downloaded into the whole body energy system using a series of different techniques that momentarily return the indicator muscle to homeostasis, so that it can once more indicate the presence of other information or imbalances.

Two other primary kinesiology tools used to ask non-verbal questions involve the use of the subtle energy systems of the chakra-nadi system, called *mudras*, and the acupoints of the acupuncture meridian system. These non-verbal questions are used to both ascertain the nature of the imbalance and the potential techniques to correct that imbalance. The mudras used in Energetic Kinesiology are called *hand modes*, and acupoints that indicate specific types of imbalance are called *specific indicator points*. A hand mode or a specific indicator point each provides a mechanism to identify a unique frequency resonance pattern.

A unique combination of hand modes and specific indicator points used in combination is called *acupressure formatting*. Every imbalance in the body has a unique frequency resonance pattern; however, more complex problems are represented at many levels and thus have more complex frequency resonance patterns. Acupressure formatting allows the practitioner to address these more complex, multicomponent imbalances directly and efficiently. The use of acupressure formatting to identify very specific contexts has greatly enhanced the effectiveness of modern Energetic Kinesiology.

Chapter 13

PAUSE LOCK

Pause lock is also called *retaining mode, circuit hold*, or simply *putting something into circuit*.[1] This technique was discovered by Dr Alan Beardall. It is used to continually hold a piece of information within neurological and energetic circuits of the body over time.

Discovery of the pause lock mechanism

Beardall was a member of the Dirty Dozen, the original 12 chiropractors who in conjunction with Dr George Goodheart developed Applied Kinesiology. Indeed, Beardall was one of the major innovators in the developing field of kinesiology and made many insightful discoveries, one of which was the discovery that he could use activation of proprioceptors to hold neurological and energetic signals over time.

Beardall made the seminal observation that if he rapidly moved his feet together and then apart while he was monitoring an 'unlocking' muscle, the muscle would remain in this unlocking state for a considerable period of time. This allowed him to activate an imbalance and then hold the electromagnetic pattern of the imbalance over time, permitting him to further investigate the nature of this imbalance.

He discovered this serendipitously while working with a patient. He was leaning over the patient and activating an imbalance when his legs happened to come together then apart as he stood up. When he next monitored the patient, he was amazed to discover that the indicator muscle was still unlocking. To his further amazement, when he brought his feet together the unlocking muscle state disappeared. Further investigation consistently revealed that if he monitored an imbalance and rapidly brought his feet together then apart, the indicator change observed in the first instance persisted over time, as long as he held his feet apart.

Beardall showed that not only could the monitor hold the information by activating the hip joint via putting their feet together and apart, this information could also be transferred to the client. This is accomplished by having the client put their feet together and apart while the monitor is touching them. Further, this permits the monitor to now put their feet together, thereby erasing the information held by their hip joint activation, and then take on new information from further testing. This allows the monitor to create a sequence of information about the original imbalance. In modern Energetic Kinesiology this is called *stacking*.

Using pause lock

This *pause and advance* technique, as Beardall originally termed it, is now called *pause lock* in most current Energetic Kinesiology modalities. It is one of the most important and useful techniques in Energetic Kinesiology, as it permits information to be held over time and for this information to be added to, creating a method for investigating the underlying factors involved with the initial imbalance observed.

Pause lock has three primary functions.

1. To isolate an imbalance so that it can be further investigated (e.g. finding the most appropriate correction for an imbalance).
2. To record an imbalance that has been accessed consciously and to allow it to be worked on without need of further conscious involvement. For example, it is difficult for a person to maintain conscious awareness of or focus on a painful site or continually think about a stressful situation without the mind wandering. If the mind wanders, there is no guarantee that you are still working on the original issue. By isolating such imbalances in pause lock, the person's conscious awareness is then free to wander to other unrelated areas. The body, as

accessed through a balanced indicator muscle, will continue to record and react to the original stressor, allowing it to be further investigated.

3. To isolate and record successive layers of compensating imbalances via stacking to reveal the underlying cause, which when corrected will also correct all these layers of compensations.

In order to place an imbalance in pause lock, you first need to locate the imbalance. This can be done by *circuit locating*, touching a specific indicator point, holding a hand mode, monitoring a muscle or thinking of a stressful situation. While this issue is being addressed, either the client or the monitor separates their legs by approximately 30 centimeters. The indicator change observed with the initial issue will *remain* in its changed state (locked or unlocked) provided that the legs are kept apart and no further stresses are addressed.

For example, when the quadriceps muscle monitors as under-facilitated or unlocking, the monitor separates his legs as the muscle unlocks. To determine the factor or factors that are associated with this under-facilitated muscle response, the monitor need only circuit locate specific indicator points such as the acupoint stomach 35 for neurolymphatic imbalance or triple heater 10 for neurovascular imbalances. Touching the involved specific indicator point will cause the unlocking muscle to relock, indicating the nature of the stressor creating the initial imbalance. The change of the indicator muscle when the specific indicator point is touched shows that there is an active match of frequencies between this specific indicator point and the imbalance in circuit.

In this example, if stomach 35 was active, i.e. the indicator changed from unlocked to locked when the monitor touched stomach 35, this would indicate that there is a neurolymphatic imbalance associated with the observed under-facilitation of the quadriceps muscle. This means that the related neurolymphatic reflex for quadriceps is a pertinent correction.

Note that a change in the indicator muscle indicates the relevance of the particular challenge, and with each relevant challenge the indicator muscle response reverses from locking to unlocking to locking, etc. Thus, it is the *change* in the indicator that identifies a frequency match, whether this be at the physical, emotional, mental or energetic level.

Transferring the circuit

The information recorded in pause lock can be transferred back and forth between the monitor and the client. This is especially important if the monitor is checking a leg muscle and then wants to move up to monitor an indicator muscle in the arm.

To transfer the circuit from the monitor to the client, the client, who is not holding any information in pause lock, simply brings their ankles together and then separates their legs while the monitor maintains physical contact with them. The monitor can now move around normally without maintaining further contact or keeping their legs apart. This can also be very handy if the monitor or client has to interrupt the work to briefly attend to something else.

Note that the monitor can hold the imbalances of the client without affecting the information being held in circuit for a considerable period of time. Two unpublished studies have shown that once pause lock is initiated and then there is no further leg movement, the signal held in pause lock will persist for 30 minutes to one hour or more without further reactivation.

Important considerations when using pause lock

As soon as both the monitor and client close their legs, the information in pause lock is lost and you will have to start again from scratch. Often, it is helpful to place some object (such as a tissue box) between the feet of the client to help them to remember to keep their feet apart. Gordon Dickson calls this the *memory box*.

Both the monitor and the client must be well hydrated, as this technique involves a lot of neurological activity. If results seem unreliable or inconsistent, recheck hydration. Hydration is discussed in-depth in chapter 22, which covers kinesiology pre-checks.

Proposed mechanism of pause lock

What follows is a speculative model based on what is known of the neurophysiology of joint proprioception combined with proposed models of human energy systems and many years of clinical observation.

First, it is pertinent to look at why the legs are so well suited for the task of storing information in pause lock. In fact, it appears that the important factor in using the legs is the vast amount of information generated by the proprioceptors of the articular capsules of the hip joints.

There are three types of nerve endings in the joint capsule and ligaments around the joints. The Pacinian corpuscles measure pressure and transient changes in pressure, and they provide information about the direction and speed of movement of the hip joint and hence where the legs are at any moment. However, they are rapidly adapting receptors and therefore provide only transitory information. The Golgi ligament organs provide information about transitory changes in tension of the ligaments of the hip joint, which can also be used to provide information about the position of the legs in relation to the hip joint.

The third type of receptor, the Ruffini end organs, are unusual receptors in that they have a biphasic response. They are arranged as overlapping arrays of receptors, and because of this structure they fire only in certain directions of tension (see Figure 13.1). Like Pacinian corpuscles and Golgi ligament organs, they have an initial phasic response that indicates the direction and speed of movement of the leg relative to the hip joint. However, they also have a secondary tonic response, which is the basis of the pause lock mechanism. The tonic response of the Ruffini end organs continues at a lower rate of firing once the leg has stopped moving. That is, once they have fired, they continue to do so at a constant rate over time.

Of these three nerve endings, the Ruffini end organs are by far the most abundant, with 8000–12,000 in the articular capsule of each hip

joint, with groups of them firing at specific angles of rotation of the joint, but not at other angles. This provides the brain with information not only on the rate of rotation but also on the direction of rotation. Once the leg has moved to a new position, the tonic response of the Ruffini end organs continues to signal the brain about the exact position of the leg. Thus, the brain receives continuous and vast amounts of information from these nerve endings, in effect saying continuously, 'Your legs are this far apart, your legs are this far apart…'

Obviously, it is necessary for the hip joints to give a lot of continuous feedback to the brain about the position of the legs, as they are so important in standing, walking and various actions. This continuous flow of neural signals to the brain

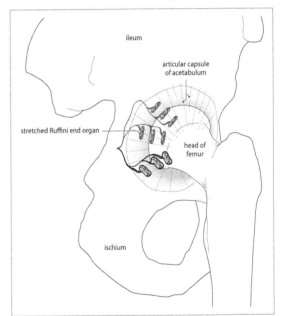

Figure 13.1 Role of hip joint proprioception in the pause lock mechanism. Ruffini end organs (REOs) are specialized proprioceptors in the fascia of complex joints (e.g. the hip and temporomandibular joints). REOs are unique because they have biphasic receptors with a transitory phasic response, followed by a long-lasting tonic response providing information on static position. REOs are highly directional, firing only in one plane of tension, but are distributed in many of planes of orientation. REOs fire with movement but then continue to fire about 100 times per second once the limb has stopped.

creates a very strong electromagnetic pattern that persists over time because of the tonic response of the Ruffini end organs. With this electromagnetic pattern created by these neural flows (e.g. your legs are this far apart), a concomitant response is created in associated energy systems in the body, for instance the acupuncture meridian system.

A muscle imbalance that creates an unlocking muscle response also creates an electromagnetic frequency pattern as measured by electromyography. This electromagnetic frequency pattern is in turn reflected as an energetic response. Thus, whenever there is a neurological response in the physical body (e.g. an unlocking muscle), there is an associated energetic response produced within the energetic body (e.g. the energy pattern of an unlocking muscle).

Furthermore, whenever two people are touching, their energy systems are joined and flow together as one energetic circuit. In the same way a person touching an electric fence becomes part of the same energy circuit as the fence, a monitor touching a client becomes part of the client's energy system. Thus, when a monitor is touching a client and an energetic-electromagnetic response is produced in the client's energy system (e.g. the energetic-electromagnetic response to an unlocking muscle), then that energetic response is also present in the monitor's energy system.

The pause lock mechanism is therefore thought to result from the vast amount of neurological information being constantly relayed from the huge numbers of proprioceptors indicating the hip joint position, creating a stable energetic-electromagnetic pattern over time. When this hip joint pattern interacts with the energetic-electromagnetic pattern of the corresponding issue (e.g. an unlocking muscle), these two energetic patterns create a higher order interference pattern. Any issue can be retained in this way (e.g. stimulating an active specific indicator point reflex, monitoring a muscle with an imbalance or even thinking a stressful thought).

The movement of the hips to this new position must be done at exactly the same time as the imbalance is addressed to create the combined interference pattern. This could be likened to the way in which a carrier wave is modulated by a signal wave in radio transmission (see Figure 13.2).

Evidence of this can be demonstrated by placing an imbalance in pause lock. The muscle imbalance will now cause the indicator muscle to unlock, creating an electromagnetic-energetic pattern of an unlocking muscle, which then modulates the electromagnetic-energetic pattern of the original hip receptor carrier wave. These subconscious responses can be considered like a 'biocomputer', and entering information into this system can be considered entering information into the biocomputer. When the legs are moved together again, the original 'Legs are apart' signal ceases and the indicator now relocks, indicating that the imbalance is no longer being held, because the message has been erased on the biocomputer.[2]

Using the computer analogy, you enter information on your computer that you can see on the screen; this is analogous to entering an unlocking muscle into pause lock. In both cases, there is a consistent electromagnetic signal recreating this information again and again hundreds of times per second. In the computer monitor, this is represented by the electron guns sweeping across the phosphorus on the screen. In the body, it is analogous to the continuous output of the tonic phase of the Ruffini end organs in the hip joint. When you turn off the electron gun by hitting the delete button, the information on the screen disappears. Likewise, when the hips are moved together again the proprioceptive signals holding the imbalance stop or dramatically reduce their firing, 'deleting' the signal of the muscle imbalance previously held in pause lock.

Using the jaw as a pause lock mechanism

While the hip joints and leg movement are generally used for the pause lock mechanism, other joints with large numbers of Ruffini end organs can also be used. Shoulder joints could be used but are not very convenient, as to suddenly raise your arms in the air limits your ability to monitor a muscle. Richard Utt introduced the use of the jaw joint (temporomandibular joint) as a second pause lock mechanism. The 5000–7000 Ruffini end organs in this joint make it ideally suited for this task. It also allows for information to be swapped between the jaw and the hips of the monitor, representing two separate pause lock mechanisms on the same person. This is very much like saving information on the hard drive of your computer, then transferring it to the A drive on the same computer. This is very important if the pause lock of the client cannot be used, for example when

working with a client with paraplegia or someone with a lot of back pain or whose pause lock mechanism is not stable.

Utt was indeed faced with this problem in one of his first Applied Physiology trainings. One of the students was paraplegic, used a wheelchair, and was unable to move his legs to activate the pause lock mechanism. Utt, in a flash of insight, realized that the temporomandibular joint has similar numbers of Ruffini end organs as the acetabular joint of the hip. In this way, this student was able to use a pause lock effectively. As he monitored a

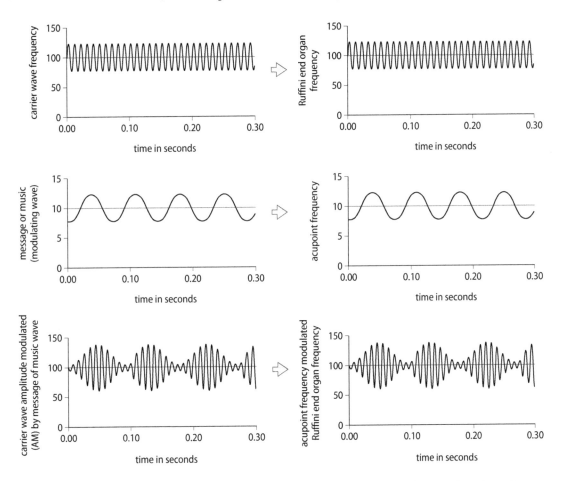

Figure 13.2 Radio transmission analogy for possible mechanism for pause lock. In a radio transmitter, the carrier wave is modulated by the message or music wave, and the modulated carrier wave now holds the information of the message or music during transmission. In an analogous way, the continuous firing of the tonic Ruffini end organ (REO) response sustains a strong electromagnetic frequency wave that acts like a carrier wave. This REO carrier wave is then modulated by interaction with the energetic frequency pattern of stress created by an imbalance or activation of an acupoint or hand mode, and this modulated REO carrier wave now holds the information of the imbalance over time.

muscle, he would open his mouth wide and keep his mouth open until his client had moved his legs together and apart to activate his hip pause lock mechanism. He could then close his jaw and talk to them.

Stacking using pause lock

Generally, the body is in a state of balanced–imbalance, with many of the imbalances really only being compensations for other imbalances. These layers of imbalance are rather like the layers of an onion. To get down to the root cause, it is necessary to peel off the various layers of imbalance to get to the root cause and correct it. If this is not done, even though we may have peeled off several of the layers, they slowly accumulate again because we have not dealt with the underlying cause.

Pause lock is one system that can isolate a particular imbalance and allow us to investigate its specific history. Once the signal is pause locked, the whole indicator muscle system is now dedicated to this particular imbalance, and other unrelated imbalances neither show up nor interfere with the subsequent investigation. This is because the context of the circuit is now the only information held in pause lock.

It is possible to correct each imbalance layer as it is presented, and eventually the primary cause (or causes) reveal itself (or themselves) for correction. Or by an ingenious method of swapping information between the monitor and the client, it is possible to identify and store these various layers of imbalances without doing any corrections until the primary imbalance is identified. This process is referred to as stacking.

Stacking allows us to add information about each layer of imbalance into the circuit, providing the context to uncover the next layer of imbalance. Each time a layer is entered into pause lock, the energetic–electromagnetic interference pattern becomes more complex. When we have entered the causal layer of imbalance into circuit, this combined interference pattern can then be matched against potential correction modalities, allowing the system to not only provide the information to identify the causal issue but also to provide the modality of correction that will be most effective.

When the primary imbalance is corrected, all the compensating imbalances will be simultaneously resolved, because the compensations disappear as soon as they are no longer required. Often, there are several imbalances that could be considered primary to various aspects of a presented condition, so it may be necessary to repeat this process several times. In addition, the body may not be capable of making the required correction to the primary imbalance through the many layers of compensating imbalances all at once. In such a case, several corrections will have to be made along the way before the primary imbalance can be identified and corrected.

The primary imbalance, and the successive layers of compensating imbalances, is collectively referred to as a circuit. Working with circuits greatly speeds up the process of correction and vastly increases its depth of penetration, even to very deep seated problems. In this way, very deep-seated imbalances in many interconnected areas of the body can be addressed by a single correction procedure.

Using stacking

As each imbalance or piece of relevant information is identified, it is entered into the monitor's pause lock. This is then transferred to the pause lock of the client, as discussed above.

The monitor can then close their pause lock and search for the next layer of imbalance (emotional imbalance, acupoint imbalance, nutritional imbalance, etc.). When this next layer is located by an indicator change, the monitor opens their legs again. This adds the new information to the imbalance already stored in the pause lock of the client, creating a more complex interference pattern in the pause lock of the monitor. The client can then 'update' the information in their pause lock by bringing their legs together and apart again. This is analogous to opening a file on your computer, making revisions in that file and then saving the new file over the top of the old one.

Note that the pause lock is a summation process. The monitor collects all the new and previously stored information, not just the newly identified imbalance, in their pause lock, while the client retains the information only up to, but not including, the last piece of information entered into the monitor's pause lock.

A more advanced application of pause lock, developed by Richard Utt, is for the monitor to put the initial imbalance into pause lock, then when there is a reciprocal indicator change on hand modes, specific indicator points, challenges, verbal questioning and other techniques, the monitor may then open their jaw widely. This enters this new piece of information into their jaw circuit. At this point, the hip pause lock is holding the initial imbalance only, while the jaw pause lock is holding both the initial imbalance and the new information. However, at this point the monitor cannot speak!

To transfer the information from their jaw pause lock to their hip pause lock, the monitor need only bring their feet together, erasing the original information, and then open them again, taking all the information that is being held in the jaw pause lock. Now the monitor is free to close their jaw and talk to the client once more. This ability for the monitor to transfer the circuit between their jaw and their hip pause lock is especially useful when working with young children or people who have difficulty activating their own pause lock because of pain or disability.

Note that each time you enter an *additional imbalance* into pause lock, the indicator changes and remains changed. Thus, the indicator keeps going from locking to unlocking to locking, etc. The identification of the next layer of imbalance will therefore create a reciprocal indicator change. An unlocking indicator will thus relock when an imbalance is identified by circuit locating an active specific indicator point or hand mode.

References

1. Dickson, GJ 1990, *What is Kinesiology?*, IHK Printing, Melbourne.
2. Beardall, AG 1982, *Clinical Kinesiology Instruction Manual*, AG Beardall DC, Lake Oswego, pp. 2–7.

Chapter 14

POWERS OF STRESS

The discovery of powers of stress

Richard Utt, founder and developer of Applied Physiology, noticed that often a balanced indicator muscle would suddenly become over-facilitated or blocked when an issue or imbalance was entered into pause lock. When he attempted to sedate the muscle, either with spindle cell sedation or using the north pole of a magnet, the muscle would remain locked. He found that if he sedated the muscle, then pause locked the over-facilitated response, the muscle would typically remain locked, but when this sedation procedure and pause locking had been repeated several times the muscle would suddenly unlock.

Now when the muscle was tonified it would relock, suggesting that all the stress in the circuit had returned to the level of homeostatic function and he had a functional indicator muscle again. Utt reasoned that the indicator muscle had over-facilitated in response to a large amount of stress that suddenly came 'online' when the issue or imbalance was pause locked. In a sense, the power of the stress was so great that the muscle circuit just could not handle it, and it was this excess of stress that caused the over-facilitation. Once this stress had been completely entered into the circuit via repetitive pause lock, the indicator muscle could again respond normally to sedation and tonification procedures.

The north pole of a standard 3000-gauss ceramic ferrite magnet can be used to sedate muscles and the south pole to tonify them. When an over-facilitated indicator muscle would not unlock when sedated by the north pole of the magnet, Utt considered this to be one power of magnetic stress. If two sedations with the magnet still did not unlock the muscle, it was two powers of magnetic stress, and if it took three applications of the magnet followed by pause locking to finally unlock the indicator muscle, then there were three powers

of magnetic stress in that circuit. Tonification of the now unlocked indicator muscle would immediately momentarily relock the muscle, suggesting that normal homeostatic muscle function had returned to the indicator muscle.

The additive nature of these magnetic powers of stress was then confirmed by further research. When three repetitive applications of the magnet fully downloaded the stress in the circuit and unlocked the over-facilitated muscle, three magnets together would also produce the same result. Likewise, if it took six applications of the magnet to fully download the stress, then six magnets together would also demonstrate the same result.

While teaching in Sweden, one of Utt's students suggested that the same might be true of an unlocked indicator muscle. Tonifying an unlocked indicator muscle should momentarily relock the muscle, if the muscle is functioning normally. If tonification does not relock the muscle, then there are powers of under-facilitated stress in the circuit. When application of the south pole of a magnet to an under-facilitated indicator muscle does not relock the muscle, you have one power of magnetic stress. If the indicator muscle does not relock after the magnet is pause locked two times, you have two powers of magnetic stress, and so on. Once the muscle relocks and can be momentarily sedated by a single spindle cell sedation or application of the north pole of the magnet, the muscle has regained normal function and all the stress in the circuit has been entered into the 'biocomputer'.

Applying powers of stress

If spindle cell manipulation rather than a magnet is used to sedate and tonify the muscle, then you have powers of stress relative to the spindle cell circuit. Utt coined the term *powers of stress* for any stress that overloads a circuit by creating over-facilitation or hyper-under-facilitation, that is, does not respond to sedation or tonification.

Powers of stress can be thought of as much like the various scales on an electrical multimeter. Because electrical resistance varies over such an enormous range, the meter scale reads only from 0 to 1 but has a selector knob that changes the amount of resistance measured. For instance, if the selector knob is set at 1 ohm (ohm is a measure of electrical resistance) then the whole dial reads 0 to 1 ohm. If the selector knob is set to 1000 ohms, then the dial reads 0 to 1000 ohms, etc. To read the amount of resistance in the circuit, it is necessary to click the selector knob to the appropriate level to bring the resistance 'on scale' before it can be 'read' on the dial.

Take an example of a circuit that has 7500 ohms of resistance. If the selector knob is set to 10 ohms, the needle of the dial will be 'pegged' against the 10 end of the scale, indicating that more than 10 ohms of resistance is present. How *much* resistance is unknown, because that scale is unable to read that level of resistance. When the selector knob is moved to the 100-ohm scale, it will again be pegged and unable to tell you how much resistance there

is in the circuit. Not until the selector has been switched to the 10,000-ohm scale will the meter be able to show you exactly how much resistance is present in that circuit (see Figure 14.1).

If there is a lot of stress in a circuit entered into pause lock and it over-facilitates the indicator muscle, then the indicator muscle can only indicate 'lots of stress', not how much stress. Sedating the indicator muscle and pause locking until the muscle can respond to sedation is much like clicking through the ohm scale on the multimeter. Once the amount of stress in the circuit has been entered to the on-scale reading, then the muscle can once again respond as a normal indicator muscle.

The significance of entering the powers of stress in the circuit via pause lock is two-fold: 1, you are then balancing a specific, identified amount of stress, not just 'lots of stress'; and 2, you have a conscious idea of how much stress is involved, in a sense the 'depth' or 'power' of the issues involved in the circuit. Because the powers of stress procedure recognizes the degree or extent of the stress caused by an imbalance, a deeper balance is achieved, as many layers of imbalance can be corrected at one time rather than requiring many circuits to correct.

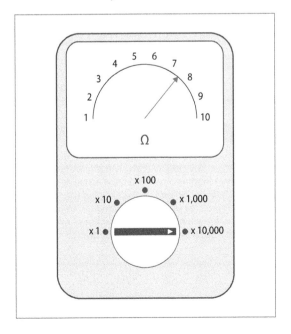

Figure 14.1 Ohmmeter for measuring electrical resistance and powers of stress in muscle monitoring. Like powers of stress in muscle monitoring, electrical resistance varies over many orders of magnitude. So the ohmmeter scale reads only from 0 to 1, with subdivisions, but it has a selector knob that changes the scale of resistance that can be measured. If set on 10, the scale can only measure up to 10 ohms, with resistance greater than 10 ohms just pegging the needle above 10; the actual resistance remains unknown. Likewise, with powers of stress it just jams the indicator muscle, leaving the actual amount of stress unknown unless this stress is 'downloaded' into the whole body energy system, bringing the indicator muscle back into homeostasis.

Alternative methods of releasing powers of stress

While either repeated spindle cell sedation or toni-fication and pause locking or the application of a magnet and repeated pause locking are means of entering powers of stress, there are other methods that may also be used to enter the powers of stress, releasing the over-facilitated state of muscle imbal-ance: 1, circuit-localization of stomach 3 right and left; 2, heart self points; 3, the Stress Indicator Points System (SIPS); and 4, modes of processing (MOP) points.

Stomach 3 right and left

The stomach 3 acupoints (see Figure 14.2) to release over-facilitated or hyper-under-facilitated states of stress generated by strong emotional responses was developed by Georg Weitsch, a German Applied Physiologist. When strongly 'charged' emotional issues are entered into circuit, they will often cause the indicator muscle to over-facilitate, or they may become hyper-under-facilitated and not be able to lock when tonified. These over-facilitated and hyper-under-facilitated responses are even more common when deep subconscious emotional areas of the limbic system and brainstem are entered into circuit. Weitsch discovered that often the entering of highly charged emotions or emotional issues into the circuit would cause a surge of stress to go

through the circuit, often causing a polarity reversal within the cellular protoplasm.

Like the liquid crystal screens of laptop computers, the cytosol, or liquid within the cell, has liquid crystal properties, such that when an electrical charge is applied there is a sudden polarity reversal. In the case of the laptop screen, polarity reversal causes the black blank screen to become white or colored in those areas of the screen undergoing the reversal in polarity, thus producing the words written on the screen. In the case of cells, this sudden polarity reversal caused by the surge of emotional energy through the circuit results in the over-facilitated or hyper-under-facilitated state of the muscle. Like a circuit breaker in an electrical circuit when a surge of electricity has passed through the circuit, the 'circuit breakers' may all pop into the *off* position, hence the circuit can no longer respond. In an analogous way, when the cells experience this surge of emotional energy, they may reverse polarity, popping into the *off* response position.

The circuit locating of stomach 3 right and left seems to reset the cell polarity, 'switching' the polarity back to its original state and releasing the over-facilitated or hyper-under-facilitated state of the muscle. This is like just switching the circuit breakers back to the *on* position resets the elec-trical circuit. Thus, whenever you have entered an issue that causes a sudden over-facilitated or hyper-under-facilitated response in the indicator

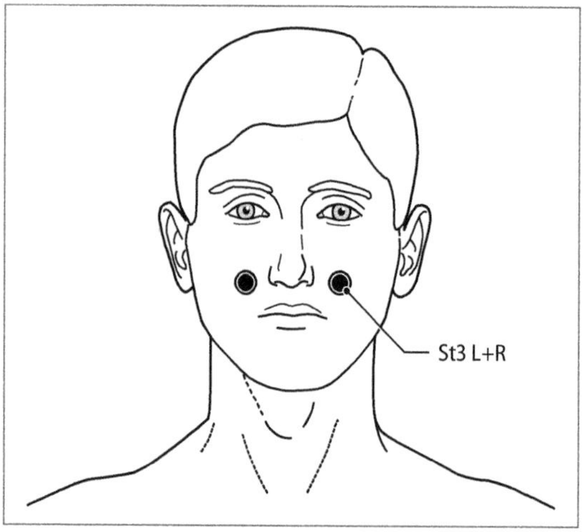

Figure 14.2 Stomach (St) 3 right (R) and left (L) acupoints. The stomach 3 acupoints (R and L) are in line with the nostrils in a notch under the cheekbone. If the indicator muscle has gone over-facilitated or hyper-under-facilitated when an emotional issue has been entered into circuit, this indicates a surge of emotional energy has 'popped' the circuit breaker and it needs to be reset. By simply circuit locating (touching) these acupoints, the powers of stress generated by the strong emotional response can be released. If this method has been effective in releasing the powers of stress, the indicator muscle will once more respond to spindle cell stimulation.

muscle, you can just circuit locate stomach 3 right and left and remonitor the muscle. If the cause of the over-facilitated or hyper-under-facilitated state was a simple polarity reversal, then circuit locating these points will immediately bring the indicator muscle back into homeostasis, as indicated by an indicator change. The over-facilitated muscle will thus unlock, but can be relocked momentarily by spindle cell or Golgi tendon organ tonification, or the hyper-under-facilitated muscle will now lock but can be sedated momentarily by spindle cell or Golgi tendon organ sedation.

Heart self points

The heart self points (see Figure 14.3) were developed by Susan Probert, an Australian Applied Physiologist, from intuitive understanding. Probert had observed that the muscle would often go over-facilitated or hyper-under-facilitated whenever an issue was entered into circuit that exceeded the person's conscious or subconscious ability to handle the stress in a homeostatic way. It seemed to occur as a splitting off or dissociative response to these types of stresses. In her words, 'It is as if the personality can just not deal with the issue and opts to split-off—leave the body to cope with the issue.' This sudden dissociation causes the over-facilitated or hyper-under-facilitated muscle state.

Holding the heart self points again appears to 'reset' the circuit and allow the person to be 'present' even in the face of these stressors. When there is an over-facilitated or hyper-under-facilitated muscle that will not respond to other release methods, we have never found the heart self points not to bring the indicator muscle back into home-ostasis. For the best results, these points should be held until they pulse, a sensation similar to feeling the wrist pulse.

Sometimes circuit locating the original heart self points (kidney 27 right and left, Central Vessel 22, Central Vessel 18 and Central Vessel 14) does not give an indicator change. The monitor can then enter all five heart self points into their jaw pause lock and have the client circuit locate Governing Vessel 20, known as spirit gate or hundred meeting points in traditional Chinese acupuncture. As this Chinese name suggests, this variation shows when the under-lying issue is more spiritual in nature. If there is an indicator change when these six points are held, the monitor need only enter this into hip pause lock, then close their jaw, and both the monitor and client continue to hold these points until a pulse is felt by the monitor. This completes the downloading of the powers of stress and indicates the muscle has returned to normal homeostasis.

Issues that cause over-facilitated or hyper-under-facilitated responses and require heart self points to release these states often create a spacey or dizzy

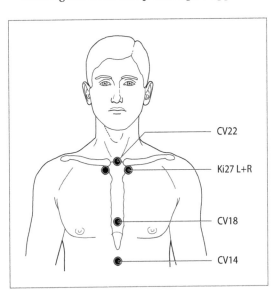

Figure 14.3 **Heart self points.** The heart self points consist of five acupoints, Central Vessel (CV) 22, Kidney (Ki) 27 left (L) and right (R), CV 18 and CV 14, that need to be held simultaneously. When there is over-facilitation or hyper-under-facilitation of the indicator muscle that will not respond to other powers-of-stress release methods, holding the heart self points all at the same time can reset the circuit. Holding these acupoints together until they pulse (like a wrist pulse) will download the powers of stress into the circuit.

CV22

Ki27 L+R

CV18

CV14

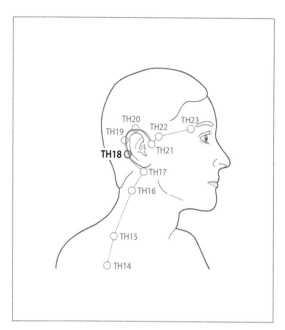

Figure 14.4 Stress Indicator Points System muscle stress point: triple heater (TH) 18. The SIPS muscle stress point is the acupoint TH 18, located posterior to the ear in the center of the mastoid process (the bone hump behind the ear). Holding this acupoint on the left side will immediately 'lock' an under-facilitated muscle, while holding TH 18 on the right side will immediately 'unlock' an over-facilitated muscle.

response in the person when the issue is balanced. This is believed to be caused by the reorganization of their energy structures in the absence of the old deep-seated imbalance. These points seem to show when there is a high level of subconscious stress or distress, which seems to be causing an 'I'm out of here' or 'I don't want to deal with this' response at the higher self or spiritual level. Sometimes just holding these points until there is a pulse or indicator change can balance the circuit, and thus this procedure may also be a correction.

The Stress Indicator Points System

The SIPS, developed by Ian Stubbings, introduces the concept of entering electrical and electromagnetic stress into the circuit for downloading powers of stress. While Utt's method of entering the powers of stress greatly enhances balances, it can be very time-consuming to perform.

In 1989, Stubbings attended Utt's brain physiology formatting course which gave energetic access to specific hypothalamic and limbic areas of the brain. These areas are predominantly involved with handling survival emotions which often create many levels of powers of stress. Relative to normal circuits for a muscle imbalance, these brainstem circuits often necessitated several minutes of sedating–pause locking, sedating–pause locking, sedating–pause locking, and so on. Thus, in a clinical situation these brainstem issues with very large amounts of stress would often take several minutes to enter into pause lock. Stubbings felt there had to be another, perhaps more efficient way of achieving the same benefit, or similar benefit, in less time.

Stubbings's search to discover another way of performing the powers of stress procedure led him to discover a specific acupoint that can be used for downloading muscle stress: triple heater 18 (see Figure 14.4). Over-facilitated muscles with high levels of stress, which would have taken many applications of a magnet to unlock, unlocked in one step by holding this specific acupoint.

For instance, if the pectoralis major clavicular (PMC) were over-facilitated and the client or monitor circuit located, that is touched, triple heater 18 on the right side, the PMC would immediately unlock, offering virtually no resistance to muscle monitoring. Likewise, if the PMC were under-facilitated when initially monitored and the client or monitor circuit located triple heater 18 on the left side, the muscle would immediately lock and often actually go into over-facilitation.

Stubbings then discovered that the SIPS was a three-part procedure: 1, locating the specific acupoint that has a frequency resonance with a specific type of tissue (e.g. muscle, tendon or ligament); 2, locating the second acupoint that relates to the amount of energy flow or 'amperage' at a specific frequency; and 3, locating the third acupoint that relates to the 'resistance' to the flow of energy at that frequency.

This is analogous to Ohm's law of electricity: voltage = amperage × resistance. What this states is that voltage or the amount of energy that can potentially flow is equal to the amount of energy flow available multiplied by the resistance to that flow. For instance, if resistance is zero, then all the energy available is flowing (voltage equals amperage); however, any resistance will clearly reduce the amount of energy that is available to flow.

However, unlike electricity, in which amperage is always a flow of electrons at the physical level, the flows of energy in the SIPS can be at any level within the body–mind–spiritual being. Indeed, these flows could be at the physical level of electrical flows or at any of the other more subtle energy levels: etheric, astral, mental or spiritual. In contrast to the simplicity of Ohm's law of electricity, that is, voltage (potential flow of electrons) = amperage (amount of electrons flowing) × resistance (resistance to the flow of electrons), the SIPS's Law of Stress is far more complex, as there are now many different frequency domains of energy flow: physical, etheric, astral, mental and spiritual, each with its own unique amperage and resistance points.

The SIPS's Law of Stress is voltage (*the potential flow within a specific frequency domain*) = SIPS point (*which identifies type of tissue or function stressed at this frequency*) + amperage point (*the flow within this frequency domain*) × resistance point (*the frequency offering resistance to the flow within this frequency domain*).

Ohm's law of electricity applies only to one frequency of flow: electrons. So while rubber, wood or glass may offer considerable resistance to the flow of electrons, they offer no resistance to the flow of microwaves, X-rays, etc. Therefore the SIPS's Law of Stress has an additional component: the type of tissue or function that is stressed within a particular frequency domain. So first you have to identify the tissue or function that is being stressed, and then you identify the domain of energy flow that is involved via the amperage point. After identifying the 'amperage', then you can identify the resistance to that particular domain of energy flow. This again is accomplished by touching a series of 'resistance' acupoints that are unique to each energy domain.

Thus, the SIPS procedure is to: 1, locate the tissue acupoint (e.g. triple heater 18 for muscle tissue), then pause lock; 2, locate the 'amperage'

acupoint, identifying the type of energy flow; 3, while holding that amperage point, touch the associated 'resistance' acupoints to identify the specific type of resistance that is blocking the flow; and 4, hold the amperage and resistance acupoints identified at the same time until they begin to pulse. This is a subtle pulse similar to a wrist pulse but is not arterial in origin, and indicates the powers of stress have been completely downloaded.

One of the most significant aspects of downloading powers of stress using the SIPS is that once the powers of stress have been downloaded, the tissue or function actually returns to homeostasis. In a sense, the excess of energy in that frequency domain has been released from this small circuit and returned to the whole body energy system, where it is now redistributed.

This is important, because as you enter more and more layers of imbalance, each with their powers of stress, at some point you exceed the capacity of the client's energy systems to process this. This is analogous to opening program after program on your computer until it becomes unstable and locks up or crashes. However, by continually downloading the powers of stress using the SIPS, you can enter far more levels of imbalance into the circuit before it is necessary to perform a correction. Therefore more layers of compensation can be dealt with in a single session than could be previously. Furthermore, the SIPS procedure permits the monitor to download the full extent of stress in each tissue and in each frequency domain into the whole body energy system. Thus, you can achieve deeper balances than just entering a lot of unspecified stress into the circuit.

The modes of processing

The MOP points were developed by Hugo Tobar as part of his Neuroenergetic Kinesiology system, and are effective for downloading stress particularly in the brain and brainstem areas. Because Neuroenergetic Kinesiology initially dealt predominantly with issues involved with the brainstem and limbic system, both areas involved with survival emotions, activation of these issues would often overload the circuit, creating many levels of powers of stress.

Tobar discovered that accessing survival emotions through his newly developed extensive and specific brain formatting created high levels of powers of stress difficult to download with conventional systems. Remember, the more specific the format, the more specific the context, and in a sense the less stress required to overload the circuit. Tobar found that he first needed to identify at what level of the spiritual body the energy flows were blocked (the atmic, buddhic or monadic level), and then identify an additional MOP point for the specific survival system (e.g. fear, rage, panic or seeking) experiencing these flows. Then, by holding Governing Vessel 20 in combination with the *spiritual level point* (atmic, buddhic or monadic) at the same time as a specific

survival system point until a pulse was felt, he could effectively download all stress. This procedure both returned the indicator muscle to homeostasis and increased the depth of balancing achieved.

The MOP points are located predominantly on the head and involve the primary brain-related acupoint in traditional Chinese medicine: Governing Vessel 20. As with the SIPS points, this acupoint is then matched against secondary acupoints that identify the spiritual level point and a survival systems point. These survival systems are involved with both individual and species aspects of survival and are largely hardwired into the brainstem and limbic system and therefore regularly cause over-facilitation and hyper-under-facilitation.

Chapter 15

HAND MODES

The discovery of hand modes

In 1983, while working with a patient, Alan Beardall noticed a unique phenomenon. When the patient touched a painful area with an open hand, the muscle he was monitoring suddenly weakened, a normal response indicating a stress condition in the painful area. In a second test on the same area, however, the patient happened to touch his thumb and index finger together. Something very odd occurred: the muscle immediately strengthened and 'locked'.[1,2]

In a flash of insight, Beardall recognized that the thumb and fingers had energy flows similar to the energy flows of the meridian system itself, and that muscle monitoring provided a means of assessing these flows. He discovered that the thumb acted like an earth or a neutral, grounding the energy flows of the other fingers. Through extensive research, he found that these phenomena represented another form of readout on the essential functions within the body.

The yogis had made a similar discovery a millennium before, when they found in a more intuitive way that touching the thumb to different fingers produced different psychoemotional effects. They called this system of thumb and finger positions *mudras*. Most people are familiar with the classic yoga mudra for meditation, where the palms are facing upward and the thumb is touching the pad of the index finger, with the other fingers extended. This is seen in many ancient Indian temple sculptures.

Beardall called this new method of using muscle monitoring to identify energy flows within the body *hand modes*. In other types of Energetic Kinesiology, they have also become known as *finger modes* or *digital determinators*.

Radio wave analogy

Hand modes are a type of electromagnetic and energetic specific frequency indicators. The thumb is considered electromagnetically and energetically neutral. Each of the fingers, however, has a specific polarity and differs from the other fingers in the bandwidth of electromagnetic and energetic frequencies that flow down it.

It is as if the index finger is AM radio frequency, the middle finger is FM radio frequency, the ring finger is shortwave radio frequency, and the little finger is microwave frequency. Thus, whenever the thumb makes contact with a point on one of the fingers, it elicits a specific frequency of electromagnetic energy, like tuning in your radio. If you should touch your thumb to your index finger, that would be like turning the radio dial to 97.5 AM, whereas shifting it to the end of your middle finger would be like tuning in to 101.5 FM.

Frequency matching

Every imbalance has a specific frequency pattern or resonates at a specific energetic frequency. When an indicator muscle is monitored at the same time a hand mode is held, it will change state (e.g. from 'unlocked' to locked) only if the frequency of imbalance matches the frequency of the hand mode. Just like tuning in your radio station, you know you have a frequency match between the frequency of the radio signal and your radio dial when you get a clear signal. Likewise, a clear response from the indicator muscle tells you that you have tuned in to a specific type of imbalance. Hand modes may, however, indicate three quite different types of information, as outlined below.

Hand modes act as frequency identifiers

Hand modes can identify or define the nature or type of frequency present in a circuit or an imbalance. When a hand mode is held at the same time as a muscle is monitored, and the circuit or imbalance resonates at the same frequency as the hand mode, then it will cause an indicator change. This indicates that the imbalance in circuit is of the same type and frequency as the hand mode being held. For instance, when holding *emotion mode* (thumb touching ring finger pad) gives an indicator change, this indicates that the imbalance being investigated is primarily emotional in nature. *Thus, hand modes can identify the nature of an imbalance held in circuit.*

Hand modes act as specifiers

Hand modes can also be used to specify the type of frequency domain to be investigated. For instance, if the specific muscle mode is held and entered into circuit via pause lock, then an indicator change while circuit locating alarm points will indicate that there is a specific muscle imbalance in one of the muscles related to that meridian energy. For example, if triple heater alarm point gives an indicator change, then one of the triple heater–related muscles, teres minor, sartorius, gastrocnemius or gracilis, will have a specific muscle imbalance when manually monitored. However, if the organ mode is entered into pause lock and the alarm points circuit located, an indicator change now indicates an active stress within the organ associated with that meridian energy. Note how it is *context* that determines the meaning of the muscle response, and the hand modes are a means of providing a particular context.

Hand modes can provide information of a general nature

There are several hand modes whose primary purpose is to provide an informational context, for example *scan mode, time mode* and *priority mode*. When using scan mode, it does not indicate any particular type of imbalance, but only whether whatever is being scanned at the time matches the frequency of imbalances currently held in the circuit. Likewise, priority mode does not indicate the type of imbalance, but only if that specific imbalance being monitored is a priority to correct rather than a compensation for some other imbalance.

Types of hand modes

There are now several hand mode systems used in the different Energetic Kinesiology modalities, for instance the hand mode system of Clinical Kinesiology developed originally by Dr Beardall, in which there are more than 2000 hand modes; the finger mode system developed by Richard Utt in Applied Physiology; and another finger mode system developed by Dr Bruce Dewe in Professional Kinesiology Practice (PKP).

In some of these mode systems, the same finger position can sometimes represent a different type of energetic imbalance. Well, if there are different hand modes using the same position in two different systems, which one is right? Usually both are! How can this be? Because hand modes are frequencies, not specific types of information, much like 101.5 FM is neither a rock station nor a classical station; it is just a unique radio frequency. When rock music is assigned to this frequency, then it is a rock station, but if a classical music station is assigned to this frequency, then it plays classical music.

Universal hand modes

This brings us to the types of hand modes. Beardall discovered the basic *universal modes* (see Figure 15.1):

- index finger pad to thumb pad relates to frequencies of structural imbalances
- middle finger pad to thumb pad relates to frequencies of biochemical or nutritional imbalances
- ring finger pad to thumb pad relates to frequencies of emotional imbalance
- little finger pad to thumb pad relates to frequencies of electromagnetic or energetic imbalance.

Assignable hand modes

Within the frequency range covered by emotions, the shortwave frequencies of our radio wave analogy, there are many different emotional stations. Different kinesiology modalities *assign* different specific emotional music to the same emotional frequency as in the classical–rock station analogy above.

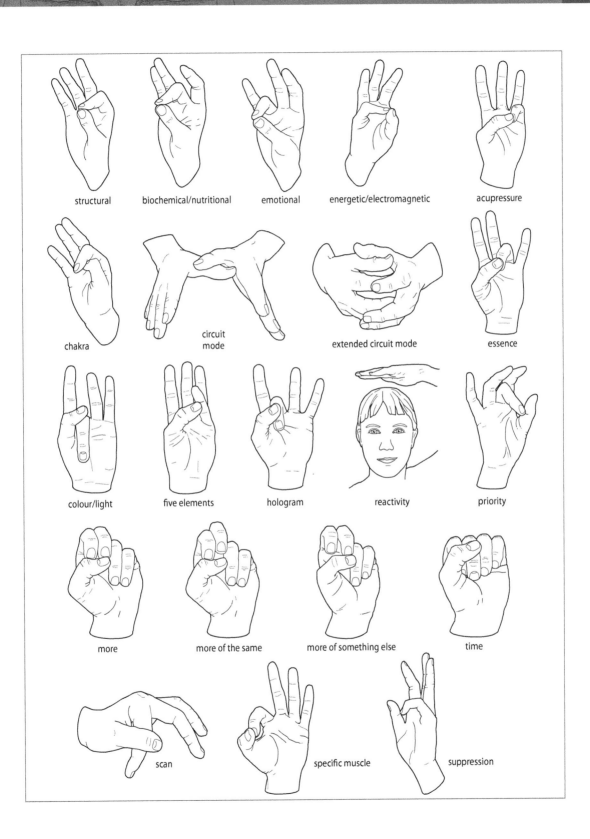

structural

biochemical/nutritional

emotional

energetic/electromagnetic

acupressure

chakra

circuit
mode

extended circuit mode

essence

colour/light

five elements

hologram

reactivity

priority

more

more of the same

more of something else

time

scan

specific muscle

suppression

Figure 15.1 **Hand modes.** The universal hand modes are made by touching the pad of the thumb to the pad of the individual fingers: 1, index finger = structural frequencies; 2, middle finger = biochemical or nutritional frequencies; 3, ring finger = emotional frequencies; 4, little finger = energetic or electromagnetic frequencies. These universal hand modes represent a primary domain with a whole set of frequencies. Other hand modes represent *assigned hand modes* within these primary domains, each of which will be described later in this book and their use in kinesiology explained.

Thus, there are two major types of hand modes: first, *universal modes* that represent a whole set of frequencies within a specific domain, for example structural, biochemical or nutritional, emotional and electromagnetic or energetic; and second, *assignable modes*. Assignable modes specify a particular frequency within a universal domain. For instance, within the emotional domain when the thumb pad is placed on the nail of the ring finger this indicates flower essence mode in most systems. Each flower essence matches a particular psychoemotional state or feeling, therefore when there is a frequency of imbalance in circuit and holding flower essence mode creates an indicator change, then the associated flower essence emotions are related to the underlying issue for that imbalance.

However, who or what did the assigning? Partly this is the intent of the person who developed the hand mode system, and the other part is the knowledge and intent of the person holding the mode. And thus if I know two systems that assign a different meaning to the same finger position, it is my intent as the monitor that makes it an Applied Physiology mode versus a PKP mode.

Indeed, in all our conceptual processing it is our intention that determines the meaning of what we observe, think and experience. If I say to you the words, 'Stop! You're killing me!' because you told a very funny joke, or 'Stop! You're killing me!' because you are choking me, there is quite a different meaning and different message behind the same words. My intent in the first case is just to acknowledge how funny your joke was, and my intent in the second case is to let you know you are doing something that threatens my life.

Even science, the most objective process that the human mind has invented, is fraught with subjective interpretation. No matter how objective the number an instrument may produce, once a particular human mind interprets its meaning it immediately has become a subjective experience. And this is because each human mind brings a different context and frame of reference, including a different intention, to this act of interpretation. Aldous Huxley expressed this beautifully as early as 1946, when he wrote, 'The scientific picture of the world is inadequate for the simple reason that science deals only with certain aspects of experience in certain contexts. All this is quite clearly understood by the more philosophically minded men of science. But most others tend to accept the world picture implicit in the theories of science as a complete and exhaustive account of reality.'[3]

This is why two scientists with different points of view (intentions) may state that the same data have two different meanings. A very clear example of this is the current debate about industry-funded scientific data versus independently funded scientific data. Consistently, data produced by industry scientists find absolutely no problem with a particular product or chemical, while independent scientists find exactly the opposite. Since they are interpreting similar sets of data, it must be their intention behind their interpretation that varies; it is obviously not the data!

Types of assignable hand modes

Assignable modes come in two types: *transferable* assignable modes and *non-transferable* assignable modes. Transferable assignable modes are ones like those used in Applied Physiology and PKP that when taught to another person always respond to the same frequencies of imbalance in a consistent and reproducible way. Non-transferable modes, on the other hand, may work very well for a particular individual with a specific energetic structure and knowledge base but are not consistent or reproducible when taught to another person without this energetic structure and knowledge base. In this textbook, we will refer only to universal modes and transferable assignable modes. See Figure 15.1 for a sample of the variety of hand modes and their meanings.

This assignation process, however, is not random or arbitrary, because hand modes are essential frequency patterns just as radio frequencies are a specific frequency pattern. So you cannot assign an FM station on an AM frequency, because these frequency domains inherently do not match. For example, in 1986 Dr Bruce Dewe, Richard Utt and Dr Charles Krebs all independently discovered that specific muscle imbalances were consistently indicated by the thumb pad placed on top of the index fingernail. Both Utt and Krebs called this *specific muscle mode* because it indicated specific muscle imbalances. This indicates that modes appear to have an essential frequency that is independent of the observer.

In contrast, Dr Dewe was working out his finger mode system, and there is a type of electromagnetic imbalance called *centering* that has three components: cloacal imbalances, gait imbalances and hyoid imbalances. In his moding system, each mode location, designated by a number, has three sublocations designated by A, B and C. So when he identified the finger mode position for centering, he assumed he would be able to assign its three components to the locations A, B and C. However, no matter how hard he tried, the finger mode would show centering only as a whole and would not partition into the three sublocations. This suggests that mode assignation is not arbitrary but is determined by the actual frequency of the hand and finger positions, and that this frequency domain limits the possible intentional assignations that can be made to each individual hand mode.

In summary, hand modes have an ancient lineage from the mudras of the yogis to the modern hand-moding system of Energetic Kinesiology. These hand modes have proved to be one of the most useful energetic tools in kinesiology, as they allow us to identify, specify and provide the context of imbalances that are often subconscious in nature.

References

1. Levy, SL & Lehr, C 1996, *Your Body Can Talk*, Hohm Press, Prescott, pp. 5–6.
2. Dickson, GJ 1990, *What is Kinesiology?*, IHK Publishing, Melbourne, p. 44.
3. Huxley, A 1946, *Science, Liberty and Peace*, Harper & Brothers, New York, pp. 35–36.

Chapter 16

SPECIFIC INDICATOR POINTS

Specific indicator points is the name given to various points on the body, most being acupoints. When these points are 'active', they will give an indicator change when circuit located (touched), indicating that a particular type of imbalance is present in the circuit. These specific indicator points 'resonate' at the same frequency as the type of imbalance that they indicate. For example, when a neurolymphatic reflex is active and the acupoint stomach 35 is circuit located while monitoring the indicator muscle, you would get an indicator change. This would inform the monitor that there is a neurolymphatic imbalance present. This further suggests that neurolymphatic reflex stimulation may be important in rebalancing the muscle or circuit being investigated. Therefore specific indicator points not only indicate the nature or type of imbalance present, which in many cases is subconscious, but may also suggest a likely therapy for correcting the imbalance.

Although there are many specific indicator points used in kinesiology, most people are familiar with the alarm points, specific indicator points for meridian energy, or meridian associated muscle–organ/gland imbalances. However, which of these is indicating is provided by the context of the hand mode that is used in conjunction with circuit locating each alarm point. For instance, if I hold specific muscle mode and circuit locate the alarm points, an indicator change indicates that there is a muscle imbalance in one of the muscles related to the meridian of the active alarm point. In contrast, if I hold organ mode and circuit locate the alarm points, an indicator change indicates there is an imbalance within that meridian-related organ.

Development of specific indicator points in kinesiology

One of the original applications of acupoints as specific indicator points was by Applied Kinesiology

chiropractors Alan Beardall and Jack Rarey, using the alarm points. Some of the tender alarm points were introduced into Applied Kinesiology as an alternative way of identifying over-energies in muscles and their related meridians. Beardall and Rarey discovered that by sharply tapping the alarm points and monitoring an indicator muscle, they could challenge the related meridian for energy imbalance. Having located an imbalance in a meridian, if the corresponding alarm point was held with light pressure and the indicator muscle again 'unlocked', this identified an over-energy in that meridian.[1]

Applied Physiology

Richard Utt then further developed this concept of acupoints as indicators of various types of imbalance. Utt systematically investigated the relationship between specific types of imbalance, both physiological and energetic, and specific acupoints. For instance, Utt would locate a neurolymphatic imbalance via Chapman points and then systematically investigate the alarm points to see which meridian points became active. For example, he would enter a Chapman neurolymphatic point into circuit and then check each of the alarm points for an indicator change. For each meridian alarm point that caused an indicator change, he then checked each individual acupoint on that meridian to locate an active point or points.

He repeated this with a large number of people, and the acupoint that reproducibly became active when a neurolymphatic imbalance was present in the body he designated as the specific neurolymphatic indicator point. This turned out to be stomach 35 on the knee. To confirm this relationship, Utt would then apply traditional neurolymphatic therapy to the original Chapman point and then recheck the specific indicator point for its state of balance. What he observed was that every time there was a neurolymphatic imbalance present, stomach 35 became active. Following application of neurolymphatic therapy, stomach 35 would no longer be active.

In a similar way, he used the neurovascular points discovered by Terrence Bennett in the 1930s and 1940s called Bennett points, to locate neurovascular imbalance and the meridian point associated with that imbalance. Again, the single acupoint triple heater 10 seemed to have a consistent frequency match with neurovascular imbalances in general. Therefore triple heater 10 became the specific indicator point for neurovascular imbalance.

Stress Indicator Points System

The Stress Indicator Points System (SIPS) was developed in early 1992 as a result of the search by Ian Stubbings to discover another, perhaps more efficient way of performing the powers of stress. Each SIPS point is a frequency match for stress in a specific tissue, which is downloaded using the SIPS procedure discussed earlier. Stubbings started at the level of the physical body first, identifying a point for muscle imbalance. He explained his idea to Krebs who used the procedure in his clinic the following week. With his logical mind, Krebs adapted Stubbings's concept for use not only with over-facilitated muscles but also directly with unlocking muscle states, to amazing effect. Leg muscles of one of Krebs's clients suffering from motor neurone disease, which had not 'locked' for 1½ years, instantly locked when the point was held and could now be balanced.

After this exciting discovery, it occurred to Stubbings that SIPS points were doing more than the powers of stress with this new procedure. He realized that certain acupoints had a special significance in relation to particular types of stress. These acupoints he called stress indicator points. A stress indicator point identifies the stress in a particular physical structure (e.g. cells, tissues or organs), as well as in energetic structures (e.g. acupuncture meridians and auric levels such as the astral or emotional plane). It then allows you to download the stress associated with the stressed structure.

The first stress indicator point discovered was the muscle stress point, triple heater 18. This point,

unknown to Stubbings, was also independently recognized by Dr. Carl Ferrari, the developer of Neural Organization Technique, as a master acupoint related to muscle function. Stubbings went on to develop a complete SIPS that provides access to most of the cells and tissues of the body as well as many psychoemotional imbalances at the primary levels of the human being: physical, etheric, astral (emotional), mental and spiritual.

Specific indicator points have thus become an important component of the modern practice of kinesiology, and are now used within almost all systems of Energetic Kinesiology.

Alarm points

Alarm points are used in traditional Chinese medicine as both diagnostic and treatment points. They are located on the trunk of the body, with at least one point relating to the state of energy balance or flow in each of the twelve regular meridians, as well as two of the eight extra meridians: Governing and Central.

In traditional Chinese medicine, the alarm points, or front *Mo* points, were predominantly used to locate chronic over-energy meridians and hence potential dysfunction associated with the meridian-related organ. Acute over-energies were generally located by using the back *Shu* points or association points. Under-energies were generally located using pulse diagnosis. In pulse diagnosis, the monitor holds the radial pulses with three fingers just above the wrist crease, similar to how the radial pulse is taken in western medicine. However, what is read is not just the heart rate but rather subtle qualities of these pulses at three different levels.[2]

At first inspection, something that seems unusual is that many of these alarm points are located on the Central Vessel and not on one of the other twelve regular meridians for which they indicate energetic imbalance. Thus, the alarm points for pericardium, heart, stomach, triple heater, small intestine and bladder are all represented by acupoints on Central Vessel. Several of the other alarm points, although not located on Central Vessel, are also acupoints of another

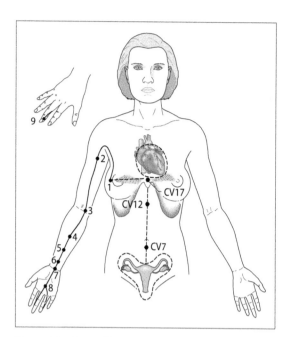

Figure 16.1 Percardium meridian alarm point: Central Vessel (CV) 17. The alarm point for pericardium, which runs from the breast to the end of the middle finger, is actually not on the pericardium meridian but rather is CV 17. This is because a secondary vessel runs from pericardium 1 directly to CV 17 such that imbalances in the pericardium meridian are directly reflected in state of balance of CV 17. After Walther DS, 1988, *Applied Kinesiology: Synopsis, Second Edition*, Systems DC, Pueblo.

meridian. For example, large intestine alarm point is stomach 25, and kidney alarm point is gall bladder 25. Why would this be?

If you remember from chapter 6, we discussed that there are secondary vessels as well as primary vessels of acupuncture. Indeed, the reason that many of the regular meridian alarm points are located on Central Vessel is because there is a secondary vessel connecting each of these regular meridians to that specific acupoint on Central Vessel. Thus, when a meridian is either under-energy or over-energy, its corresponding alarm point on Central Vessel will reflect the state of balance of the associated meridian. This is shown clearly for the pericardium meridian in Figure 16.1.

Many acupoints that need treatment often become spontaneously tender and are therefore referred to as *Ah Shi* points or sensitive points by

the Chinese. The alarm points (Figure 16.2) were originally discovered largely because they are *Ah Shi* points when active.[3] This tenderness is so exaggerated in the case of alarm points that they can be used as a palpatory method of diagnosis. If when they are palpated they are more tender than the surrounding tissues, a functional disturbance of the organ that they represent may be deduced.[4] When a person complains of spontaneous pain at an alarm point, the meridian is probably over-energy. When there is tenderness with palpation, but no spontaneous pain, the associated meridian is probably under-energy.[5]

Traditionally, the alarm point is considered a

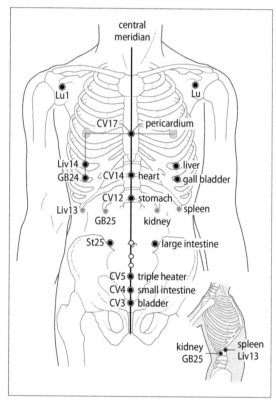

Figure 16.2 The alarm points or front mo points. When a meridian is either under-energy or over-energy, its corresponding alarm point will reflect the state of balance of the associated meridian. The alarm points have been used in traditional Chinese medicine as both diagnostic and treatment points for thousands of years, and today they are used in Energetic Kinesiology to locate imbalances within the muscle–organ/gland–meridian matrix. CV, Central Vessel; GB, gall bladder; Liv, liver; Lu, lung; St, stomach.

point of tonification, which if stimulated increases the energy in the meridian that it subserves. Hence, when touched with normal pressure the alarm point momentarily tonifies the meridian with which it is associated. If the associated meridian already contains an excess of energy, then the additional tonification by alarm point stimulation will exaggerate this imbalance and create an indicator change if an indicator muscle is monitored at the same time. When deeper palpation is required to elicit a painful response, the corresponding meridian is under-energy.

Using modern muscle-monitoring procedures, Gordon Stokes of Three In One Concepts discovered that the Chinese alarm points could be used in conjunction with a balanced indicator muscle to identify under-energies as well as over-energies.[6] A change in the response of an indicator muscle (e.g. locked to unlocked) when light pressure was applied to an alarm point indicated over-energy in the related meridian, as previously observed in Applied Kinesiology. If deep pressure on the alarm point caused an indicator change, however, then under-energy was indicated in the related meridian.

Therefore alarm points can be used to detect both over-energies and under-energies. This response to alarm point stimulation is used extensively today in Energetic Kinesiology to locate imbalances within the muscle–organ/gland–meridian matrix.

It must be noted that many developers of Energetic Kinesiology modalities have developed a number of specific indicator points that are unique to their individual systems. The use of their specific indicator points, together with muscle monitoring, allows them to rapidly identify imbalances relevant to their systems.

References

1. Dickson, GJ 1990, *What is Kinesiology?*, IHK Publishing, Melbourne.
2. Kaptchuk, TJ 1983, *The Web That Has No Weaver: Understanding Chinese Medicine*, Ryder, London.
3. Chaitow, L 1988, *Soft Tissue Manipulation*, Thorsons Publishers, London.
4. Mann, F 1972, *Acupuncture: The Ancient Chinese Art of Healing and How It Works Scientifically*, Vintage Books, New York.
5. Walther, DS 1988, *Applied Kinesiology: Synopsis*, Second Edition, Systems DC, Pueblo.
6. Utt, RD 1985, *The Seven Chi Keys*, Applied Physiology Printing, Tucson.

Chapter 17

ACUPRESSURE FORMATTING

A unique concept in modern Energetic Kinesiology, once again developed by Richard Utt, is the application of hand modes and specific indicator points used together to identify more complex imbalances. As stated previously, hand modes are a way of identifying domains of energy imbalance, for example structural or emotional, while specific indicator points are a means of identifying specific physiological and/or energetic imbalances within the body. The combination of these two indicator systems provides a mechanism to ask far more complex and specific non-verbal questions of the 'biocomputer'.

If the monitor uses only a specific indicator point or hand mode, then they are basically asking a very short or one-word question. This is very powerful, but unfortunately it limits your ability to gather information about the full extent of imbalances within the body. Using Utt's concept of acupressure formatting, and relating the frequency imbalance of a hand mode with a specific type or system of imbalance via the specific indicator points, generates a far more complex energetic interference pattern. This in a sense presents the biocomputer with a far more complex question.

Development of acupressure formatting

Utt's development of acupressure formatting happened over time from simple two-component formats to considerably more complex formats. Utt had the initial idea of acupressure formatting when working with muscle–organ/gland matrices that allowed him to specify more directly which component of these multicomponent systems he was working with.

Utt's initial applications of acupressure formatting were quite simple. When you circuit locate an alarm point with no other context, it basically indicates a state of imbalance within the meridian directly related to that alarm point. However, the imbalance causing the alarm point to be active may originate at one or even several levels. For instance, the imbalance may originate from a state of muscle imbalance, a state of organ or gland imbalance, a state of meridian-related emotional imbalance, or even an unresolved mental or spiritual issue. Any one or a combination of these factors could be the primary reason for the imbalance observed in that meridian, as indicated by the active alarm point.

In order to clarify the meaning of the active alarm point, it was necessary to provide a specific context before the alarm point was circuit located to select individual domains for investigation. For instance, when specific muscle mode was held at the same time as an alarm point was circuit located, an indicator change now would indicate that there was a muscle imbalance in one of the meridian-related muscles. While if organ mode was held at the same time as an alarm point was circuit located, then the indicator change would now indicate a meridian-related organ imbalance, etc. Hence the monitor is now making an a priori choice as to which domain and which components of that specific system they wish to investigate.

As an analogy using words, the words *may* and *be* each have a specific and unique meaning when used separately in a question. However, the word *maybe* has a unique and separate meaning from its individual components. *Maybe* provides a different context for the sentence in which it is used than its individual components do. In a similar way, holding organ mode at the same time as you circuit locate the heart alarm point is not just asking a question about any organ but rather the specific organ associated with this alarm point. So before you were asking the body a specific question, such as 'Is there a stress in an organ?' or 'In a meridian?' Now, using the organ mode × alarm point acupressure format, you are asking 'Is there a stress in the organ related to this specific meridian?', for example 'Is there stress in the heart organ?' Let us be clear: this does not mean that there is a medical pathological issue with the heart, but rather that there may be physiological or energetic stresses that affect the heart and that may over time lead to heart issues.

When Utt decided to investigate stresses in brain structures and functions, he was confronted with a highly complex multicomponent system. For this, simple two-component formatting was clearly not enough, because in the brain there are systems within systems. For instance, in the limbic system you have cortical components such as the cingulate gyrus and hippocampus, subcortical components such as the amygdala, and even hypothalamic components such as the mammillary bodies. Clearly, to identify a limbic structure and investigate it for stress first requires identifying that it is in the limbic system and then giving it a specific address within that system. This required Utt to create an acupressure format for the limbic system and then a more specific format within that system to identify, for instance, the amygdala.

This is very much like describing the location of a building within a city. First, you have to state which city it is in, then the specific street address at which the building is located. Normally, at each building specific functions are performed, therefore if you wish to specify a specific function you first have to identify the building where that function is performed. Once in that building, you can then access that particular function, which may mean you need to locate a specific room or office.

To develop the specific acupressure formats, or 'addresses', of specific brain areas and functions, Utt employed a rigorous, logical procedure. He used a set of histology slides of sections of the human brain, which provided the actual physical structures of the human brain. In order to hold the energetic frequency pattern of these structures, he would shine a laser through the histology section of that specific structure into the apex of a modified quartz crystal. As we are all aware, crystals can hold information, for example silicon crystals in computers.

At first, Utt used flawless quartz crystals, but he found that the energetic information imprinted by the laser was not stable in a clear quartz crystal and dissipated rapidly, as confirmed by muscle monitoring. By having the end of the crystal opposite the apex polished to a flat surface and coated with leaded paint, he now found that the energetic information transmitted into the crystal via the laser was stable over a period of minutes to hours, which was enough time for him to use it to investigate these brain formats. He then found that a specific mineral called sugalite, a rare mineral from one mine in South Africa, when cut into a parabolic cap for the quartz crystal would hold the information loaded by a laser over long periods of time. He called these sugalite–quartz crystals *loading crystals*, and they provided him with an effective way to hold or load energetic frequency patterns of the various brain areas into the crystal for future investigations.

Utt would select a particular area of the brain, for example the amygdala, then he would hold the apex of a loading crystal on the region of interest in that structure and shine a ruby laser through the histology section of the tissue into the loading crystal. He would then balance the area of interest on the test subject as best as he could so there appeared to be no overt imbalances in this system. Then he would place the apex of the loading crystal on Governing Vessel 24.5, called the glabella, and shine the laser through the sugalite and out of the apex onto this acupoint, at which point he would pause lock the information 'downloaded' from the crystal into the acupuncture meridian system. Then he would investigate which alarm point or points became active and determine which specific acupoint(s) on the alarm point–related meridian had become active and record these.

Utt then repeated this procedure on 25–50 different people and recorded his findings. Inspection of his findings would generally reveal a specific acupoint related to the specific brain area whose energetic pattern had been stored in the loading crystal. There would normally have been several active acupoints, even on different meridians, for each test subject. However, there was usually a single acupoint that appeared in almost every test subject's results. This acupoint was then taken as the specific indicator point for that particular brain area. Once he knew the specific acupoint, he could then check another 25–50 people to validate that this acupoint consistently represented the energetic frequency resonance pattern of the original brain area on the histology slide.

It must be noted that Utt often had to initially use a broader acupressure format such as 'limbic system' or 'cortex' in order to provide the context to locate an indicator point (or points) for a more specific brain structure or area. For instance, when investigating the amygdala, a subcortical component of the limbic system, Utt found that he had to first enter the limbic format into pause lock, and then in this context enter the amygdala's energetic frequency pattern into the biocomputer via downloading the stored pattern from the loading crystal. Only then could his procedure of using alarm points to locate specific acupoints be employed.

Utt discovered that after loading the energetic frequency pattern of the amygdala into the energetic system of a 'neutral' subject, the following pattern of active acupoints might appear for this specific individual: bladder 2, Central Vessel 14, small intestine 3 and kidney 14. For the next subject, the pattern may be lung 9, small intestine 12 and Central Vessel 14. For the next individual, the pattern may be triple heater 5, Central Vessel 14 and bladder 9. Clearly, there was a single acupoint, Central Vessel 14, which reproducibly appeared for all the test subjects, but other acupoints appeared to be unique to each subject because of their personal circumstances.

Armed with this new information, Utt could now investigate the acupressure format for the amygdala in a new way. First, he would be sure that the amygdala point was not active by entering the amygdala format limbic format + Central Vessel 14 into pause lock. He would now activate a specific component of the amygdala physiology, for example fear, by pause locking the subject's response to closing a book loudly close to their head when it was unexpected. Then he would once again check the amygdala format to find that it was now active. He would then perform an acupressure emotional stress release by holding both gall

bladder 14 acupoints on the forehead until the stress was resolved (indicated by gentle synchronous pulsations of these points). Then once again he would assess the amygdala format and now find that it was no longer active. This clearly demonstrated the link between the amygdala format and actual amygdala-generated reactions and their resolution by application of an acupressure technique.

Krebs further developed brain area formatting based on Utt's original model in his Learning Enhancement Acupressure Program (LEAP). Then Hugo Tobar, Krebs's former student and now colleague, went on to employ similar procedures to develop acupressure formats for the brainstem, the limbic system and the cortex, including many brain pathways, which is now the basis of his Neuroenergetic Kinesiology program. Other types of Energetic Kinesiology, for instance the Stress Indicator Points System, also employ acupressure formatting as part of their protocols.

The validity of acupressure formatting

Although there has been no external validation of activation of specific brain structures via acupressure formatting, two types of information provide practical and theoretical support for this technique. First of all, there is ample anecdotal evidence to demonstrate that specific brain functions found to be deficit by standard psychometric testing, for example digit span assessment of auditory short-term memory, demonstrate stress with the acupressure format for the relevant brain area, in the case of digit span the hippocampus. The hippocampus is indeed the primary brain area involved in short-term memory. Following the resolution of stress identified by acupressure formatting to be associated with the hippocampus, the same subjects now demonstrated age-appropriate scores. When the hippocampus was once again assessed for stress via muscle monitoring and acupressure formatting, the stress observed before treatment was no longer observed, and this important function had been normalized.[1]

Second, acupressure formatting makes the implicit assumption that brain areas and functions can reliably and specifically be activated by acupoint stimulation. There have been a number of studies that show that activation of verum, or 'real', acupuncture points, as compared to sham points, produce different patterns of subcortical and cortical activation in the brain.[2] Patterns of brain activation relative to specific acupoints have been verified in several studies.[3]

In contrast to the more variable results with pain, using functional magnetic resonance imaging and positron emission tomography, Lewith and colleagues found that there are indeed specific and largely predictable areas of brain activation and deactivation attributable to specific acupuncture points associated with hearing and vision that stimulate the visual and auditory cortices, respectively.[4] Thus, there is consistent evidence, especially for direct, sensory-related brain areas, that there is a strong correlation between acupoint stimulation and brain area activation. There is also relatively strong evidence in multiple studies to verify that verum acupoint stimulation consistently produces brain activation not seen with sham point stimulation.[5]

These correlations then support the hypothesis that acupressure formatting could access specific brain areas and functions. Thus, matching the frequency resonance pattern of the acupressure format with activity in specific brain areas and pathways, in conjunction with muscle biofeedback, may provide a mechanism to detect disruption of neural flows within these brain areas and pathways.

For example, as stated above, digit span is a standard measure of auditory short-term memory that is highly dependent on integrated hippocampal function. When people demonstrate deficit digit span performance, stress is always found in the hippocampus and/or other memory areas of the brain via acupressure formatting and muscle monitoring. Once these stresses are resolved by various acupressure techniques, people's auditory short-term memories reproducibly improve to normal or in some cases to better than normal as measured on standard psychological testing. This

is despite the fact that millions of digit span tests performed by clinical psychologists have shown that digit span does not improve spontaneously and is basically stable over your lifetime.[6]

In a similar way, even highly complex functions such as reading comprehension show measurable improvements after acupressure formatting to access stress caused by attempting this activity, followed by acupressure therapy (J Paphazy, unpublished data from children who pre- and post-tested with the Wechsler Intelligence Scale for Children—Revised before and after they received the LEAP treatment from 1986 to 1991). Thus, even though the exact nature of the activation of cortical and subcortical neural substrates via acupressure formatting is not understood, reproducible observable and measurable normalization of the functions directly reliant on these neural substrates strongly suggests that these specific brain structures are indeed targeted by acupressure formatting.

A recent paper demonstrates the effectiveness of acupressure formatting in producing highly statistically significant improvements in four different types of standard speed-of-processing tasks for auditory and visual processing.[1] This paper presents a full description and discussion of acupressure formatting, and supporting evidence with regard to its application to normalizing speed-of-processing tasks in a controlled study. You are referred to this paper for an extensive discussion of the scientific basis for acupressure formatting.

There have also been direct clinical observations of the effect of acupressure formatting on physiological function. An Austrian anaesthesiologist, Dr Sylvester Klaunzer, had completed the 2-year integrated LEAP training program at the university in Saalfelden, Austria, a private institution that runs this training in conjunction with the University of Salzburg, Austria. He recently reported the following anecdote with regard to acupressure formatting.

Dr Klaunzer was working in intensive care, and a cardiac patient suddenly developed atrial fibrillation and unstable blood pressure that was not responding to drugs; the patient was in a very serious condition. Because the drugs had not worked, and the patient was close to death, Dr Klaunzer decided to just enter the acupressure format for the limbic system and then applied acupressure to Central Vessel 14, the specific indicator point for the amygdala. Within seconds, Dr Klaunzer observed the heart and blood pressure monitors begin to show stabilization of function. If he released the acupressure on Central Vessel 14, the fibrillation and blood pressure irregularities returned immediately. But after 15 minutes of continuous acupressure, both the heart rate and the blood pressure were totally stabilized and remained so over the next few days! (Dr S Klaunzer, personal communication, 2008).

Dr Klaunzer has now repeated this with six additional patients with the same results. What should be noted is that the amygdala specifically controls arterial blood pressure and heart rate, the very conditions that were dysregulated and out of control. These functions, overtly controlled by the amygdala, normalized when he held the specific acupressure format for the amygdala.

Using acupressure formatting

A convention was established to distinguish between acupressure formatting and the normal sequential use of hand modes and specific indicator points. When an acupressure format is written, an 'x' between a specific hand mode and another hand mode or specific indicator point indicates that these modes and/or indicator points should be held at the same time as entered into pause lock, because together they represent a single integrated format. On the other hand, if there is a '+' between the hand mode and the specific indicator point, this indicates that these modes and/or indicator points can be pause locked sequentially—first one, then the other.

One of the things that make acupressure formatting very powerful is that it allows the monitor to ask questions of varying degrees of complexity. The format itself represents an interlinked, interactive set, and thus it creates a much more complex energetic interference pattern containing much more information. An acupressure format may be as simple as organ mode × alarm point, or more complex when addressing specific brain areas, such as the limbic system, which requires the acupressure format organ mode × gland mode × Central Vessel 23 × Central Vessel 24. Then, by merely adding a specific indicator point, + Central Vessel 14, to the limbic system format, it now specifies the amygdala. Clearly, to specify just a simple organ system requires less information than to specify a specific component of a complex multi-component structure such as the amygdala within the limbic system.

The most powerful way of working with these tools is to sequentially use individual hand modes and specific indicator points in combination with acupressure formatting. In Energetic Kinesiology, this process of sequentially entering information into the biocomputer via pause locking hand modes, specific indicator points and/or acupressure formats is termed *building a circuit*. This is a mechanism of gathering information from stressors at the physical, energetic, emotional and mental levels that relate to the presenting issue. The end result of this process at the energetic level is a complex frequency interference pattern.

Acupressure format waveform analogy

In the same way that many frequencies of sound of a musical instrument are summed as a single waveform by the ear, the many different frequencies resonance patterns of an acupressure format, the hand modes and specific indicator points, are summed to form a unique energetic frequency signature. When looking for the relevant technique (or techniques) to balance or resolve the presenting issue, it is just a question of matching the frequency signature of the acupressure format with the frequency signature of a specific correction technique.

We will use an analogy of the frequencies of a musical instrument and their resultant waveform to help you visualize how acupressure formatting can be used to identify a specific stressor affecting a specific brain area, and then extending the analogy further, to show how the same acupressure formatting can be used to locate the appropriate acupressure technique to resolve the original stressor.

Figure 17.1a presents the individual frequencies of a musical instrument. However, what strikes the eardrum is not all those individual frequencies but rather the single resultant waveform. The complex individual frequencies of the musical instrument are reduced to a single waveform by constructive and destructive interference. When the individual frequencies are out of phase, troughs cancel out peaks to the degree that they are out of phase, and peaks in phase add to other peaks to the degree

that they are in phase, etc. The end result is a frequency interference pattern represented by a single waveform: the waveform of the musical instrument in Figure 17.1b. Figure 17.1c is an analogous presentation of the different frequencies comprising an acupressure format composed of the frequencies of different hand modes and various acupoints, which then undergo the same constructive and destructive interference interactions to produce a coherent single-frequency interference waveform of the combined acupressure format in Figure 17.1d.

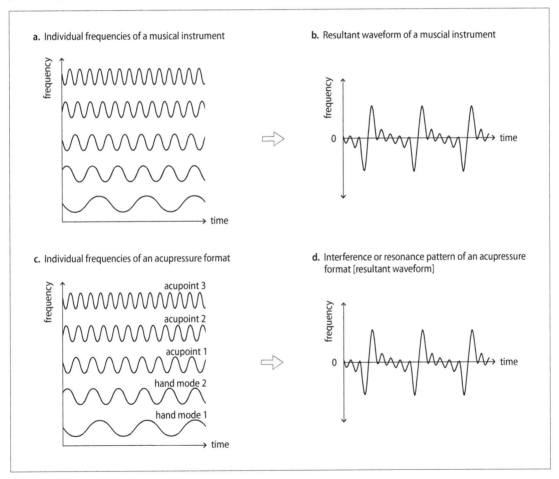

Figure 17.1 Musical instrument and waveform or frequency resonance pattern. a, Different sound frequencies. A musical instrument produces many different frequencies of sound, but this is not what enters the ear. **b, Waveform or frequency resonance pattern.** This is produced by constructive and destructive interference of all frequencies of the musical instrument is what actually strikes the eardrum. **c, Acupressure format.** Holding an acupressure format composed of a number of hand modes and acupoints creates many different separate subtle energy frequencies. **d, Waveform or frequency resonance pattern.** This is produced by constructive and destructive interference, all frequencies of an acupressure format.

To use another musical analogy, even if our current instrumentation could measure sound-waves only to the level of low C, we could still know of the existence of high C via frequency resonance between the two C notes, as the high C is a supra-harmonic of low C. So if you banged strongly on the high C key, this strong vibration in the C note range would begin to vibrate the low C string via frequency resonance. The actual movement of the high C string, however, would remain unknown to you but can be surmised by the effect that it had on the low C string whose frequencies we can measure.

The difference between the musical instrument and the acupressure format is that we *do* currently have instrumentation to accurately measure the frequencies of the musical instrument, and thus directly observe its resulting waveform, which is within the electromagnetic domain of the positive space/time dimension. In contrast, we do not, at present, have instrumentation to directly measure the magnetoelectric frequencies of a hand mode or acupoints, because they appear to be expressed in the negative space/time dimension. However, the measurement of biofields is developing rapidly,

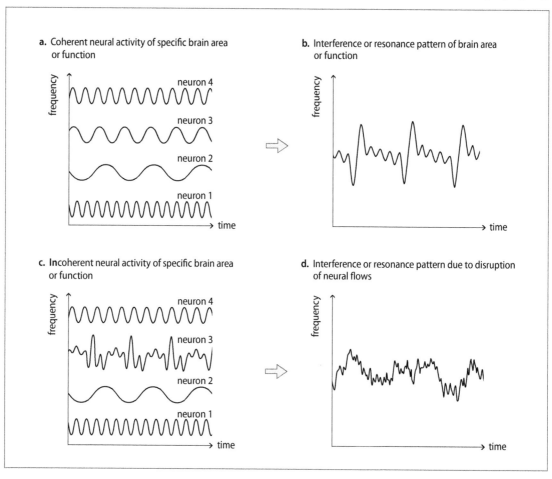

Figure 17.2 a, Coherent neural activity of a specific brain area or function. Firing of individual neurons in a specific brain area in synchrony creates coherent neural activity. **b, Coherent waveform or frequency resonance pattern.** This is created by all frequencies of neurons firing coherently and interacting by constructive and destructive interference. **c, Incoherent neural activity of a specific brain area or function.** Firing of individual neurons in a specific brain area when desynchronized creates incoherent neural activity. **d, Incoherent waveform or frequency resonance pattern.** This is created by all frequencies of neurons firing incoherently and interacting by constructive and destructive interference.

and it seems likely that within half a decade there will be instrumentation to directly measure the frequency resonance waveforms of acupoints and hand modes.

Likewise, the interaction of the various neurons firing in a specific brain area will create an electromagnetic frequency interference pattern or integrated resonance waveform that in recent years we have developed the instrumentation to measure directly, like the vibration of the low C string in our musical analogy. However, similar to the high C frequencies that cannot be measured directly in the previous analogy, an acupressure format will create a frequency interference pattern or integrated resonance waveform because of the activation of frequencies associated with the hand modes and specific indicator acupoints held. But the frequency resonance waveform of hand modes and acupoints will be a supraharmonic of the frequency resonance waveform of the electromagnetic frequencies generated by the specific brain area. Thus, activating the specific brain area acupressure format by holding the hand modes and acupoints simultaneously will create a supraharmonic waveform that matches the electromagnetic frequency waveform of the actual brain area via frequency resonance.

Coherent neural activity of specific brain areas and/or functions, as in Figure 17.2a, generate coherent frequency resonance waveforms, as shown in Figure 17.2b. Likewise, incoherent neural activity of specific brain areas and/or functions, as in Figure 17.2c, generate incoherent frequency resonance waveforms, as shown in Figure 17.2d. Thus, the frequency resonance waveform generated by the activity of this brain area can interact either coherently or incoherently with the acupressure format for that brain area. Because the original acupressure format developed for this specific brain area was for its balanced state, the acupressure format has a coherent frequency resonance waveform. Therefore when a specific brain area's activity creates a coherent frequency resonance waveform, it will match the coherent acupressure format's suprahamonic frequency waveform for this brain area. The interaction of two coherent frequency waveforms is always additive, with one

sustaining the other (Figure 17.3a). Because there is no stress generated by two coherent waveforms interacting, the indicator muscle will remain 'locked', indicating coherence of function within this brain area, with no active stressor(s) affecting this area or function.

In contrast, if there are disturbed, desynchronized neural flows in this particular brain area, this will alter the brain area frequency resonance waveform, shifting it out of phase with the coherent frequency resonance waveform of the acupressure format for this brain area. The altered frequency resonance waveform for this specific brain area will now create dissonance or incoherence when matched against the coherent frequency resonance waveform of the acupressure format (Figure 17.3b). Indeed, it is this dissonance or incoherence that results in an indicator change. The indicator change informs the monitor that there is disruption of coherent function within this brain area as a result of loss of synchrony or timing of neural flows within this area, or between this area and other brain areas.

Likewise, each type of stressor creates a specific pattern of incoherence in brain function, which is represented by a specific incoherent frequency resonance waveform. So once a specific brain area has demonstrated desynchronized neural flows caused by some stressor, the incoherent frequency resonance waveform created by the stressor can then be matched against the frequency resonance waveforms of hand modes and specific indicator points. A frequency match between this specific stressed frequency waveform and the frequency resonance waveform of a specific hand mode or indicator point can then be used to either add more information to the circuit, by entering this indicator change into pause lock, or to identify the type of corrective technique needed to resolve the stressor that desynchronized the neural flows.

Therefore once all the information has been entered into the circuit that is required to resolve the presenting problem, via the same frequency resonance waveform matching process, the monitor can quickly determine the appropriate type of therapy to apply. Following application of this therapy, the efficacy of the therapy can then be assessed by re-entering the original acupressure formats in the original context. If there is no longer an indicator change, the factors that formerly disrupted the neural flows underlying that specific dysfunction have been resolved and coherent neural flow re-established.

You will note that the waveform of the frequency interference patterns of the brain area acupressure format and the frequency interference pattern of the electromagnetic activity in that brain area can either match coherently, causing no indicator change, or match incoherently, resulting in an indicator change. Acupressure formatting thus permits the practitioner to select a priori a specific brain area as the site of interest. If there are currently no stressors acting on or affecting this brain area, then there would be no indicator change.

However, when the acupressure format is entered into circuit, it now designates a specific brain area or system as the context and reference point for the identification of stressors in other more specific brain areas or functions within this larger brain area or system. Therefore a stressor that disrupts a more specific function may not create enough stress to give an indicator change

when the acupressure format for an overall brain area or system is entered into circuit, and in a sense it becomes a hidden stressor. In order to locate these hidden stressors that may disrupt only an aspect of certain brain functions, you would then need to use more specific acupressure formatting to specify exactly which components of this overall brain area have lost integrated function.

For example, entering an acupressure format for a more general brain area such as the limbic system will often show a coherent frequency resonance match with the overall limbic system and therefore no indicator change. However, once this general limbic system format has been entered into circuit, the format for the limbic system now provides a context for more specific acupressure formats of more specific areas or functions within the limbic system. For instance, once the limbic system acupressure format has been entered into pause lock with no indicator change, by adding a more specific limbic format, for example adding the amygdala format, an indicator change will now signal that one or more stressors are indeed affecting the coherence of amygdala function, even though this stress in the amygdala was not enough

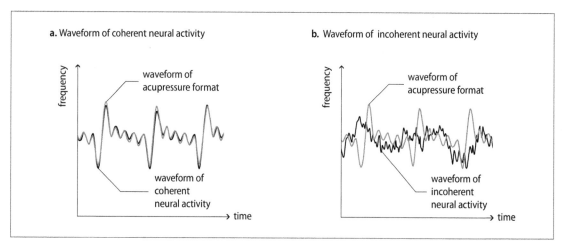

Figure 17.3 a, Interaction of an acupressure format's waveform with a waveform of coherent neural activity in a specific brain area or function. The waveform of the acupressure format derived from balanced brain function matches the waveform of coherent neural activity in a specific brain area or function. There is no indicator change, indicating that no active stressors are affecting integrated brain function. **b, Interaction of an acupressure format's waveform with a waveform of incoherent neural activity in a specific brain area or function.** The waveform of the acupressure format derived from a balanced brain area does not match the waveform of incoherent neural activity in a specific brain area or function. This creates an indicator change, indicating that one or more active stressors are disrupting integrated brain function.

to cause an indicator change at the level of the limbic system as a whole.

In summary, when the brain area has integrated coherent neural flows, and the acupressure format for that brain area is activated, the frequency resonance waveforms of the brain area and the acupressure format are coherent and the indicator muscle locks. If there are desynchronized neural flows within the brain area, this will create incoherence between the brain area frequency resonance waveform and that of the acupressure format. This, in turn, causes the indicator muscle to 'unlock', indicating loss of integrated function within this brain area.

We have used stress in brain areas as our initial example because they are complex and require acupressure formatting in order to detect, but the same logic applies to locating and balancing other types of imbalances affecting more specific structures and functions of the body. For less complex structures and systems than brain areas, however, you may not need to use acupressure formats, and simple individual hand modes and specific indicator points will suffice. Also, whether the technique used to identify an imbalance is based on acupressure formatting or simply on individual hand modes or specific indictor points, the procedures to balance or correct the imbalances found are basically the same and follow the same protocol.

While many single system or less complex systems imbalances can be addressed without acupressure formatting, requiring only the use of individual hand modes or specific indicator points, *only* acupressure formatting provides access to the many complex organ systems of our body, including the most complex of all—the human brain. Indeed, the ability to work effectively with brain-based problems was what led to the initial development of acupressure formatting, and the continuing development of progressively more complex systems of acupressure formatting to provide access to ever more specific brain functions, opening up almost undreamt of possibilities for improvement in sensory–motor and cognitive functions, even following traumatic brain injury. Dr Krebs is one of the hundreds of thousands of people whose life was dramatically changed from the use of acupressure formatting. In Dr Krebs's case, the change was from paralysis and brain damage to functioning again as a whole person!

References

1. Frankel, T & Krebs, CT 2013, Acupressure formatting: a novel acupressure-based technique to access brain and re-integrate functions (in press).
2. Fang, JL, Krings, T, Weidemann, J, Meister, IG & Thron, A 2004, Functional MRI in healthy subjects during acupuncture: different effects of needle rotation in real and false acupoints, *Neuroradiology*, Vol. 46, No. 5, pp. 359–362.
   Zhang, WT, Jin, Z, Luo, F, Zhang, L, Zeng, YW & Han, JS 2004, Evidence from brain imaging with fMRI supporting functional specificity of acupoints in humans, *Neuroscience Letters*, Vol. 354, pp. 50–53.
   Hu, KM, Wang, CP, Xie, HJ & Henning, J 2006, Observation on activating effectiveness of acupuncture at acupoints and non-acupoints on different brain regions [in Chinese], *Zhongguo Zhen Jiu*, Vol. 26, pp. 205–207.
   Wenjuan Qiu, Bin Yan, Jianxin Li, Jin Zhang, Jianping Du, Jian Chen, Baoci Shan, Kewei Chen 2011, A resting-state functional MRI study of the post-effect of acupuncture, *2011 IEEE/ICME International Conference on Complex Medical Engineering*, pp. 103–108.
3. Hu, KM, Wang, CP, Xie, HJ & Henning, J 2006, Observation on activating effectiveness of acupuncture at acupoints and non-acupoints on different brain regions [in Chinese], *Zhongguo Zhen Jiu*, Vol. 26, pp. 205–207.
   Hui, KK, Liu J, Makris, N, Gollub, RL, Chen, AJ, Moore, CI, Kennedy, DN, Rosen, BR, Kwong, KK 2000, Acupuncture modulates the limbic system and subcortical gray structures of the human brain: evidence from fMRI studies in normal subjects, *Human Brain Mapping*, Vol. 9, pp. 13–25.
   Yan, B, Li, K, Xu, J, Wang, W, Li, K, Liu, H, Shan, B, Tang, X 2005, Acupoint-specific fMRI patterns in human brain, *Neuroscience Letters*, Vol. 383, pp. 236–240.
   Yuanyuan Feng, Lijun Bai, Wensheng Zhang, Yanshuang Ren, Ting Xue, Hu Wang, Chongguang Zhong, Jie Tian 2011, Investigation of acupoint specificity by whole brain functional connectivity analysis from fMRI data. In: *Conference Proceedings: Annual International Conference of the IEEE Engineering in Medicine and Biology Society*, pp. 2784–2787.
   Siedentopf, CM, Golaszewski, SM, Mottaghy, FM, Ruff, CC, Felber, S & Schlager, A 2002, Functional magnetic resonance imaging detects activation of the visual association cortex during laser acupuncture of the foot in humans, *Neuroscience Letters*, Vol. 327, pp. 53–56.
   Kong, J, Kaptchuk, TJ, Webb, JM, Kong, JT, Sasaki, Y, Polich, GR, Vangel, MG, Kwong, K, Rosen, B, Gollub, RL 2009, Functional neuroanatomical investigation of vision-related acupuncture point specificity—a multisession fMRI study, *Human Brain Mapping*, Vol. 30, pp. 38–46.
   Lee, H, Park, HJ, Kim, SA, Lee, HJ, Kim, MJ, Kim, CJ, Chung, JH, Lee, H 2002, Acupuncture stimulation of the vision-related acupoint (Bl-67) increases c-Fos expression in the visual cortex

of binocularly deprived rat pups, *American Journal of Chinese Medicine*, Vol. 30, No. 2–3, pp. 379–385.

Li, X, Xu, G, Shang, X, Yang, S & Yufang, W 2008, Development of acupuncture-reading with EEG, MRI and PET. In: *Proceedings of the International Conference on Technology and Applications in Medicine.*

Li, G, Cheung, RT, Ma, QY & Yang, ES 2003, Visual cortical activations on fMRI upon stimulation of the vision-implicated acupoints, *NeuroReport*, Vol. 14, No. 5, pp. 669–673.

Beissner, F & Henke, C 2011, Methodological problems in fMRI studies on acupuncture: a critical review with special emphasis on visual and auditory cortex activations, *Evidence-Based Complementary and Alternative Medicine*, Vol. 2011, Article ID 607637.

Cho, Z, Oleson, T, Alimi, D, Niemtzow, R 2002, Acupuncture: the search for biologic evidence with fMRI and PET techniques, *Journal of Alternative and Complementary Medicine*, Vol. 8, pp. 399–401.

Pariente, J, White, P, Frackowiak, RSJ & Lewith, G 2005, Expectancy and belief modulate the neuronal substrates of pain treated by acupuncture, *Neuroimage*, Vol. 25, No. 4, pp. 1161–1167.

White, P, Bishop, FL, Prescott, P, Scott, C, Little, P, Lewith, G 2012, Practice, practitioner, or placebo? A multifactorial, mixed-methods randomized controlled trial of acupuncture, *Pain*, Vol. 153, No. 2, pp. 455–462.

4. Lewith, GT, White, PJ & Pariente, J 2005, Investigating acupuncture using brain imaging techniques: the current state of play, *Evidence-Based Complementary and Alternative Medicine*, Vol. 2, No. 3, pp. 315–319.

5. Fang, JL, Krings, T, Weidemann, J, Meister, IG & Thron, A 2004, Functional MRI in healthy subjects during acupuncture: different effects of needle rotation in real and false acupoints, *Neuroradiology*, Vol. 46, No. 5, pp. 359–362.

Zhang, WT, Jin, Z, Luo, F, Zhang, L, Zeng, YW & Han, JS 2004, Evidence from brain imaging with fMRI supporting functional specificity of acupoints in humans, *Neuroscience Letters*, Vol. 354, pp. 50–53.

Hu, KM, Wang, CP, Xie, HJ & Henning, J 2006, Observation on activating effectiveness of acupuncture at acupoints and non-acupoints on different brain regions [in Chinese], *Zhongguo Zhen Jiu*, Vol. 26, pp. 205–207.

Wenjuan Qiu, Bin Yan, Jianxin Li, Jin Zhang, Jianping Du, Jian Chen, Baoci Shan, Kewei Chen 2011, A resting-state functional MRI study of the post-effect of acupuncture, *2011 IEEE/ICME International Conference on Complex Medical Engineering*, pp. 103–108.

Hui, KK, Liu J, Makris, N, Gollub, RL, Chen, AJ, Moore, CI, Kennedy, DN, Rosen, BR, Kwong, KK 2000, Acupuncture modulates the limbic system and subcortical gray structures of the human brain: evidence from fMRI studies in normal subjects, *Human Brain Mapping*, Vol. 9, pp. 13–25.

Yan, B, Li, K, Xu, J, Wang, W, Li, K, Liu, H, Shan, B, Tang, X 2005, Acupoint-specific fMRI patterns in human brain, *Neuroscience Letters*, Vol. 383, pp. 236–240.

Yuanyuan Feng, Lijun Bai, Wensheng Zhang, Yanshuang Ren, Ting Xue, Hu Wang, Chongguang Zhong, Jie Tian 2011, Investigation of acupoint specificity by whole brain functional connectivity analysis from fMRI data. In: *Conference Proceedings: Annual International Conference of the IEEE Engineering in Medicine and Biology Society*, pp. 2784–2787.

Siedentopf, CM, Golaszewski, SM, Mottaghy, FM, Ruff, CC, Felber, S & Schlager, A 2002, Functional magnetic resonance imaging detects activation of the visual association cortex during laser acupuncture of the foot in humans, *Neuroscience Letters*, Vol. 327, pp. 53–56.

Kong, J, Kaptchuk, TJ, Webb, JM, Kong, JT, Sasaki, Y, Polich, GR, Vangel, MG, Kwong, K, Rosen, B, Gollub, RL 2009, Functional neuroanatomical investigation of vision-related acupuncture point specificity—a multisession fMRI study, *Human Brain Mapping*, Vol. 30, pp. 38–46.

Lee, H, Park, HJ, Kim, SA, Lee, HJ, Kim, MJ, Kim, CJ, Chung, JH, Lee, H 2002, Acupuncture stimulation of the vision-related acupooint (BI-67) increases c-Fos expression in the visual cortex of binocularly deprived rat pups, *American Journal of Chinese Medicine*, Vol. 30, No. 2–3, pp. 379–385.

Li, X, Xu, G, Shang, X, Yang, S & Yufang, W 2008, Development of acupuncture-reading with EEG, MRI and PET. In: *Proceedings of the International Conference on Technology and Applications in Medicine.*

Li, G, Cheung, RT, Ma, QY & Yang, ES 2003, Visual cortical activations on fMRI upon stimulation of the vision-implicated acupoints, *NeuroReport*, Vol. 14, No. 5, pp. 669–673.

Beissner, F & Henke, C 2011, Methodological problems in fMRI studies on acupuncture: a critical review with special emphasis on visual and auditory cortex activations, *Evidence-Based Complementary and Alternative Medicine*, Vol. 2011, Article ID 607637.

Cho, Z, Oleson, T, Alimi, D, Niemtzow, R 2002, Acupuncture: the search for biologic evidence with fMRI and PET techniques, *Journal of Alternative and Complementary Medicine*, Vol. 8, pp. 399–401.

Pariente, J, White, P, Frackowiak, RSJ & Lewith, G 2005, Expectancy and belief modulate the neuronal substrates of pain treated by acupuncture, *Neuroimage*, Vol. 25, No. 4, pp. 1161–1167.

White, P, Bishop, FL, Prescott, P, Scott, C, Little, P, Lewith, G 2012, Practice, practitioner, or placebo? A multifactorial, mixed-methods randomized controlled trial of acupuncture, *Pain*, Vol. 153, No. 2, pp. 455–462.

6. Lezak, MD 1995, *Neuropsychological Assessment, Third Edition*, Oxford University Press, New York.

Chapter 18

METHODS OF GATHERING INFORMATION

Muscle monitoring as a biofeedback tool provides powerful access to stressors at both conscious and subconscious levels. The use of pause lock to retain electromagnetic and energetic patterns of stress, coupled with the information provided by hand modes and specific indicator points, provides a mechanism to gather information about the specific stressors involved. In addition, it provides the context of these stressors and the factors underlying this contextual information.

Information can be gathered in several different ways using muscle monitoring and pause lock. Based on the client history, the monitor has several choices on how to go about gathering information. The three most common types of approaches to gathering information are: 1, the use of acupressure formatting and specific indicator points, a non-verbal, subconscious approach; 2, challenging an indicator muscle for relevant associations and frequency match; and 3, asking the person overt 'yes' and 'no' questions while monitoring the indicator muscle.

We have previously discussed the use of hand modes and specific indicator points as a mechanism for defining the domain and specific areas related to an issue experienced by the client. Challenging an indicator muscle for frequency match has certain advantages over asking 'yes' and 'no' questions, because the muscle response is an all-or-nothing phenomenon; it either locks or unlocks. When 'yes' and 'no' questions are used, the questions must be extremely clear and stated in such a way that they have only one of two answers: 'yes' or 'no'.

'Yes' and 'no' questioning

How does the body notify us that the answer to a question is 'yes' or 'no'? It does this because of the nature of neuroprocessing in the brain. Any information presented to the brain is rapidly assessed initially by subconscious and normally subcortical areas of the brain, before it is passed on for higher processing at the conscious level. The survival system inspects this incoming information and rapidly scans its data banks for relevant associations from past experience. The amygdala and other components of the survival system then activate survival emotions it has associated with these past experiences. And it does this automatically, based on the subconsciously assigned emotional charge associated with pleasure and reward and with pain and punishment. Indeed, this is what gives information valence or emotional charge to be remembered in the first place.

Therefore, when the monitor asks the client to state the word 'yes', they are normally having a consciously neutral experience and just doing what they are asked. No particular conscious emotional state is involved. However, when they state 'yes', the subconscious emotional system rapidly assesses its past experiences with this word. 'Yes' has very limited negative emotional charge associated with it; indeed, it normally has a very highly positive charge, as it is associated with getting what you have asked for, resulting in reward, or being allowed to do what you want to do, resulting in pleasure. There is no conscious or subconscious stress on this!

However, when a client is asked to state the word 'no', the subconscious likewise scans both conscious and subconscious experiences for associations with this particular word. Unlike 'yes', 'no' has generally very strong conscious and subconscious associations with negative emotional states, such as frustration, anger, pain and punishment, which then generate a subconscious state of stress in the person.

Just think of when you were two years old. How many times were you told 'no' with great emphasis when you wanted to hear 'yes'? The 'no' was basically an abnegation of your wants and desires at that moment, which you wanted and desired with every fiber in your being, as you only lived in that *now* moment. Hence, 'no' almost always has a certain degree of subconscious stress associated with it because of our past experiences, often in early childhood, but which are *now* for the subconscious survival systems scanning this data. Therefore merely stating 'no', or being told 'no', will generate enough stress to cause an indicator change.

These responses to 'yes' and 'no' can therefore be used as a mechanism to gather information. It is thus possible to ask the person's 'biocomputer' what their association with a particular issue is, and it can respond with a 'yes' or 'no' response. However, two things must be understood: 1, the subconscious is totally literal in its interpretation of this information and does not get the gist of what you meant, so it will only answer exactly the question you asked; and 2, the question asked must unequivocally lead to only a 'yes' or a 'no' answer.

Regarding the first point, Krebs has the following anecdote from his early days as an Energetic Kinesiologist. He was working with a woman who had an emotional issue, as identified by emotion mode in circuit. The issue involved a male, as determined by circuit-localization of kidney 27 on the right side, but the person was not identified by the context of the emotion. Therefore Krebs asked the woman the following question: 'Is this person someone you are currently interacting with?' The reply was 'No!' Therefore Krebs discounted the possibility that her husband might be the person involved in this emotional issue. Further investigation failed to reveal who the male that was causing stress in her life might be (he even tried 'her lover'). Finally, Krebs asked another question: 'Is this person a member of your immediate family?' The answer was 'Yes', and because she had only daughters, it left her husband as the only male possible. Then Krebs asked, 'Is this male your husband?' to which her biocomputer indicated 'yes!'

This seemed to represent a paradox, as the biocomputer had stated it was not someone she was interacting with, and yet it was her husband. Krebs then asked the woman verbally, 'How can it be your husband when your biocomputer says you are currently not interacting with him?' And she stated that he was in the USA, 12,000 miles away, and that she had indeed had little interaction with him in the past week and no physical interaction at all! The biocomputer was literally answering the question. When Krebs asked the direct question 'Is it your husband?' it gave him the correct answer, 'yes', but when asked the question that *inferred* it could be her husband, the answer was 'no' because she literally was not interacting with him. This highlights how literal the biocomputer is in answering questions. Indeed, it is very much like an actual computer: it does not infer, it does not get the gist, it does not get the implied meaning; it only answers directly in a very literal way.

Therefore when asking 'yes' and 'no' questions, you need to literally have only one of two possibilities: 'yes' or 'no'. If the question is open-ended, like the one Krebs asked, you will often be lead down the garden path, because the muscle has to do something and it can only lock or unlock. If it unlocks, the monitor will interpret this as 'no', whereas if it locks the monitor will interpret this as 'yes', but neither of these interpretations is correct, and therefore the monitor will be deluded into making incorrect associations and interpretations of the information provided by the muscle response.

Therefore while 'yes' and 'no' questions may have a role to play in kinesiology, they have to be used extremely precisely and with overt caution to be sure there is only a single possible answer.

Challenging

Challenging is the term used to describe making a statement to the client or having the client make the statement out loud and then observing the indicator response. The indicator response is the result of a frequency match with whatever issues are involved in that person's conscious and subconscious association with the statement made. As with stating 'yes' and 'no', the subconscious scans relevant past experiences, giving more weight to those experiences that affected physical or ego survival.

The advantage of challenging over 'yes' and 'no' questions is that there will be a response only if the statement creates a frequency match with the energetic pattern of the imbalance being addressed and is therefore relevant. Therefore questions that are either irrelevant or do not generate a frequency match for the imbalance do not change the indicator. In a sense, the biocomputer is now stating that the challenge is not a frequency match for the stated issue and hence not of interest.

So when there is a frequency match between the stated challenge, for example 'mother', 'father' and a particular negative past or present stressor, the indicator will change, disclosing the existence of this stressor. However, if on making the challenge statement there is no indicator change, it confirms that this challenge statement is not related to any relevant stress.

SECTION V

Client assessment

A kinesiology session usually involves the kinesiologist working in a clinic room with the client lying fully clothed on a massage table. This section opens with a discussion of the important factors involved in working with clients, including what constitutes ethical behavior and how to take a thorough client history. It then discusses how to assess the client and determine the most appropriate treatment to apply, a process completed every time a client comes for a kinesiology session.

Before beginning the kinesiology balance itself, the practitioner must perform a series of manual pre-checks to ensure the accuracy of the information the client's 'biocomputer' can provide. There are a large number of pre-checks that are used in different Energetic Kinesiology modalities; however, we have included just five pre-checks that we believe are essential in order for the biocomputer to provide accurate and reliable biofeedback.

After completing the pre-checks, the kinesiology balance itself begins, and we have termed the first phase of the balance *setting the context*. Kinesiology by its very nature is totally context-dependent, and the results of a kinesiology balance are directly related to the initial context set for that balance. There are several approaches to setting the context for a session, and all these are discussed in this section.

Pain is one of the most common presenting issues or contexts observed in kinesiology. There are three primary factors that must be assessed:

1. the intensity of the pain, usually assessed on a subjective 0-10 scale
2. the quality of the pain (throbbing, aching, stabbing, etc.)
3. the location of the pain.

This assessment of the pain is extremely important, as one or all three of these factors may or may not change during the session, and hence the client may say, 'The pain's still there!' But is it the same intensity of pain, the same type of pain and/or is it in the same location? Once resolved, it is hard to remember the original pain and what it was like, unless it was benchmarked in the initial client assessment.

Chapter 19

WORKING WITH CLIENTS

Legal and ethical behavior

As an Energetic Kinesiologist, you will need to be aware of the regulatory guidelines that govern the complementary health care industry in your country. It is your responsibility to access and follow all legislation that is relevant to your work as an Energetic Kinesiologist. This will usually include guidelines relating to occupational health and safety, infection control, privacy and confidentiality of information, and child protection, as well as all guidelines relating to working with clients.

Sample codes of ethics

The following code of ethics is taken from the American Energy Kinesiology Association website: In my willingness to promote awareness of ethics within the energy kinesiology community, and myself, I will:

- Conduct business and professional activities with integrity, in a professional, honest, and fair manner.
- Perform only those services for which I am qualified and represent my education, certifications, professional affiliations and other qualifications honestly. I will make a referral, when appropriate and if possible.
- Acknowledge the inherent worth and individuality of each person by honoring clients' and students' religious, spiritual, health, education, political and social views, and life choices, not discriminating against race, creed, color, gender, and sexual orientation.
- Accept responsibility to maintain my physical, mental, emotional and spiritual well being.
- Refrain from diagnosing, prescribing, or treating any medical disorder unless licensed to do so.
- Strive for professional excellence through ongoing assessment of personal strengths,

limitations and effectiveness, and by continued education and training.
- Abide by all applicable laws governing Energy Kinesiology. I shall consider working for the repeal or revision of laws detrimental to the legitimate practice of Energy Kinesiology.
- Acknowledge the confidential nature of the professional relationship with my client. I will respect each client's right to privacy, disclosing confidential information only when either authorized by the client or mandated by law.
- Respect the professional status of other Energy Kinesiologists and other health care practitioners.

Another code of ethics is taken from the Australian Kinesiology Association Web site.[1]

- I set a credible, honorable and ethical example for my profession as a kinesiologist.
- I conduct my work with the highest integrity.
- I honor the confidentiality of my clients.
- I encourage clients to be self-responsible in realizing their own truth.
- I honor my financial responsibilities by being fair and honest in all areas of my business.
- I regard as imperative the financial success, stability and growth of my business in alignment with this code of ethics.
- To my client, I do not defame or criticize other models of medicine or healing.
- I acknowledge the need to refer my clients to other professionals whenever necessary.
- I continue to expand and update my kinesiology skills.
- I continue to explore my own self-development through kinesiology and other modalities.
- I recognize the importance of my role as a professional kinesiologist and continue to

promote the expansion of kinesiology in the community.

Responsibilities of practitioner and client

The responsibilities of the practitioner and the client within the session strategy need to be clarified.

Practitioner responsibilities may include:

- appropriate hygienic behavior
- appropriate client relations
- appropriate sexual behavior
- commitment to the treatment plan
- providing treatment and follow-up
- discussing relevant contraindications or possible complicating factors to treatment
- reviewing the treatment plan
- adjusting the treatment plan when necessary.
- Client responsibilities may include:
- following advice during and after sessions
- sharing with the practitioner all known information regarding their presenting issues
- advising the practitioner of any relevant contraindications or possible complicating factors to treatment
- advising the practitioner of compliance issues
- commitment to the treatment plan.

Maintaining integrity

It is important that you always maintain a high level of integrity in your kinesiology practice. This means that in every interaction with a client you need to ensure you are motivated by what is in your client's best interests and not by what is in your own interests. This is often a difficult task and requires you to always reflect on your actions, being honest with yourself. If on reflection you find yourself to have been lacking in integrity, have the courage to learn from the experience and alter your future actions accordingly.

Being always honest is often a difficult task, and it is important to keep the following points in mind.

- Have the courage to be honest.
- If you do not know the answer to something, say so.
- Do not make up answers or give an answer just to placate someone.

- Value honesty over being nice.
- Being honest does not mean being critical or cruel.
- Always deliver honest advice with loving kindness.

Communicating with clients

To ensure that the client receives maximum benefit from their kinesiology sessions, it is important that the lines of communication remain open. A client will feel safer and return more often for treatment if they feel that they can ask questions whenever they need to and that those questions will be answered promptly and clearly.

During kinesiology sessions, you need to answer client queries with clarity, using the appropriate language. To aid in this, keep the following points in mind.

- Remember that all queries are about the client; do not take them personally.
- Avoid using kinesiology jargon that clients may not be familiar with.
- Avoid using new age jargon and concepts, which may confuse or offend clients.
- Do not presume prior knowledge on the part of the client.
- Assume the client knows nothing about kinesiology and you are less likely to confuse them.
- Assume the client knows nothing about counseling, self-awareness, personal development, spiritual evolution or any other paths or models.
- Respect every client's personal belief system, and make sure you frame your questions and explanations in terms of their belief system and not yours.
- Respect the client's right to understand the process you are taking them through.
- Respect the client's right to forget things you have told them before!

Responding to reactions

You need to ask clients to monitor their reactions during sessions and to provide you with feedback when necessary. In addition, it is important that you maintain client-focused attention throughout the session and respond to any reactions that you observe. Responses to reactions during a session may include adjusting application intensity or the positioning of the client, discussing responses with the client, and adhering to clinic guidelines for response to accidents and emergencies, using first aid procedures.

If a client communicates severe reactions that are not usual to experience during kinesiology treatment, you need to evaluate whether you have the experience and/or expertise to help them. If not, it is essential that you refer them to the appropriate health care practitioner immediately. Should the client need immediate medical care, do not delay in contacting the appropriate local or emergency service.

Reference

1. Australian Kinesiology Association 2013, *Code of Practice* [online] Available at: <http://www.aka.asn.au/Resources/Documents/doc2.pdf> (accessed 13 August 2013).
   Energy Kinesiology Association, Code of Ethics [online]. Available at: <http://www.energyk.org/index.php/trainingworkshops/27-pages/about-us/9-code-of-ethics> (accessed 20 August 2013)

Chapter 20

TAKING A CLIENT HISTORY

Initial discussion

When beginning a session with a client, you must clearly establish their purpose for the session. As the practitioner, it is your responsibility to ensure you clearly understand the client's presenting issue and have gathered all information necessary to effectively deal with their issue. You also have a responsibility to explore the client's expectations of the session and clarify their expectations to ensure they are realistic.

In these discussions and exploration of the client's presenting issues, it is extremely important that you actively listen to your client. This may take the form of feeding back information they have said to clarify that information. For instance, if the client says, 'Every morning I wake up I have back pain', you may then say back to them, 'I understand that in the morning you have pain in your back'. This may lead to clarifying the nature and location of the pain, or maybe even extremely relevant information that they had failed to indicate on the client form, such as, 'Yes, ever since my operation on my back...' This is obviously extremely pertinent information for the session that you will provide to them!

It is also very important for you to ask them if there are any other issues going on in their life, perhaps even of a very different nature, that they feel may impact on their presenting issue. You should also question them about information you feel may be relevant from their health history.

The client should be aware of the model of health care that you are providing. In this model, both the practitioner and the client have a role to play. It is not a model of the practitioner 'fixing' or 'curing' the client's issue but rather an interactive process of unveiling the basis and causal factors of the presenting issue. The client needs to be aware of the fact that they are actively participating in their health care and may be required to take certain actions, such as avoiding certain foods or performing particular exercises to assist in the resolution of their issues.

You must also clearly explain the techniques you will use and the limits of your services.

Determining a client's eligibility

Once you have clarified the client's purpose and expectations, you need to determine the client's eligibility to receive your service. If the client fits the eligibility requirements of the clinic, then you can begin the consultation.

You must refer the client to another health care professional if:

- their needs are beyond the services you are able to provide
- they want diagnosis and treatment for a possible medical condition (or conditions)
- they want to be tested medically to determine a pathological cause or to establish parameters beyond the scope of your practice, for example pregnancy, blood count, blood cholesterol or blood sugar.
- they present with a known or possible infectious disease suggested by fever, nausea and/or lethargy
- their symptoms do not have a logical explanation and they have not been medically evaluated
- the client is underage and does not have parental consent
- in your opinion, their needs will best be met by referral to another health care professional.

Obtaining a client's history

When taking a client's history, you need to ensure that you seek information in a respectful way. Your manner should make the client feel comfortable enough to share their personal information, while always maintaining a professional relationship. You should make all enquiries in a purposeful, systematic and diplomatic manner.

As you take the client's history, the information must be recorded in an accurate, relevant and well-organized manner. Once collected, you must ensure that you manage all information in a confidential and secure way so that you maintain compliance with all the regulatory requirements of the area in which you operate.

While there is a lot of different information that you could collect when taking a client history, what information you include and how you organize that information will depend on how you prefer to operate and/or the policies of the clinic in which you work. An example of a client history form is shown in Figure 20.1.

Information you could collect when taking a case history includes:

- date of presentation
- identifying personal details
- source of referral
- presenting issue or reason for session
- subjective evaluation of current issue
- previous occurrence of current issue
- maternal or paternal genetic predispositions
  - general state of health
  - physical
  - emotional
  - sensitivities
  - diet and appetite
  - sleep patterns
  - bowel and urinary habits
  - exercise
  - lifestyle
  - menstrual cycle
- childhood and adult illnesses
- accidents, injuries or operations
- vaccinations
- root canal work
- hospitalizations
- occupational history and environment
- family history and relationships
- cultural background

- religious beliefs and whether the client is currently practising
- other current medical or alternative health care
- vibrational remedies, medications or supplements (current and previous) and their perceived side effects
- known allergies to medications or supplements
- social lifestyle, including social drug usage
- primary health care provider.

Identifying inhibitory factors

Before beginning a health assessment or session, you need to identify any factors that are likely to inhibit your work with the client. These could include language difficulties, an inability to understand the principles of kinesiology, other treatments and/or activities they are undertaking, disabilities, emotional trauma, lack of privacy or focus because of additional people being present, and cultural or gender factors.

If you identify any inhibitory factors, then it is necessary to implement strategies to minimize the impact of these factors, if that is possible. For example, if a client has a disability you may need to adjust your muscle-monitoring technique, use surrogate muscles during the balance, or avoid changes of position on the table that may prove difficult or uncomfortable for the client. If a client has language difficulties, you may need to have a family member or friend present to provide translation between yourself and the client. Or if the client's presenting issue is a very personal, gender-related issue that the client may be uncomfortable discussing or having treated by you, you may need to refer them to another same-gender practitioner.

At all times, it is very important to be sensitive to a client's cultural and religious context, for example age recession takes you to preconception. This does not mean it is a past life issue, but only that this issue has a contextual component that originated before their conception. If the client's belief system contains the concept of past lives, then you may suggest that this issue has a past life component. However, if the client has strong religious beliefs that include the traditional Christian

Example of a Case History Form

PERSONAL PROFILE

Name: _____ Date: _____

DOB: _____ Referred by: _____

Phone: home _____ work _____ mobile _____

Address: _____ Suburb: _____

Postcode: _____ email: _____

Occupation: _____ How long in this work: _____

Family GP: _____ Other health professional: _____

Siblings (name, age, gender): _____

_____ Your place in family: _____

Spouse/Partner's name: _____

Children (name, age, gender): _____

Cultural background: _____

Religion (are you currently practicing?): _____

HEALTH HISTORY

Past trauma (inc. date, age): _____

_____

Past surgery (inc. date, age): _____

_____

Childhood and other illnesses (inc. date, age): _____

_____

CURRENT LIFESTYLE

Current medication: _____

Current supplements: _____

Food preferences: 'meat & 3 veg'   vegetarian   vegan   macrobiotic   high protein
(*circle one*)   wheat free   gluten free   dairy free other: _____

Daily intake: coffee _____   tea _____   alcohol _____   water _____

Frequency of: Bowel movement _____   Passing urine _____   Hours of sleep per night: _____

Exercise: _____

Figure 20.1 **Client history form.** An example.

PHYSICAL PAIN *(tick relevant boxes and describe the pain in each area)*

☐ Neck & shoulder: _____

☐ Back: _____

☐ Knee & Feet: _____

☐ Elbows & Hands: _____

☐ Any other pain: _____

OVERALL WELLBEING

Energy Level: High ☐   Medium ☐   Low ☐   Variable ☐

Emotions: High ☐   Medium ☐   Low ☐   Variable ☐

Describe your relationship to the following area of your life

Emotional / mental state: _____

Finances: _____

Relationship with partner: _____

Parents: _____

Siblings: _____

Work: _____

Self esteem / personal power: _____

Reasons why you are here (inc. history of current problem): _____
_____
_____
_____
_____

Is there anything else the practitioner should know? _____

❖ I have stated all conditions that I am aware of and this information is true and accurate.

❖ I agree to keep the practitioner updated as to any changes in my medical profile and understand that there should be no liability on the practitioner's part should I forget to do so.

❖ I understand that kinesiology only balances energy and it does not treat disease.

❖ I understand that kinesiology should not be construed as a substitute for medical examination, diagnosis, or treatment of any medical condition, and that I should see a physician, or other qualified medical specialist for any physical or mental ailment I am aware of.

❖ I understand there is a cancellation policy. I may cancel or change my appointment time up to 24 hours in advance of my session. If I do not show up for my appointment, I will be charged a penalty fee.

Signed: _____   Date: _____

or Islamic belief that you experience only one life, you must reframe the need to explore information originating before conception in a way that is acceptable to their beliefs.

For instance, preconception is indicated in an age recession and you know from your client history that the person is a devout Christian. You can reframe this concept by explaining that there is information necessary to assist the resolution of their presenting issue that has its origin before their birth. Indeed, we are all the result of many past lives: your grandfather's life, his grandfather's life, etc. Genetic mutations or even deeply ingrained personality traits can be passed on from generation to generation, and these inherited patterns may be the source or a component of the client's presenting issue. Reframing in this way allows the client to feel comfortable with the concept that there is information needed that pre-dates their conception and birth.

Chapter 21

ASSESSING THE CLIENT

Preparing for assessment

Throughout the health assessment process, make sure you respect the client's boundaries. Everyone has different levels of comfort, so be sure to give clients permission to openly express their discomfort any time during a session. Then make sure you adjust your application of techniques whenever a client communicates discomfort. This includes adjusting your questioning if a client is uncomfortable with disclosing some personal information. It is important to take care when touching acupoints in potentially sensitive areas, and in these cases it may be necessary to have the client touch these points.

Before beginning a health assessment, you need to prepare the client for the session. The first step is to seek feedback from the client on their levels of comfort, comprehension and participation. It is also necessary for you to inform clients that whenever they experience discomfort they should immediately communicate this to you.

Once the client is settled, you can begin performing the kinesiology pre-checks. While performing all assessment techniques, make sure the client understands what is happening by explaining clearly what you are doing and by giving them ample opportunity for questions and feedback.

Informed consent

It is essential that you have your client sign an informed consent form before beginning any work with them. In addition, you also want to obtain verbal consent before conducting the health assessment and/or performing any technique that may be uncomfortable or invasive for some clients. In the case of a minor or ward of the state, you must ensure that an appropriate adult be present during all assessment and treatment.

Please note that clients have the legal right to withdraw consent for treatment at any time during your work with them.

Potential sensitivities

While performing a health assessment, you need to anticipate potential sensitivities of the client and adapt your approach accordingly to take these into account. Potential sensitivities may include gender, ethnicity, language, religious beliefs, cultural heritage, sexuality, mobility, presenting disease state and personal history.

For example, a client may have physical pain that severely restricts their ability to move on the table. You will need to adjust your methods to ensure that you do not cause them unnecessary pain or discomfort while working with them. Alternatively, a client may have a cultural background in which they do not discuss their feelings openly; again, you will need to adjust your methods to ensure the client does not feel uncomfortable. In addition, a client who has experienced physical or sexual abuse in their past may find being touched on some areas of their body very uncomfortable, and you need to accommodate their sensitivity.

Assessment methods

Throughout the client assessment, you need to maintain clinical and practitioner hygiene. An example of this would be if assessing the client involves contact with any area of the body that may be unclean or infectious. In this case, you would need to wash or disinfect your hands before proceeding with the assessment or treatment.

If a client presents with an issue that has been investigated by a medical practitioner or another health care professional, you need to request that they bring all the information relating to the issue with them to their appointment. Information that a client may provide you with includes diagnostic reports from a specialist, X-rays or other scans, blood test results, hair analysis results, reports containing details of their issue, or a referral note from another complementary health care practitioner. Reports from another practitioner could take the form of a naturopathic report or a homeopathic assessment.

Once you have obtained client consent and prepared for any potential sensitivities, then you are ready for the health assessment to begin. The client may be assessed via:

- discussion and/or questioning
- indicator muscle monitoring
- stress challenge with an indicator muscle
- pain assessment
- observation of body posture
- a range of motion tests
- determining their current ability to perform an activity
- stress challenge against a goal statement
- stress challenge against a nutrient or toxin
- any method in which you have been trained to a competent standard.

To determine the scope of the health assessment you will perform with your client, you need to combine all the information you have gathered from the client history form with your initial discussions and observations of the client. Results of all assessments should be recorded in the case notes in an accurate and well-organized manner so that they can be interpreted readily by other health professionals.

Identifying contraindications

Once you have assessed the client, you need to identify any contraindications to the kinesiology session and modify your session strategy accordingly. Contraindications to kinesiology balances and possible complicating factors may include:

- the presence of an infectious disease, as suggested by fever, nausea and lethargy, until a diagnosis has been received from a medical practitioner
- acute surgical and medical conditions, such as cardiac arrest and loss of consciousness

- traumatic injuries or conditions requiring immediate medical attention
- pain that has not been medically investigated
- swelling, inflammation, lumps and tissue changes that have not been medically investigated
- rashes and changes in the skin that have not been medically investigated
- severe mood alterations, for example depression and anxiety, unless the client has sought medical treatment
- bleeding and bruising
- nausea, vomiting or diarrhea
- temperature (hot or cold)
- sudden loss of weight that has not been medically investigated.

This list of contraindications is meant only as general guidelines for working as an Energetic Kinesiologist. It is important that you are informed of the rules and regulations that apply in your country and the area in which you practice.

Planning treatment

While you are assessing the client, it is necessary to analyze and interpret the information you receive so that you can prepare an appropriate treatment plan for them. This process involves correlating the information you have gathered in the assessment process with the client's case history. You will need to take into consideration the client's presenting issue and desired outcomes, how long they have had the issue, the severity of the issue and its impact on the client, the client's age and mobility, all information gathered through assessment of the client, the client's progress since beginning treatment, and any effects from previous sessions, as well as their ability and willingness to follow your suggestions and make changes in their life.

In addition, you must be able to recognize the signs and symptoms of the client's issue and determine if they are indications for balancing or contraindications. When contraindications are identified, you will need to refer the client to another health care professional or wait until their condition has been medically investigated.

Once you have gathered all the health information from your client, you will need to assign priorities to it in consultation with the client, and determine which issue is the priority to be balanced in the current session. Clients always have a purpose or reason for seeking kinesiology treatment. It is important to remain focused on the *client's* desired outcomes throughout each session and ensure you select techniques that are appropriate for meeting those outcomes. A treatment plan is formulated to provide the client with their desired outcomes within the time you have allocated, therefore any unnecessary deviations from that plan may result in the client's expectations not being met.

Once you have decided on the order of balancing that you intend to follow for this client's issues, you will need to discuss with the client your rationale for the treatment plan. It is important that clients are fully informed of the treatment they will be receiving, because it is their life and/or health that will be affected. Throughout all discussions, make sure the client has ample opportunity to ask questions, and respond clearly to all their enquiries using language the client will understand.

Finally, your treatment plan should be recorded in the client's case notes and organized in such a way that it can be readily interpreted by other kinesiology practitioners.

While muscle monitoring is always used to guide you during a session, it is still essential for you to use techniques that follow your treatment plan and are appropriate for the client's presenting complaint. Going off track from your treatment plan just because 'the muscle monitoring told me to do it' is not appropriate. As a health care practitioner, you must be able to determine when muscle monitoring is guiding you in an appropriate direction for your client's desired outcomes and when the muscle response is inappropriate. Remember: an indicator muscle can respond only

to the questions you ask, and as the practitioner it is your responsibility to ask questions that are appropriate for the treatment plan you have discussed with the client.

Evaluating progress

At the beginning of each session, you need to evaluate progress with the client. Evaluating progress includes discussion of presenting symptoms and changes since the last session, the duration and location of symptoms, sensations, and progress toward desired outcomes.

The effects of the previous session need to be identified at the beginning of each session and recorded in the client's case notes. Effects of previous sessions may be as simple as 'Client is better', 'Client is worse', 'No change' or 'New state is emerging'. Alternatively, the client may have experienced more complex effects that have had a significant impact on their life, either positive or negative.

Keeping in mind the client's progress and the effects of previous sessions, you then need to review previous treatment plans and decide whether the client is progressing as expected toward their desired outcomes or not. If progress is as expected, you would simply continue with your plan for the client. However, if progress is not going as expected, then you need to evaluate what changes to make.

If a client is not progressing as you expected, or new information is provided by the client, then you may need to make changes to your original treatment plan. These changes may include using a different method to set the context of the session, altering the techniques you apply or giving the client different strategies to follow between sessions.

Changes you make to the treatment plan need to be discussed with the client and negotiated to ensure that optimal outcomes are achieved from the kinesiology treatment.

Chapter 22

CONDUCTING PRE-CHECKS

As with any computer, before you can effectively use the 'biocomputer' there is a series of pre-checks that must be performed. When you turn your computer on, the very first thing it does is go through a whole series of pre-checks of all the systems operating within the computer. If any of the systems do not pass these pre-checks, you are not allowed to operate the computer until the basic operating systems are in working order.

Unfortunately, in the human body a kinesiologist cannot just press the belly button and wait for the person's eyes to blink to know the biocomputer is 'online' and ready to provide accurate data. Instead, there are a series of manual pre-checks that must be performed to ensure the accuracy of the information the biocomputer is providing.

There are a large number of possible systems checks that could be made before using the biocomputer. Indeed, different Energetic Kinesiology modalities use different combinations of these. However, we feel that the following five systems checks are essential in order for the biocomputer to provide accurate and reliable biofeedback.

The five primary systems checks we deem essential are: 1, the relative degree of hydration of the tissues of the body; 2, a concept in kinesiology called *electromagnetic switching*, represented in the brain by polarity reversals in which output becomes 'switched' and therefore feedback is not reliable; 3, a check for the stability of the Central and Governing Vessels, as these midline meridians are involved in the stability of the other 12 primary meridians and hence the energetic stability of the body as a whole; 4, the state of ionization of the body, which if unstable may cause irrelevant indicator changes when circuit locating acupoints; and 5, a check for the stability of the pause lock mechanisms, as imbalances within these mechanisms may cause irrelevant data to be included in circuits.

Hydration

For optimum performance, clarity of thinking and proper mind–body integration, the body depends greatly on having adequate hydration, that is, enough water. Without pure water, the body's electromagnetic and physiological systems are impaired, for instance the lymphatic drainage and organ function are impaired. The body needs sufficient water to hydrate the tissues so that they maintain their proper electromagnetic potential and physiological function.

Water is essential for all metabolic processes, because it is the primary solvent in the body and is necessary for electrical, electromagnetic and neurophysiological signaling. It is also essential that the body be adequately hydrated both to be able to accurately access information and for the indicator muscle to operate properly.

Water and hydrogen bonding

Each water molecule consists of two hydrogen atoms and one oxygen atom. These three atoms are bonded together by the sharing of electrons, and this type of bonding is classified as *covalent bonding*. Furthermore, water molecules are bonded to each other by a special form of intermolecular bonding called *hydrogen bonding*, which is extremely important in biological systems. Hydrogen bonding is a special form of dipole–dipole attraction, and it is found in systems where a hydrogen atom is bonded to an atom of oxygen, nitrogen or fluorine.

Because oxygen is highly electronegative, that is, has a strong affinity for electrons, while hydrogen has relatively low electronegativity, the resulting bond is very *polar*, and the shared electrons are strongly attracted toward the oxygen atom. In contrast, in hydrogen gas (H_2) there are two identical hydrogen atoms and the electrons are shared equally, making it a *non-polar* molecule. In water molecules, the shared electrons spend much more time around the large oxygen atom and less time around the very tiny hydrogen atoms. This makes the oxygen end of the molecule slightly more negative, as electrons have a negative charge (see Figure 22.1).

These partial charges on water molecules mean that the negative oxygen ends of molecules will attract the positive hydrogen end of other water molecules. This attraction between positive hydrogen ends and negative oxygen ends of water molecules causes them to align with each other and is called a *hydrogen bond*. This is much like moving the north pole of a magnet past the south pole of another magnet will cause the south pole to move to align with the north pole. So the hydrogen bond is not a physical bond but only an attractive force. Each individual hydrogen bond is weak, but thousands together are powerful enough to control the shape of proteins and hold big molecules such as DNA together.

Because of its polarity, water spontaneously arranges itself into interlocking patterns as the negative hydrogen ends of two water molecules attract the positive oxygen end of another water molecule. This pattern repeats with other water molecules, creating an interlocking sheet of water molecules, which when located at the surface is called the *surface tension* of water (see Figure 22.2). Thus, surface tension created by the hydrogen bonding of water molecules is so strong that many insects, such as water striders, can literally walk on water. This surface tension also accounts for capillary action, the tendency for water to climb up the tip of the towel hanging into the sink and then drip out of the other end onto the floor.

Water can have a number of three-dimensional patterns supported by hydrogen bonding, which have only recently been described by Roy and Tiller.[1] Roy and Tiller propose that these

a. water molecule showing electron orbits

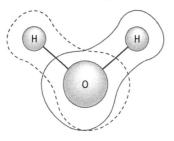

b. water molecule showing partial charges

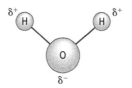

H = hydrogen
O = oxygen
δ^+ = delta + partial charge on the hydrogen atoms due to shared electrons spending more time around the bigger oxygen atom
δ^- = delta − partial charge on the oxygen atom due to its much larger size such that the shared electrons spend much more time around the bigger oxygen atom

Figure 22.1 The water molecule.
a, Water molecule showing electron orbits. Pathways of electrons orbit both the tiny hydrogen atoms and the much larger oxygen atom. Shared electrons spend considerably more time moving around the large oxygen end of the molecule, making it slightly negative, and less time moving around the hydrogen end, making it slightly positive.
b, Water molecule showing partial delta charges. Water molecules have an uneven sharing of electrons such that the hydrogen end of the molecule develops a partial positive charge (δ^+) and the oxygen end of the molecule develops a partial negative charge (δ^-). This makes water a *polar* solvent, giving it important unique properties.

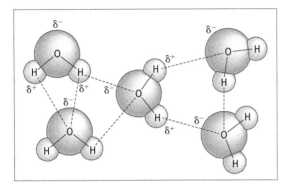

Figure 22.2 Hydrogen bonds in water. Because of the partial delta positive and negative (δ^+ and δ^-) charges of water molecules, they spontaneously arrange into interlocking patterns as the negative oxygen end of one water molecule is attracted to the positive hydrogen end of another water molecule via hydrogen bonding (dashed lines). H, hydrogen atom; O, oxygen atom.

three-dimensional structures of water can provide a mechanism for holding or storing information and may be the basis of homeopathy and the memory of water described by Emoto.[2]

Spheres of hydration

Amino acids are polar organic molecules with a partial positive charge on the carboxylic acid end and a partial negative charge on the amine end. These partial charges occur because the two oxygen atoms pull the electrons closer to the acid end, leaving the amine end with a partial positive charge (see Figure 22.3).

Amino acids form long chains called proteins by joining together with peptide bonds. In the peptide bond, the carboxylic acid end of one amino acid gives up an OH$^-$ and the amine end of another amino acid gives up an H$^+$. This forms a covalent bond between the carboxylic acid group and the amine group, the peptide bond, while the H$^+$ and OH$^-$ join to form water (H_2O) (see Figure 22.4). Proteins formed by a series of peptide bonds therefore have a series of partial positive and negative charges along their length, slightly positive at each carboxylic acid group and slightly negative at each amine group (see Figure 22.5).

The intracellular fluid is composed mostly of water, but this water interacts strongly with the proteins inside the cell because of the partial

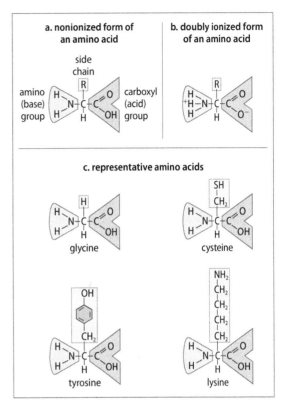

Figure 22.3 a, Non-ionized form of an amino acid. Amino acids vary in the number of carbon (C) atoms between the amine group (NH_2) on one end and the carboxylic acid group (COOH) on the other end. They also vary in the presence of side chains (R)—from a single H atom to long chains of CH_2 groups to aromatic rings. **b**, Ionized form of an amino acid. An amino acid that has been dissolved in water loses the H ion (H$^+$) of the carboxylic acid to water, leaving the carboxylic group (COO$^-$) slightly negative and the amine group (NH_2) slightly more positive, or it may even double ionize, taking on an additional hydrogen ion (H$^+$) on the amine end and increasing the positive charge and therefore the negative charge of the carboxyl end. **c**, Representative examples.

charges distributed along the length of the protein. The polar water molecules align themselves with the partial charges along the proteins: two hydrogen atoms facing each negative charge on the protein, and one oxygen atom facing each positive charge on the protein. Then the next layer of water molecules orients to this first layer, with the two hydrogen atoms of one water molecule aligning to the oxygen atom of another water molecule to form a second layer of water molecules. This layering of

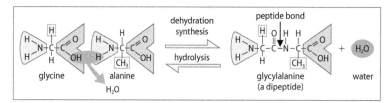

Figure 22.4 Dehydration synthesis: the formation of the peptide bond. The carboxyl group of one amino acid gives up one hydroxyl group (OH⁻), and the amine group of another amino acid gives up one H ion (H⁺), resulting in the formation of a covalent bond between the carboxyl and amine groups. The result is the formation of a peptide bond between two amino acids and one molecule of water (H_2O). C, carbon atom; N, nitrogen atom; R, side chain.

oriented water molecules continues until the positive and negative charges of the protein are totally covered. These layers of charge-oriented water molecules around the protein are termed the *spheres of hydration* (see Figure 22.6).

Structure of cytosol and role of hydrogen bonding

In the cytosol (cell fluid), the water molecules between two proteins surrounded by their spheres of hydration is relatively unstructured and therefore quite fluid. It forms a layer of lubricant between the two protein molecules, which are then free to fluidly slide past or over each other. Thus, when the skin is stretched and released it rapidly returns to its original shape.

As water is removed from cells because of dehydration, the water molecules are first removed from the lubricant layer of unstructured water molecules, then progressively more and more from the water molecules forming the sphere of hydration around the proteins. This progressively exposes the charged sites on the proteins (see Figure 22.7).

Soon, the charged sites on one protein begin to 'see' or respond to the charged sites on the other protein and begin to form hydrogen bonds directly with the other protein. This now causes the two proteins to stick to each other and thus resist movement. So instead of sliding smoothly over or past each other with their spheres of hydration covering the charge sites, they stick and slide only slowly. When this is in skin, the skin is

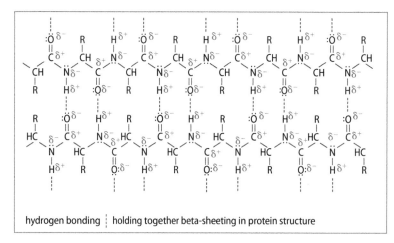

hydrogen bonding ┊ holding together beta-sheeting in protein structure

Figure 22.5 Primary and secondary structure of proteins via hydrogen bonding. The primary structure of proteins is simply a chain of amino acids linked by peptide bonds. Because of the distribution of delta positive and delta negative charges along the length of the protein molecule, proteins spontaneously form secondary structures as the delta negative and positive charges of two proteins align themselves via hydrogen bonding. The simplest structure is beta sheeting between adjacent proteins, where the delta positive charges of one protein molecule directly align with the delta negative charge of another protein molecule, creating a folded sheet–like structure. While each individual hydrogen bond is weak, thousands between two proteins create strong tissues.

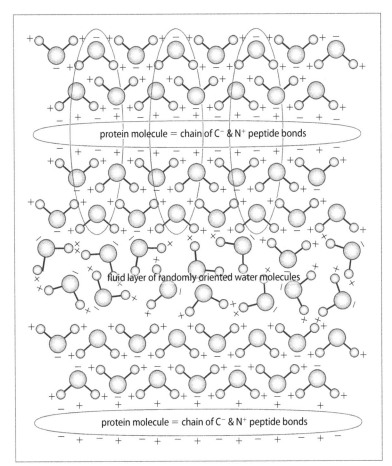

Figure 22.6 Spheres of hydration. Polar water molecules are oriented by charge around charged proteins because of the delta negative charge of the carboxylic (COO$^-$) and delta positive charge of the amine groups (NH$_3^+$). The first few layers of water molecules are highly structured, forming a sphere of hydration, but as the protein's charge sites become increasingly covered, the water molecules become progressively more unstructured, and the unstructured water between the spheres of hydration of two proteins acts like a lubricant between the protein molecules, allowing them to slide easily past each other.

now stretched instead of snapping back into place; you can actually see the skin form lumps and only slowly return to its original shape.

Hair tug test

Free nerve endings are found infiltrating between the cells. When the body is well hydrated, molecules slide smoothly and easily past each other, but as the proteins lose their layers of hydration they begin to interact. The molecules now resist movement and pull or stretch these free nerve endings, firing a volley of nerve impulses into the central nervous system. This spurious and erratic input to the spinal segment interferes with the muscle proprioceptive feedback and causes an indicator change if the muscle is monitored immediately after stretching the skin. This is the basis of the hair tug test.

Why pull the hair? The roots of the hair have free nerve endings wrapped around them, one of the reasons it hurts to pull on hair. Hair is also more convenient to tug on rather than trying to grab skin. When the tissues are dehydrated, pulling on the hair both stretches the skin and activates numerous free nerve endings, creating a strong burst of erratic input to the central nervous system.

Certainly one of the most incredible observations in kinesiology is to have someone perform this hair tug test and find that they are dehydrated via the indicator change, then to drink a glass of water and find that they now test hydrated! How can you be hydrated in less than a minute?

The sensors 'reading' the osmolarity (viscosity) of the blood are located in the circumventricular organs of the hypothalamus that directly contact the blood. So as your water volume decreases with dehydration, these hypothalamic sensors 'know'

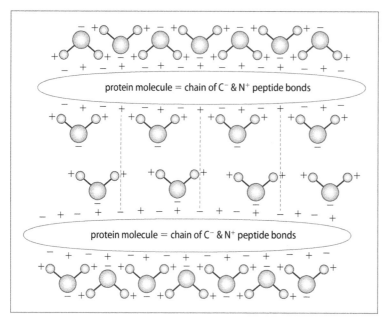

Figure 22.7 Dehydration: the loss of water molecules from the cell fluid. As dehydration progresses, fluid water between the spheres of hydration is lost first, followed by progressive loss of water molecules from the sphere of hydration. As the structured water molecules covering the charges on the protein molecules are lost, the delta charges on the proteins begin to 'see' each other, causing the proteins to stick together, which pulls on the free nerve endings between the proteins when the skin is stretched. This sends a volley of electrostatic signals into the spinal segments that inhibits the indicator muscle. C, carbon atom; N, nitrogen atom.

how many milliliters of water you are deficient by. As you drink water, the capillaries of the roof of the mouth directly beneath the hypothalamus absorb water and immediately relay this information to the circumventricular organs monitoring osmolarity. By the rate of decrease in the viscosity of the blood, these sensors know if you have drunk enough water to satisfy your hydration status.

These sensors can then immediately send an autonomic nerve signal directly to the sphincter muscles controlling the capillary beds of the tissues that are dehydrated. This opening of the sphincters rapidly rehydrates these tissues by taking water out of the blood. However, the hypothalamic sensors will do this only when sufficient water has been drunk to replace the water that will be lost to the tissues from the blood volume.

Hidden dehydration

Whenever some physiological function is imbalanced for a period of time, the body creates a state of physiological compensation to allow it to function at the maximum level it can under the continuing stress. Because this compensation represents a new homeostasis, it will resist change and also often monitor as 'no problem here' when challenged with kinesiology.

For hydration, this compensated state often causes the hydration hair tug test to show no indicator change and thus indicate that all is well. However, tapping along the sagittal suture (the center line of the skull) and immediately challenging by tugging the hair will expose this compensated state.

Directly under the sagittal suture is the longitudinal sagittal sinus, where the arachnoid villi project into this sinus to absorb the cerebrospinal fluid back into the venous system, returning this fluid to the blood. The viscosity of the cerebrospinal fluid in the sagittal sinus is determined by the state of hydration, so if the body is dehydrated it has a higher viscosity. So when you tap, you create a shock wave that stretches the arachnoid villi, which then activates nerve output to the central nervous system. When the blood in the sagittal sinus is relatively fluid, this output does not create enough electrostatic to cause an indicator change. However, when the blood is too viscous this will cause enough electrostatic to cause an indicator change, indicating that there is a hidden state of compensated dehydration. Once this indicator change is entered into pause lock, then the hair tug test will now cause an indicator change showing that there really is a hydration problem in the body.

Types of hydration stress

While often lumped under dehydration, there are several different aspects of hydration that may be problematic.

Overt dehydration stress

Overt dehydration stress is the state in which there is an absolute deficiency of water in the body. It is usually created by not drinking enough water over time, or drinking powerful diuretics such as alcohol and coffee without drinking enough water. This is the type that normally shows with the hair tug test, but it can also be hidden because of physiological compensation.

Hydration stress

Hydration stress results when enough water is consumed but it is not able to be uniformly distributed. In fact, there may be an excess in some tissues while other tissues can be dehydrated and lack enough water for optimum function. This is possible because the autonomic nervous system controls the sphincter muscles controlling the hydrostatic pressure in the capillary beds. When these are too tight, then the blood pressure in the capillary beds is reduced and less water is pushed into the tissues, leaving the tissues partially dehydrated. Because these capillary sphincters are controlled independently, one tissue can be dehydrated while another may be well hydrated, even in the same organ.

While dehydration is generally a body-wide condition, hydration stress often affects only specific tissues; for example, you can have hydration stress in the kidneys. In this case, the kidney tissues can be dehydrated relative to homeostasis, while the body as a whole has sufficient water and thus is not dehydrated. So in hydration stress, it is more a distribution problem than an absolute deficiency problem.

When 'water' is a stress

When just stating the word 'water' causes an indicator change, it may mean that there is an emotional issue blocking water consumption, which may then lead to overt dehydration. Some people are dehydrated only because they almost never drink water—partly because they are just seldom thirsty! Why would you drink water if you are not thirsty?

There are hypothalamic centers for thirst and the desire to drink water, and if these centers are imbalanced then you will not be thirsty or desire to drink water, although you may drink many other fluids, often diuretics! Resetting these hypothalamic centers, or addressing the underlying emotional context, will usually resolve these water problems.

Depending on the type of hydration stress present, there may be different approaches to resolving the hydration problems.

Recommended daily water intake

It is recommended that anyone receiving energy or sending energy drink a minimum of 2 liters of pure water daily. Receiving healing energy, which balances the body and opens and clears energy pathways, may cause toxins to be released into the bloodstream and the lymphatic system, which then need to be flushed out. Also, working with healing energy, which passes through the practitioner to the client, can be dehydrating for the practitioner.

A guide to determine the correct amount of water for the individual is to calculate the body weight in kilograms multiplied by 25, which gives the number of milliliters of water needed per day. Generally speaking, six to eight glasses per day are required under normal conditions. More water should be consumed in hotter climates or conditions and when extra physical demands are made on the body.

Switching

The concept of switching or neurological confusion in body and brain processing was originally developed by Dr George Goodheart in Applied Kinesiology.[3] Even though the switched behaviours had been observed for a long time, there had been no coherent explanation for these confused behaviors. For instance, everyone is familiar with the phenomenon of someone saying 'Turn right!' while pointing vigorously to the left, or when you ask the client to lie down on their back and they lie down on their stomach instead, thinking they are doing exactly what you asked them to do. These are clearly confused switched behaviors.

From the perspective of Applied Kinesiology, this neurological confusion is the result of cranial faults that then perturb the neurological flow to or from the brain. When the cranial fault is corrected, the associated switching is observed to disappear in most cases. In later Energetic Kinesiology modalities, switching is considered an energetic polarity reversal which then results in neurological confusion. When this energetic reversal is corrected by stimulating specific acupoints, such as kidney 27, the associated switching disappears and the person would now say, 'Turn right!' and point to the right.

A person's perception of their body's orientation in space is dependent on vestibular processing and the body maps that they generate in the parietal cortices. The vestibular system provides a point of reference for your orientation in physical space, and the parietal cortex then constructs mental maps that represent this location of you and your body parts in physical space. Normally, the left hemisphere of the brain and right front quadrant of the body have a slightly greater positive than negative charge and hence are said to have a positive polarity. Likewise, the right hemisphere of the brain and the left front quadrant of the body have a slightly greater negative than positive charge and hence are said to have a negative polarity.

Mental processing uses this body polarity with respect to its orientation to the external world. Because the right side of the front of the body is positive, the brain's reference to the right side is to positive polarity, and likewise its reference to the left side of the body is to its negative polarity. However, brain processing can be affected by the orientation of the polarity of the brain and the body. Should this polarity become reversed for any reason, the brain will still reference with respect to the orientation of the polarity rather than to the actual side of the body. Thus when a person says 'Turn left' but is vigorously pointing

toward the right, they have suffered switching with regard to their polarity orientation. In this case, the body's orientation is still to the correct physical side of the body: their right arm is vigorously pointing right but the mental representation that is based on polarity orientation has become reversed and 'Turn left' comes out of their mouth.

In the context of pre-checks, it is only this physical body orientation and mental polarity reversal that is in conflict. There is, however, a deeper type of switching that has to do with the survival emotions and your psychoemotional perception of your world, which Dr Charles Krebs termed *survival switching*. This is not dependent on body polarity orientation but rather on activation of specific survival emotions that shut down various brain areas as a mechanism of physical and/or psychoemotional survival. A full description of these is beyond the scope of this textbook, but you are referred to Krebs's book *A Revolutionary Way of Thinking* or papers he has written for further information on this topic.[4]

The neurology of switching

As pointed out above, switching comes in two distinct forms: superficial switching and survival switching. However, the neurological substrates of these two types of switching are totally different, as are their effects on your function and behavior. In this textbook, we will discuss only projection switching, which is often termed *superficial switching*.

Projection switching results from how the brain processes sensory information. All sensory input starts as a nerve impulse at a sensory receptor, then travels via the peripheral nerves to the dorsal root ganglia of the spinal nerve just outside the spinal segment receiving that spinal nerve. From there, the axons of the dorsal root ganglia go up the spinal cord to the thalamus. Relay neurons from the thalamus cross over to the opposite hemisphere and send the nerve impulse to the area of the cortex which then processes these sensory impulses and turns them into a conscious perception of that sensory experience. However, this conscious perception is not perceived as being located in the head; rather, it is then projected mentally back to the receptor that generated the original signal.

To understand sensory processing, you first have to understand that all nerve impulses are identical, no matter what receptor creates them. Thus, the 'bip!' (the sound of a nerve impulse) of the photophore in the retina, the 'bip!' of the hair cell in your inner ear, or the 'bip!' of a pain receptor in your toe are the same until they reach the primary sensory cortex, where each 'bip!' is then interpreted as the type of sensory experience processed by that part of the cortex. Thus when a 'bip!' arrives at the part of the parietal cortex processing pain, the conscious experience is pain. So pain 'bips!' go to the pain association cortex of the parietal lobe and elicit the conscious sensation of pain.

A simple example will clarify what may seem a very complicated system. When you are walking along and suddenly stub your left big toe on a rock, the nociceptors (pain receptors) in your big toe fire a stream of nerve impulses up the peripheral nerves to the spinal nerve, where the 'bip! bip! bip!' is relayed into the spinal cord and up the spinal cord to the thalamus of the brain, from which the 'bips!' are once again relayed to the right parietal sensory cortices that process the pain. It is only in the parietal cortex that the 'Ow!', the pain of stubbing your toe, actually exists. However, people do not say, 'Ow! My right parietal cortex hurts', but rather, 'Ow! My left big toe hurts!'

Why? Because the 'Ow!' is projected mentally back to the pain receptor in the big toe that created

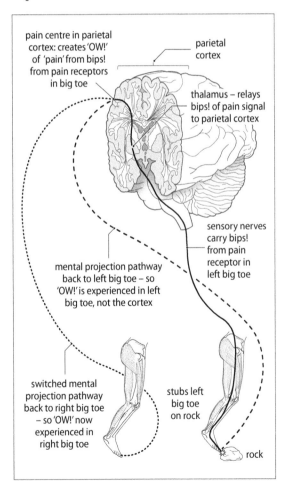

pain centre in parietal cortex: creates 'OW!' of 'pain' from bips! from pain receptors in big toe

parietal cortex

thalamus – relays bips! of pain signal to parietal cortex

sensory nerves carry bips! from pain receptor in left big toe

mental projection pathway back to left big toe – so 'OW!' is experienced in left big toe, not the cortex

switched mental projection pathway back to right big toe – so 'OW!' now experienced in right big toe

stubs left big toe on rock

rock

Figure 22.8 Projection switching. All sensory input from any receptor is the same, that is, a nerve impulse, but it is then converted into a sensory experience in the sensory cortex. So when you stub your right big toe on a rock, the left parietal cortex generates the 'Ouch!' of pain. However, you experience the 'Ouch!' of pain in your right big toe via mental projection back to the source of the incoming nerve impulse. When switching is present, the signal is projected back to the wrong location. Solid line, nerve pathway into the cortex; dashed line, normal mental projection pathway back to the receptor; dotted line, switched mental projection pathway back to the receptor.

the 'bips' in the first place (see Figure 22.8). The same is true of all other senses. So when I look at you, the 'you' I see out there is merely a projection of the 'you' created in my occipital cortex from 'bips' from my retinal photophores (light-sensitive cells).

This is the basis of projection switching. Information enters the brain from a receptor is delivered to the correct cortical primary sensory area to be processed, and is processed correctly to create the conscious perception, but it is then incorrectly projected to the wrong place in the body, or the wrong place with respect to body orientation. For example, I mean to tell you turn right, but when I mentally reference my body orientation, my right was correctly referenced as my right side but because of a polarity reversal in my mental orientation, I find my mouth saying, 'Turn left!' I may immediately recognize my error, or be totally unaware that I said the wrong direction.

An excellent real life example is the following. Krebs was once sharing a house with several people, and one morning one of his housemates came out of her room and said, 'Charles, this is really strange. I've just woken up and I can see the welts on my left arm from sleeping on it, but it feels normal. It's my right arm that is asleep. How the hell could that happen?' Krebs told her to massage her kidney 27 acupoints, which she said were indeed tender, until the sensitivity disappeared. This only took 30–40 seconds. She then said, 'This is weird. As the tenderness of the points disappeared, suddenly my right arm felt normal and now my left arm has pins and needles!'

What this demonstrates is the true nature of brain function, which is to project back to the source of stimulation the nature of the experience the brain is having. In this case, the sensory receptors in her left arm were sending a stream of impulses to areas in her right parietal cortex that then interpreted this as a feeling of pins and needles. In the normal course of events, it would have correctly projected this sensation back to her left arm. But because of confusion on the part of the brain, a polarity reversal, the signals of the feeling were switched and projected to the wrong side of the body. So she was consciously feeling the sensation in the wrong arm.

This illustrates how the brain references itself and may become confused with respect to itself. Right becomes left, top becomes bottom, and front becomes back—and vice versa. A sensation coming from here is perceived as coming from another place. In fact, the brain creates its own reality from the sensory information it receives. Its creation may be true to the world of the sensory input, or it can just as easily be an illusion based on its confusion.

A well-known phenomenon that exemplifies this propensity for illusion is the case of the phantom pain in amputated limbs. People who have lost an arm or a leg will often still feel sensory events in that missing limb. One of Krebs's clients, who had lost his left leg above the knee, was still feeling pain in his left foot. The nerves that had gone to his left foot were clearly still firing sensory information into his brain after the amputation, perhaps because of the physical trauma and the scar tissue formed in the stump of his leg. His brain then correctly projected the 'pain' back to where the pain receptors of his missing foot used to be, the original source of nerve impulses in that nerve. But because the foot was no longer there, this pain appeared to be only an illusion of pain, hence the name *phantom pain*. When Krebs used muscle monitoring to locate the active acupoints on his stump, and balanced them, the client's phantom limb disappeared, probably because the stress of the trauma or scar creating the stream of nerve impulses to his parietal cortex had ceased.

It is important to recognize and rectify projection switching, because it perturbs the responses or 'answers' the body gives through muscle monitoring. It is usually a transitory state of confusion that will correct itself over time; however, if you want to muscle monitor a client right now, and they are switched, you must first clear this switching to get clear and correct responses from the body. Therefore correcting switching allows clearer and more accurate feedback from the biocomputer.

Types of projection switching

Projection switching comes in three types, which relate to the types of neurological fibers through which the switching occurs. The primary white matter tracks in the brain are the commissural fibers connecting the right and left hemisphere; the association fibers connecting the back of one hemisphere to the front of the same hemisphere, and vice versa; and the projection fibers, which connect the brain stem and spinal cord to the overlying cortex, and vice versa. You will notice that these are indeed the three axes of our physical orientation as well as the three axes of body polarity.

As we have stated, the front right quadrant of the body has an overall slight positive polarity, the front left a slight negative polarity, the back left a slight positive polarity and the back right a slight negative polarity. And as we have said, in the brain the right hemisphere has a slightly negative polarity and the left hemisphere has a slightly more positive polarity, which may be caused by the crossing over neurons carrying both sensory and motor signals. Likewise, the top half of the body tends to be slightly more positive than the lower half of the body.

Therefore, when using the body polarity for mental orientation there may be switching in the commissural fibers, which can create concomitant confusion about left and right; or switching in the association fibers, which can create concomitant confusion about the location of front and back; or switching in the projection fibers, which can create concomitant confusion in the orientation of top and bottom.

If there is any type of switching present in any orientation, it can create inaccurate feedback from muscle monitoring such that the biocomputer may indicate a muscle imbalance on the left side of the body when it is actually on the right side. Or it can create an imbalance on the front of the body when the muscle with imbalance is actually located on the back of the body. Or muscle feedback may indicate a muscle imbalance in the top half of the body when it is actually located in the lower half of the body.

To make this more concrete, we will illustrate with physical examples. With right–left switching, the biocomputer may indicate that the right pectoralis major clavicular (PMC) is under-facilitated, but when you monitor the right PMC it is actually in homeostasis, and on monitoring the left PMC you find it under-facilitated. Clearly, the biocomputer is confused. Likewise, muscle monitoring may indicate the biceps muscle as having an imbalance when actually the imbalance is in the triceps muscle, or muscle monitoring may indicate the biceps muscle of the arm when the imbalance is actually located in the hamstring muscle in the leg. This puts paid to the concept 'The body doesn't lie.' Indeed, this is technically true, but the body certainly can fib a lot! Or, more correctly, it can demonstrate confusion because of switching.

Other than providing inaccurate biofeedback to the monitor, what are the other common consequences of this confusion to the person with this switching?

Left–right switching (commissural fibers):
- is often observed in people who have reading and learning problems
- causes confusion between the left and right of the body
- underlies the dyslexic tendency to confuse 'd' and 'b'.

Top–bottom switching (projection fibers):
- causes confusion about the top and bottom of the body
- results in difficulty walking up or down stairs
- causes disorientation looking down from heights (or looking up)
- underlies the dyslexic tendency to confuse 'd' and 'p'.

Front–back switching (association fibers):
- causes confusion about the front and back of the body
- results in difficulty reversing a car, using the rear vision mirror
- underlies the dyslexic tendency to have handwriting drift up or down as the writing progresses across the page.

The above three forms of switching must therefore be cleared in order for the biocomputer to provide accurate and reliable information for accurate indicator muscle biofeedback.

Central and Governing meridian energies

The Central and Governing Vessels are two of what are called the eight extraordinary meridians or simply eight extra meridians in Chinese medicine. These meridians are unusual in that they have their own unique acupoints. The other six extra meridians are flows that connect acupoints on the other 12 primary meridians. Central and Governing Vessels are also unique in that they constitute a single integrated figure 8 flow within the body. Central Vessel runs up the body from Central Vessel 1 on the perineum to the last external point of Central Vessel 24 in the labial groove just below the bottom lip. Governing Vessel likewise runs from the tip of the coccyx up along the spinal vertebrae and over the head to end at the frenulum of the upper lip, that is, the flap of tissue that connects the inner surface of the upper lip to the middle of the gum.

While these are the external points on the Central and Governing Vessels conducting ch'i, this is only part of the story. The Central Vessel flow continues into the mouth and then down through the core of the body, where it is transmuted from yin energy of the Central Vessel to yang energy as it enters Governing Vessel 1. Then it flows up Governing Vessel as yang energy over the head and enters the mouth and flows down through the core of the body, where it is transmuted into yin energy entering Central Vessel 1. Then it flows up Central Vessel as yin energy. Clearly, this is a closed figure 8 of oscillating polarity, as yin is electromagnetically negative and yang is electromagnetically positive. To indicate its importance in traditional Chinese medicine, it is called the *Heavenly* or *Celestial circuit*.

The other 12 bilateral regular meridians all connect to these integrated Central and Governing flows. Thus, instability in either the Central or Governing Vessel may perturb the stability in one or more of the other 12 primary meridians. These meridian disturbances may produce spurious or irrelevant indicator changes when a muscle is monitored. Therefore for accurate muscle monitoring you must check the balance of yin and yang energy flows in the Central and Governing Vessels and then rebalance these flows.

Ionization

Air ions are molecules with atoms attached that have gained or lost an electron. If an atom loses an electron, it becomes a positive ion or an *anion*, if it gains an electron it becomes a negative ion or a *cation*. Because the earth is negatively charged, and thus repels negative ions, the air you breathe normally has slightly more positive ions than negative ions. The normally accepted ratio of positive to negative ions is five positive to four negative ions. In open, well-ventilated natural spaces on a clear day, the healthy number of air ions should be 1000–2000 ions per cubic centimeter at a five positive:four negative ion ratio.[5]

However, both ion numbers and the ion ratio can change, often dramatically, in different environments, and these changes can have perceptible effects on people's health, behavior and even emotional or mental states. You may have heard of the 'sick building syndrome'. In recent times, in an attempt to promote energy conservation, more and more buildings are built with hermetically sealed windows that cannot be opened, and all the air exchange is through miles of metal ducting. While indeed very energy-efficient, these buildings have highly altered numbers and ratios of air ions. Metal ducting for air conditioning and heating are positively charged, so they tend to strip the negative ions out of the air and often greatly reduce the number of air ions delivered to the offices and work areas. The altered ion ratios and numbers then often result in changes in people's behavior, health and even emotional states, hence the name *sick building syndrome*, although it is not the building that is sick but rather the people that work there!

Numerous studies have now shown that when there is a reduction in overall ionization and an increase in positive to negative ratio, this has many effects on our health.[6] As reported by Soyka and Edmonds, Kornbleuh researched applying negative ions to burn victims and found it effective at relieving pain and increasing the speed of healing. But ion ratio and numbers can also impact strongly on our emotions as well as our physiology, and alteration in ion ratios is associated with changes in our moods as well as our physical health. With an increase in positive ions, people tend to become more irritable and short-tempered, while as negative ions increase, people tend to feel calm and overall, just plain better! This is why Soyka and Edmonds state, 'Negative ions are being called "happy ions", in contrast positive are called "grouchy ions".'

The ratio of negative and positive ions in the air around you has been found to affect your psycho-emotional states as well as your overt physiology. Environments with an excess of positive ions often activate the sympathetic nervous system, putting us in a heightened state of alertness, which may border on irritability or grouchiness. There are a number of places in the world in which winds blow off high dry land and are enriched with positive ions. The föhn winds blowing out of the Alps of Switzerland in early spring and autumn are associated with misfortune and unhappiness, and they have been traditionally called the 'witches' wind'. In California there is the Santa Ana, and there are the Chinook winds of the Rocky Mountains of the northern USA and Canada. All these ill winds contain high levels of positive ions and are notorious for creating irritable people. In fact, when these winds blow, people become tense and aggressive; suicides, murders and crime rates increase, as do traffic and other types of accidents.[7]

In contrast, when the air is enriched with negative ions this tends to activate the parasympathetic nervous system and results in feelings of calmness and contentment. A major mechanism for generating negative ions is shearing water. When water breaks up, the positive ion stays with the larger drop of water, while the negative ions are delivered to the air in the fine mists. The excess of negative ions produced by shearing water, such as occurs at waterfalls and waves breaking on a beach, are one of the reasons people almost always find these environments relaxing and calming.

However, it is not only the external ionization of the air that affects our health and moods, but also the airflow through our nostrils. The flow of air through your nostrils is not, as most people imagine, simple 'in' and 'out', with basically the same amount of air flowing through each nostril. Research of breathing patterns has shown the existence of a nasal cycle in which one nostril breathes more than does the other. This results from the swelling of the tissues of the right nostril and then the left nostril such that as the tissue in one nostril swells it reduces the airflow through that nostril. This cycle periodically shifts dominant breathing sides about every 20 minutes, with the turbinates of the nasal passages acting as ionizing chambers.

Indeed, Shannahoff-Khal discusses the nasal cycle and research associating hemispheric dominance shown in humans and dolphins, and its apparent relationship with the alternating nasal cycle.[8] Right nostril–left hemisphere dominance corresponds to increased activity, and is associated with more positive affective states (happiness), and left nostril–right hemisphere dominance represents decreased activity or rest, and is associated with more introspective, affective states (sadness).

The nasal cycle and the production of negative and positive ions in the turbinates indeed appear to be the source of our overall body polarity. The air flowing through the right turbinates appears to be positively ionized, while air flowing through our left turbinates is negatively ionized, and these correlate with polarity of the anterior body as described by Davis and Rawls.[9] Thus, proper ionization of airflow through the nasal cycles sustains the proper ionization of the anterior body surfaces: left nasal flows generating more negative ions, supporting the slightly more negative left anterior surface of the body, and right nasal flows generating the slightly more positive right anterior surface of the body. Indeed, this would appear to be the positive and negative currents that the eastern physiologists propose are in fact the real basis on which body polarity is maintained.

Thus, only recently has western science confirmed[10] what the yogis have understood for millennia: that the air flowing in through the left nostril is ionized, resulting in a greater number of negative ions, and activates predominantly the right hemisphere. Likewise, air flowing in through the right nostril is ionized positively and activates predominantly the left hemisphere. This is the basis of a classic yogic brain-balancing technique called *nadi shodan*, or alternate nostril breathing.[11]

From the Energetic Kinesiology perspective, this is the basis of the ionization pre-check. Because the nasal cycle ionization controls the body polarity, imbalances within these air flow cycles will alter body polarity, and these alterations in body polarity may well result in an indicator change when an acupoint (e.g. an alarm point or other indicator point) is circuit located. Thus, the indicator change may have nothing to do with the acupoint being touched, but rather be an artifact of the polarity imbalance created by the altered nasal cycle! This is the reason it is necessary to check for proper ionization, and why aberrant ionization needs to be balanced before using acupoints as specific indicator points.

In Applied Kinesiology, Goodheart observed the following with regard to ionization of each nostril,[12] and what an indicator change with each test means:

- indicator change on breath in through the left nostril indicates excessive negative ions
- indicator change on breath out through the right nostril indicates deficient positive ions
- indicator change on breath in through the right nostril indicates excessive positive ions
- indicator change on breath out through the left nostril indicates deficient negative ions.

To assess the ionization balance, the monitor first blocks the right side nostril and has the person breathe *in* through their left nostril; the monitor checks for indicator change. Then the monitor blocks the left side nostril and the person breathes *out* through their right nostril; the monitor checks for indicator change. Then the monitor blocks the left side nostril and has the person breathe *in* through their right nostril; the monitor checks for indicator change. Then the monitor blocks the right side nostril and has the person breathe *out* through their left nostril; the monitor checks for indicator change. The indicator muscle should remain locked on all four tests. If it does not, then corrections need to be instituted to reset the nasal ionization, and with it the

imbalances in body polarity. Once the ionization and body polarity are reset, the monitor knows that when they circuit locate an acupoint the indicator change is not indicating a spurious polarity imbalance but rather a real imbalance in the acupoint itself.

Checking the pause lock mechanism

Because the pause lock mechanism is central to the practice of modern Energetic Kinesiology, it will be used repeatedly throughout each session. Therefore it is essential that this mechanism is checked for its state of balance before it is used. How might it be out of balance?

Activation of the hip joints and their associated receptors will not create an indicator change unless there is some type of structural or muscular imbalance disturbing hip joint function and proprioception. However, there are circumstances, the result of structural misalignment or imbalances in hip joint proprioception, in which movement of the legs generates an indicator change. This indicator change created by activation of the imbalanced pause lock mechanism creates information that is not only irrelevant to the information being stored in pause lock but more importantly may disturb the information already stored in pause lock.

In addition, if a mode or specific indicator point causes an indicator change but activation of the imbalanced pause lock mechanism also causes an indicator change, these indicator changes would cancel each other out and no indicator change would be observed. This would lead to the monitor missing valuable pieces of information. Therefore it is essential that the pause lock mechanism be checked for its state of homeostasis to ensure that it is in a fully functioning state before you begin using muscle monitoring and storing information in pause lock.

Before using pause lock, the monitor must check both their own pause lock and the pause lock of the client. If this is not done, information can be lost from pause lock or erroneous information can be added, confusing the information that is being held.

The following procedure is used to check for

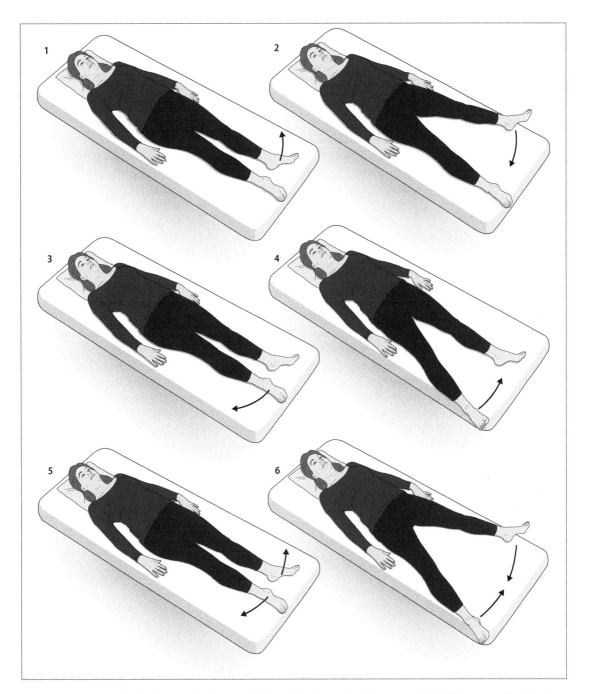

Figure 22.9 Checking for imbalances in the pause lock mechanism. 1, The client moves their left leg out to the side of the table and a balanced indicator muscle is monitored. 2, The left leg is brought back to the center and the indicator muscle is monitored again. 3, The client moves their right leg out to the side of the table and the indicator muscle is monitored. 4, The right leg is brought back to the center and the indicator muscle is monitored again. 5, The client separates both legs simultaneously and the indicator muscle is monitored. 6, Both legs are brought together again and the indicator muscle is monitored.

imbalances in the pause lock mechanism (Figure 22.9).

1. The client moves their left leg out to the side of the table and a balanced indicator muscle is monitored.
2. The left leg is brought back to the center, and the indicator muscle is monitored once more.
3. The procedure is repeated, with the right leg being moved out to the side of the table, the indicator muscle monitored, and the leg returned to the center and the indicator muscle monitored again.
4. Finally, both legs are separated simultaneously and the indicator muscle monitored, then both legs are brought together again and the indicator muscle monitored.

If there is any change in the indicator muscle in any of these cases, you must locate and correct the imbalance involved. You must *not* use a faulty pause lock, as the information may be perturbed by this faulty pause lock mechanism.

The monitor must complete the same pause lock check procedure on themselves using the balanced indicator muscle of the client. Should you get an indicator change when checking the balance of the pause lock mechanism, you must correct this imbalance or not use that pause lock mechanism. A way to rapidly correct a pause lock imbalance in the short term, often long enough to use in a session, is to rub the posterior superior iliac spines, the bumps on either side of the spine at the top of the sacrum (Figure 22.10). If the problem persists, then the person may require structural work to stabilize their pelvis.

Of course, the same considerations need to be applied to the temporomandibular joint, or jaw pause lock, so that the monitor can confidently use this for jaw stacking. The monitor uses the balanced indicator muscle of the client, and while touching the client then opens their own jaw widely and monitors the client's indicator muscle. If there is no indicator change, then the monitor closes their jaw and remonitors the client's indicator muscle. If there is still no indicator change, the monitor can now use their jaw pause lock to hold information when stacking. However, if there is an indicator change with the opening or closing of the monitor's jaw, they cannot use their jaw pause lock during the session and must endeavor to have their temporomandibular joint balanced to be able to use jaw stacking in future sessions.

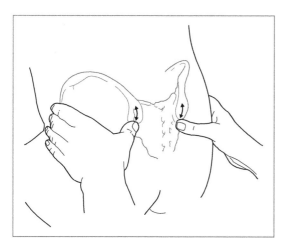

Figure 22.10 Correction for the pause lock mechanism. To correct a pause lock mechanism imbalance in the short term, usually for the duration of a treatment session, rub firmly on the posterior superior iliac spines, the bumps on either side of the spine at the top of the sacrum, while the person breathes in and out deeply.

References

1. Roy, R, Tiller, WA, Bell, I & Hoover, MR 2005, The structure of liquid water; novel insights from materials research; potential relevance to homeopathy, *Materials Research Innovations* 9-4: 1433-075X

2. Emoto, M 1999, *Messages from Water, Volume 1*, Hado Publishing.

3. Walther, DS 1988, *Applied Kinesiology: Synopsis*, Systems DC, Pueblo, pp. 149–152.

4. Krebs, C 1998, *A Revolutionary Way of Thinking*, Hill of Content Publishing, Melbourne.
   Krebs, C 2004, *Understanding Switching in the Body and the Brain: What Does it Mean?*, Melbourne Applied Physiology, Learmonth.

5. Walther, DS 2000, *Applied Kinesiology: Synopsis, Second Edition*, Systems DC, Pueblo, p. 545.

6. Soyka, F & Edmonds, A 1977, *The Ion Effect*, EP Dutton, New York.

7. Soyka, F & Edmonds, A 1977, *The Ion Effect*, EP Dutton, New York.
   Beasley, VR 1978, *Your Electro-Vibratory Body, Second Edition*, University of the Trees Press, Boulder Creek.

8. Shannahoff-Khalsa, DS 2008, *Psychophysiological States: The Ultradian Dynamics of Mind–Body Interactions*, Academic Press, San Diego, p. 283.

9. Davis, AR & Rawls, WC Jr 1974, *Magnetism and Its Effects on the Living Systems*, Exposition Press, Hicksville, p. 105.

10. Shannahoff-Khalsa, DS 2008, *Psychophysiological States: The Ultradian Dynamics of Mind–Body Interactions*, Academic Press, San Diego, p. 283.
    Davis, AR & Rawls, WC Jr 1974, *Magnetism and Its Effects on the Living Systems*, Exposition Press, Hicksville, p. 105.

11. Swami Satyananda Saraswati 1997, *Asana, Pranayama, Mudra and Bandha*, Bihar Yoga Bharati, Munger.

12. Goodheart, GJ, Jr 1987, *Applied Kinesiology 1987 Workshop Procedure Manual*, privately published, Detroit.

Chapter 23

SETTING THE CONTEXT

Kinesiology by its very nature is context-dependent, and the results of any treatment rely on awareness of this context dependence. Therefore the results of a kinesiology balance always arise from the initial context set for that balance. There are several approaches to setting the context for a session:

1. discussing the issue and potential outcomes
2. performing one or more activities to activate a system or systems within the body
3. setting an overarching verbal goal for the outcome of the session
4. activation of an acupressure format relevant to a particular physiological system or structure
5. assessment and activation of a pain or structural imbalance.

It should be noted that these approaches are not necessarily used individually but are more often used in combination with each other.

While context is important in any form of therapy, it is perhaps more important in Energetic Kinesiology because of the nature of muscle biofeedback. Muscle monitoring is always a summation process in which the muscle will respond with a 'locked' response, indicating lack of stress for that particular context, or an 'unlocked' muscle response, indicating stress in that context. However, this response is the result of summing all the positives and negatives relative to that context and thus is not a statement of absolute absence or presence of stress. Rather, it merely indicates that in this case the negative contextual stressors have or have not exceeded 50%. Even a slight change in context can reverse this outcome from positive to negative or from negative to positive.

If the context provided is the whole body or an overarching issue, it may be very different from the context of a specific body part or specific details of that overarching issue. For example, if someone asks, 'How are you today?', you have to consciously and subconsciously sum all the negative and positive factors going on in your life at that moment and either answer 'Good' (locked muscle) or 'Not good' (unlocked muscle). If you have twisted your right ankle and it hurts when you stand on it, your response will be dependent on whether you are standing or sitting. Further, if I should slightly change the context to 'How is your right ankle today?' your response would clearly be 'Not good'. So are you good or not good? The response is totally context-dependent.

Because the origin of muscle responses to context is often in subconscious areas of our brain, the client cannot consciously compensate for contextual responses. That is, the client's muscle response cannot say 'Oh, but...' or elaborate on its response. Therefore it is critical for the practitioner to provide a clear context at the beginning of the session so the meaning of the muscle biofeedback is clear and unambiguous. This is also important to ensure that the outcomes of the treatment will meet the client's expectations.

Discussing the issue and potential outcomes

Clients come with presenting issues, and these are often multicomponent issues that will not be resolved by a single Energetic Kinesiology treatment. Therefore it is necessary to discuss the different components of each issue and which of these components is the priority to address in that session. To do this requires discussion of the issue with the client and then identifying the outcome the client wants for that particular session.

This method for setting context is a component of every Energetic Kinesiology session. In sessions that have more general issues this may be all the context setting that is required, while more specific issues may then need to be defined by more specific methods of setting context, for example acupressure formatting or activation of a pain.

Performing pre-activities

A client might present with an issue that involves difficulty in performing a particular activity or activities. For example, they might be having difficulty with reading or with coordination when kicking a ball. By performing an activity before balancing, you will establish a baseline against which changes can be measured. Performing a *pre-activity* freezes a movement or activity in time so the client can clearly experience its effects. Repeating the activity after the balance will then help the client notice the changes, such as an ability to read more fluently or an ability to kick a ball with greater ease and accuracy.

For some forms of Energetic Kinesiology, such as Brain Gym, pre-activities are a major component of the goal-setting process, and conscious focus on the goal set is the primary form providing context.[1]

Setting a goal

A goal is the desired outcome of the kinesiology session and normally focuses on a positive change desired by the client. The goal expresses the desired outcome with confidence and focuses the attention on a positive outcome to supplant the previous negative patterns that have prevented them from achieving this goal. A goal is stated as if the goal has been accomplished and the problem or imbalance is already gone. In this way, goal setting is used to create conditions to attract future outcomes.[2] The stated intention of the goal often then brings up or activates the current negative experiences and perceptions because of the incongruity between the stated positive goal and past negative experience.

For example, a client presents with pain that prevents them from doing physical exercise, which in turn means they have put on weight and do not feel good about themselves. Their desire may be expressed as 'wanting to get rid of the pain'. However, setting the context for the session in a positive statement, such as 'I am now pain-free and able to exercise', may then allow the client to begin exercising to achieve their desired weight and feel good about themselves once more.

A way to help clients set their goal is to ask them, 'If this problem were gone, how would your life look?' and 'What could you then do differently?' This then shifts the focus from their current situation to what their life could be like if that goal is achieved. That is, it shifts their focus from the negatives in the present to the positive future outcome desired.

Activating an acupressure format

Another direct form of setting context is to enter an acupressure format for a specific physiological, emotional or energetic issue. The acupressure format provides a subconscious context selecting this particular system as the focus of the session. For example, if you enter the acupressure format for the immune system, then the muscle monitoring and biofeedback obtained will all relate to various aspects of immune function.

As previously discussed, acupressure formatting allows the practitioner to set a very specific context relative to the presenting issue of the client. Based on the practitioner's and client's discussion about the desired outcomes of the session, the practitioner must make choices about which type of context setting to employ. For example, a specific allergy reaction, which is directly an immune system problem, may be more effectively addressed via acupressure formatting for allergies than by setting an overarching goal of 'I want to be well'. In the latter case, the immune system may or may not be the primary focus of the session, but because the immune system is the underlying cause of the allergies, a less effective outcome may be observed.

Activating a pain or structural imbalance

The most specific form of setting context is to directly activate the most overt factors involved in the presenting issue. Activation of pain or a structural imbalance sets the limits of the context to the systems that are directly involved in creating these problems. While it is the narrowest form of setting context, it can be extremely effective when the presenting issue has a very clear origin or causal factor(s).

Clearly, the way context is set for any session will be unique to the outcomes desired and will often involve using multiple methods of context setting. Discussion of the issue and potential outcomes will be necessary at the beginning of every session. This will then help to determine what other context-setting methods may be necessary for this client to achieve their desired outcomes.

For instance, it may well be that an overall goal, such as 'being pain-free', is an appropriate context for the client. But to achieve this outcome may require the practitioner to employ specific context, such as acupressure formatting for a particular system or muscle, which in turn may require pain or muscle and structural activation. But in this case, setting the goal provides the context not only for the whole balance but also for the acupressure format and pain activation. Therefore issues may arise to be resolved that relate to an overall goal that would never have appeared if a more specific context had been set first.

Clearly, choosing the correct form for setting the context is an important part of any Energetic Kinesiology balance. It must be thoroughly thought through to determine the appropriate type or types of context setting to be used.

References

1. Dennison, PE & Dennison, GE 1992, *Brain Gym: Simple Activities for Whole Brain Learning*, Edu-Kinesthetics, Ventura.
2. Topping, WW 1990, *Success Over Distress*, Topping International Institute, Bellingham.

Chapter 24

ASSESSING PAIN

Probably the most common presenting issue in any kinesiology practice is pain of some type. It is important to initially address the likely origin of the pain and whether this is best treated by an Energetic Kinesiologist or another health care professional, for example a medical doctor, surgeon or chiropractor. With pain, it is extremely important that this has been thoroughly investigated by a medical professional, and that either the origin has been identified and is appropriate for a kinesiologist to work with or the medical professional can find no indication or reason for the pain.

For instance, a man presented to Krebs with pain, and intense pain when palpated, under his left rib cage. When asked if he had seen a medical professional, he stated 'No'. Krebs requested that the client see his primary health care provider immediately. As it turned out, the client had fallen on a chair and had ruptured his spleen and was bleeding internally. His doctor immediately referred him for surgery after brief evaluation of this painful condition. Indeed, if Krebs had proceeded with a kinesiology session the client might not be alive today!

How to assess pain

With pain, there are three things that need to be assessed before beginning any treatment. First is the type of pain: acute pain, such as sharp, excruciating or stabbing pain; or chronic pain, which tends to be more aching, burning, throbbing, etc. Second is the location of the pain and whether the location is constant or varies over time. Third is the intensity of the pain. For this, you need to establish a subjective scale of pain, because pain is one of these unusual things that once it is gone you almost immediately cannot remember how intense it was.

The type of pain informs you about several possibilities. Acute pain that has just appeared informs you that the origin of the pain probably relates to something that happened recently, and questioning will often reveal what this factor was. In cases of acute pain, usually the location of the pain relates to the causal factor. Knowledge of the causal factor may very well determine the treatment you will perform. Chronic pain, on the other hand, often has origins that are far removed from the current location of the pain and as such may be *referred* pain.

A classic example of this are what are called active *trigger points*, which while painful are usually well removed from the actual source of the pain.[1] Indeed, trigger point therapy is a well-recognized therapeutic technique that is often very successful with chronic pain. Chronic pain is very often the result of long-term unresolved skeletal muscular issues that through a series of compensatory muscle reactivities are no longer related to the region of the body in which the pain originated.

Krebs recently had a client who was an avid right-handed tennis player and was suddenly having difficulty returning her forehand volleys. However, she presented at his clinic with pain in her left elbow. So the desired outcome for the session was to resolve the chronic pain in this elbow. When the pain in the left elbow was put into circuit through a series of acupressure formats and several reactive muscle circuits (to be discussed in Chapter 34), the final correction was a muscle reactivity in which one muscle actively inhibits another muscle. The hallucis longus muscle of the left big toe was inhibiting the opponens pollicis muscle of the right thumb, as determined by muscle biofeedback. Opponens pollicis is a muscle used in gripping the handle of the tennis racket. When acupressure therapy was applied, not only was the reactivity resolved but the pain in her left elbow totally disappeared and her forehand was as good as ever!

It is absolutely critical that the kinesiologist

identifies specifically the location of the pain and whether that location is persistent over time. If the pain is persistent over time, it may suggest the type of activity or origin of this pain. If its location varies over time, this may suggest there is a more complex relationship between the origin of the pain and its location. Therefore your focus would be less on the location of the pain and more on possible factors generating this pain.

To establish the intensity of pain, which by its very nature is subjective, you need to create a pain scale that the client can relate to. One of the most common is the 0-10 scale, with 0 indicating absolutely no pain and 10 being the worst pain of that particular type and location that they remember. The client is then asked to give a number of the pain as it is currently being experienced, for example it is now '7 out of 10'. This clearly provides a benchmark against which future improvement in pain can be registered. This is important, because when pain disappears you tend to forget, almost immediately, how intense it actually was.

Without this measure of initial intensity, you may perform a very successful treatment but there may still be some pain left and the person will say, 'But there's still pain there.' However, if you had benchmarked the intensity of the original pain with this 0-10 scale, and they had said it was initially 7 and it is now 3, the pain has been more than halved and they will become aware of that change. Therefore it is important to rate the level of pain both before and immediately after treatment so the client has a comparison to assess the change that has occurred.

One of the most common observations of kinesiologists following treatment for pain is that the client will suddenly say, 'But now there's pain in another place!' And this is indeed true. This is much like me pinching you on one arm and biting you on the other arm. While the pinch hurts, it is totally ignored because the bite is much more intense and all your conscious attention will be drawn to the area of greater pain intensity: the bite. As soon as I stop biting you, you will say, 'Ow! My other arm hurts!' because it is still being pinched. Very often, it is useful to inform the client, specifically the client with lower back pain, that

once the pain is resolved, pain may appear somewhere else in the body. In the case of lower back pain, it is almost always in the neck, because of the structural relationship between the cervical and lumbar vertebrae.

Activating a pain

One of the most important approaches to resolution of pain is to activate the pain before beginning treatment. This is because within the body at any point in time there are hundreds of thousands of different processes occurring, each of which requires some degree of both your conscious and subconscious attention. Therefore the signal-to-noise ratio for a particular signal, such as pain, may be largely overridden by the very large 'noise' resulting from the operations of the rest of your body. Richard Utt developed an effective technique, based on a technique developed by Dr Nogier, the founder of an ear acupressure method.[2] In this technique, pain is activated momentarily and then immediately entered into pause lock. This means the client suffers only a momentary increase of pain but has exaggerated the pain, increasing the signal-to-noise ratio. This means you have more data about the pain in circuit and therefore can do a deeper and more effective balance.

Another concept developed by Richard Utt is for the person to physically locate the pain by touching it, if that is possible, and focusing on that pain as you pause lock. If they cannot touch the location of the pain, they can just intently focus on it with their mind as you activate pause lock. This focuses their conscious attention on that pain or area of pain, again greatly enhancing the signal-to-noise ratio. Attending to pain or any other issue brings 'online' your conscious perception of this issue again, selecting this issue out of all the other noise or processing that is occurring in the background. This is like opening a specific file on your computer so that it now occupies the whole screen and your awareness. The file was always there in the computer, you just were not attending to it.

Once the type or quality of the pain, its location, the consistency of its location and its intensity have been benchmarked, then the monitor must decide how best to activate the pain to provide the most effective context for balancing this pain. Note that often pain, especially chronic pain, may require several circuits to resolve it completely.

Following a treatment for pain, the monitor needs to assess the quality, location and intensity once more. They should note any change in any of these three factors. If any of these three factors improves, this is a positive outcome because even though pain may persist, one or more aspects of it are showing positive change. If the pain changes location, especially for pain that had a consistent location before balancing, you can tell the client, 'You have it on the run!' However, if the pain does not change in quality, location or intensity after treatment, this suggests there may be a 'real' physical or structural origin to the pain, and referral to a medical or another complementary health practitioner, for example a chiropractor, may be in order.

References

1. Simons, DG, Travell, JG & Simons, LS 1998, *Travell & Simons' Myofascial Pain and Dysfunction: The Trigger Point Manual (2-Volume Set), Second Edition,* Lippincott Williams & Williams, Philadelphia.
2. McGee, CT 2000, *Healing Energies of Heat and Light: A Quantum Leap in Health Care,* MediPress, Coeur d'Alene.

SECTION VI

Set-up: information gathering

The set-up phase of a kinesiology balance comes after setting the context and before applying any correction techniques. It involves identifying important information that relates to the client's presenting issue. Most forms of modern Energetic Kinesiology incorporate a very thorough set-up phase into their balances. This usually involves entering into circuit a series of hand modes, specific indicator points and/or acupressure formats that are related to the physiological, emotional, mental and psychospiritual aspects of the client's presenting issue.

The set-up procedures in Energetic Kinesiology are necessary to decompensate the balanced/imbalance state causing the client's current issue. The set-up releases the blocked energy in the client's multidimensional being and creates an increasingly chaotic state as decompensation proceeds. It is from this chaotic decompensated state that reorganization may occur. The more thoroughly decompensated the system becomes, the greater the chaos and the greater the possibility for a reorganization of the system closer to optimal homeostasis. That is, the more thorough the set-up phase of the balance, the greater potential for reorganizing the client's system back toward homeostasis.

Because this book is intended as an introduction to the field of Energetic Kinesiology, we have chosen to include only the set-up procedures that are commonly applied in every kinesiology session. We have included how to use hand modes to access information; a mechanism to access subconscious emotions involved in the stressor; age recession to identify the exact time in the past when the stress program was created; ways of identifying ancillary factors involved; and hand modes, specific indicator points and acupressure formatting to access subconscious fear-based emotional memories.

The basic set-up procedures presented in this book do allow the practitioner to decompensate the client's imbalance and thus provide an opportunity for healing to occur. However, utilizing more sophisticated set-ups, such as acupressure formatting, permits more thorough decompensation of the client's imbalance and hence are able to consistently produce longer lasting clinical results. In recent years, a number of very sophisticated acupressure formatting systems have been developed for working with the body and the brain and often produce remarkable results.

Chapter 25

USING HAND MODES TO GATHER INFORMATION

Recording information

Originally, kinesiologists gathered information about the stress in a circuit by using the change in an indicator muscle, which is an all-or-nothing response, and hence it is a binary system. This is similar to the way a computer works using a binary code. For a computer, '1' or '0' are the only possible responses. Likewise, in kinesiology the muscle can only 'lock' or 'unlock' and therefore has only one discrete piece of information it can gather at any one time.

Later, the discovery of pause lock by Alan Beardall allowed kinesiologists to gather and store information such that you could build a circuit by an additive process. As described previously, the monitor could move their feet together then apart when they got an indicator change on a vibrational indicator, challenge, verbal question or other technique. This indicator change would then be held in circuit along with the signals telling the body that the legs are apart. At this point, the monitor would ask the client to bring their legs together and apart while they were touching them. This transferred the information held in the hip pause lock mechanism of the monitor to the hip pause lock mechanism of the client, like backing up a file to an external hard drive. This alternating of information exchange between the monitor and the client became known as *stacking*.

As noted earlier in the discussion on pause lock, the temporomandibular joint of the jaw has a similar number of Ruffini end organs that create the pause lock signal and can thus be used as a second pause lock mechanism on the monitor. So instead of having to transfer the data collected to the client's pause lock each time, the monitor can simply use alternating of the jaw and hip pause

lock mechanisms to continually stack information. This is called *jaw stacking*.

Jaw stacking was the next big leap forward in building circuits. Stacking allows the monitor to build more sophisticated circuits that carry complex and related information about the client's issue. This information is held as a complex interference pattern of all the interacting frequencies of information; remember that the indicator changes because the new frequency of a vibrational indicator, verbal challenge or question matches the frequency of the information already held in circuit. As this new piece of information is added, these frequencies interact, creating a new, more complex interference pattern that represents all the data contained in the circuit.

Development of continuous recording mode

Ian Stubbings, the developer of the Stress Indicator Points System, noticed that there was still a great deal of information being missed even in these more sophisticated methods of pause locking. Physical activity or trains of thought are not separate movements or processes, but rather all human activities are sequences of individual actions and thoughts that occur at discrete points in time. However, using the traditional pause lock mechanisms, even with stacking, you are only digitally sampling this sequence of physical and mental actions.

Therefore if you do not happen to sample during the time window of a particular action or thought, the stress contained with that action or thought will be lost. Stubbings felt that there must be a way to record this continuous flow of biofeedback. When we enter only discrete pieces of information about the imbalance, we have lost critical links or components of these continuous actions and thought streams. This reduces the amount of detail available and may even leave critical components out of the circuit, reducing the depth or detail available for balancing.

The only information that can be stored in a circuit by an indicator change is an imbalance that creates a stress level greater than 50% of the capacity of a client's electromagnetic–energetic circuit. What happens to those components that only create less than 50% stress in the client's circuit? These stresses clearly will not create an indicator change and therefore will not be recorded by traditional digital pause lock mechanisms. In addition, there may be a series of relatively small stressors that when added together over time exceed the 50% threshold and thus when taken together would create an indicator change. These stressors would also be missed by traditional pause lock mechanisms, and the information they contribute about the stressors in the circuit as a whole would be lost. Therefore these many minor stressors may prove to provide significant information about the imbalance, but because they individually never exceed 50% stress they will not be recognized or entered into circuit, and thus information will be lost (see Figure 25.1).

For example, when moving an arm through its range of motion there is a sequential activation of the individual prime movers involved in this action, with some active for only a short period of time. However, their contribution to the action may be critical if it is to be performed correctly. Think of a tennis player who goes off their serve. It may

be only one or two muscles whose transitory activation changes the timing of the serve sufficiently to cause the ball to go into the net.

A method for recording continuous information in a circuit was conceived and developed by Stubbings in 1997. He called this method *continuous recording mode*, and it involves holding large intestine 16 on the back of the right shoulder blade, as shown in Figure 25.2, then opening pause lock. What Stubbings discovered was that as long as he maintained contact with the large intestine 16 acupoint, every stressor involved with an action or thought process was continuously recorded until he opened his mouth, taking the total information into his jaw pause lock then bringing his legs together and apart as he released the circuit-localization of large intestine 16. This transferred the information to his hip pause lock and stopped the continuous recording. What he now had in circuit were not only the individual stressors that exceeded 50% on their own, but all the stressors, including those that when added together may exceed 50%.

Continuous recording mode recognizes and captures the dynamic aspects of imbalances throughout the full range of motion or thought stream. Some imbalances, such as muscle reactivity, may exist only when the reactor muscle is activated, which may be for only a fraction of a second during an action. However, in that fraction of a second there is overt muscle inhibition that may be involved in this action; remember that muscles involved in the same action can often become reactive to each other. Clearly, this has huge significance for sports and mental performance, as these transient but significant stressors

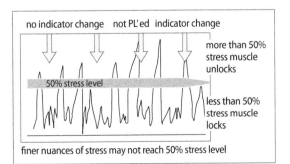

no indicator change   not PL'ed   indicator change

50% stress level

more than 50% stress muscle unlocks

less than 50% stress muscle locks

finer nuances of stress may not reach 50% stress level

Figure 25.1 Continuous recording mode (CRM) versus pause locking. When pause lock (PL) is activated, it records only whatever event(s) happened at or near the time that pause lock was activated, and it can record only information causing more than 50% stress. In contrast, once the indicator point for CRM is pause locked and held, all imbalances or stressful information, including those that individually create less than 50% stress, are recorded until the indicator point is released and pause lock is activated once more. All the stressors activated while CRM was held are recorded, including those that do not exceed 50%. After Stubbings, I 2004, *SIPS 2 Manual*, SIPS Kinesiology.

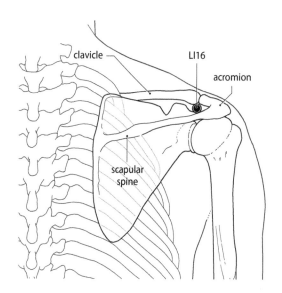

Figure 25.2 Continuous recording mode (CRM) a specific indicator point: large intestine 16 right. CRM is started by holding the acupoint large intestine (LI) 16 on the back of the right shoulder blade, then opening pause lock. To end the continuous recording, you take the information into your jaw pause lock then bring your legs together and apart as you release LI 16 on the right. As long as you maintain contact with the acupoint LI 16 right, every stressor involved with an action or thought process is continuously recorded.

would not normally be identified and entered into pause lock.

An analogy can be made with a spectrographic analysis of the chemical components of lemons. There are hundreds of major and minor peaks in the chemical subunits that comprise natural lemon flavor. When scientists created artificial lemon flavoring, they blended up the 30 or so of the chemicals represented by the major peaks on the spectrograph in similar ratios. Human taste buds distinguish very clearly the difference between natural and artificial lemon flavor. The richness of the taste of natural lemon is contained in the detail of the minor peaks, the nuances of the more subtle chemical structure of the natural lemon flavor. Thus, the real essence of lemon flavor is clearly contained in these nuances. Likewise, many of the nuances of a kinesiology balance may go unrecognized because only the major peaks are recorded.

Continuous recording mode appears to create a carrier wave that continuously records all stresses that may occur between the indicator change initially pause locked and the indicator change that ends the recording. This simple technique can greatly enhance the depth and power of your balancing by addressing the full dynamic nature and context of the imbalance and ensuring that you gather all the relevant information in the circuit.

Identifying relevant information

Once you have set the context for the session, the next step in a kinesiology session is to set up the balance by gathering information that is relevant in that context. There are a number of pieces of information that may need to be identified: an associated emotion; the age at which the issue originated; people, circumstances or other factors involved in the issue; amygdaloid reactive emotional programs underlying the issue; etc.

There is, of course, a lot of information you could gather about any one issue. So how do you know what information is most relevant for balancing the person's issue? Issues in our lives tend to be multidimensional, and they often create stress at several different levels within our being and are often related to multiple times within our lives. How are we to know when we have gathered enough information and covered the relevant context to balance the issue in circuit?

As you collect information with regard to the issue in circuit, it is possible to check whether you have gathered all the information relevant to that particular circuit. This can take the form of knowing you need more of a specific type of information or more of a different type of information, or finally if there is information that needs to be addressed but is currently suppressed. For each piece of information, it is also possible to check whether this plays an essential role to the issue in circuit or if there are collateral issues related to the issue in circuit but that are not active at that time.

The use of priority mode

How are we to know whether a stressor identified by an indicator change from holding a vibrational indicator, making a verbal challenge or asking a question is truly relevant and an essential part of the issue being addressed? In Applied Kinesiology, Dr. Goodheart recognized that while he had a powerful biofeedback tool, like doing a search on Google today, it often provided too much information of varying quality. So he sought a way to separate the truly relevant information from the not so relevant.

Initially, he used a technique that involved drawing the patient's attention both consciously and subconsciously to each piece of new information uncovered using muscle monitoring by placing a rubber band around their wrist and snapping it, then immediately remonitoring the indicator muscle. If there was another indicator change, then Goodheart considered this new information to be truly relevant and entered it into the circuit. If there was no indicator change with the rubber band snapping, then the information was not considered of primary relevance and was therefore not entered into the circuit.

In 1988, Alan Beardall developed a hand mode for priority, which greatly expedited this procedure for determining whether the information identified is relevant and should be entered into circuit. This mode involves placing the nail of the middle finger on the thumb crease, as shown in Figure 25.3. If this mode is held following the identification of a factor causing stress, then a reciprocal indicator change indicates that this information is indeed relevant and should be entered into the circuit.

Priority mode is therefore an extremely useful and now well-established way of selecting data to enter into circuit based on its relevance. Information that does not give a change with priority mode is generally a compensation for other relevant information that is within the circuit. When the causal issues are addressed, the compensations largely disappear, as there is no further need to compensate!

It is important to realize that priority mode relates specifically to the context and time within which you are working, as priorities are constantly changing within the framework of the energy patterns in the body. Priority mode can be used to find: 1, the priority goal or issue to address at this time; 2, the priority information needed for the

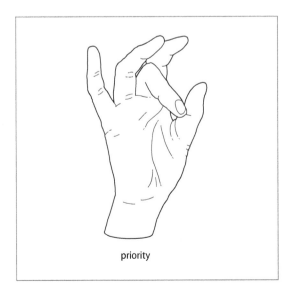

priority

Figure 25.3 **Priority mode.** The priority hand mode involves placing the nail of the middle finger on the thumb crease. If this mode is held following the identification of a factor causing stress, then a reciprocal indicator change indicates that this information is indeed a priority to be entered into the circuit. If there is no indicator change with priority mode, the issue just identified is only a compensation for a deeper issue and need not be entered into pause lock.

balance to be effective; 3, the priority correction to apply; and 4, the priority order in which corrections should be applied.

The use of more mode

Once an issue has been entered into circuit and information relevant to this imbalance has been accumulated, when do you know if you have accumulated all that is needed to effectively balance this circuit?

Two chiropractors, T Franks and M Cohen, developed the basic more mode. The pad of the middle finger is placed on the edge of the thumbnail and the pad of the index finger on the edge of the nail bed. A change in an indicator muscle shows that the circuit is not complete. There is either additional information needed about what you are currently doing, or additional information of another type is required for this circuit to be fully developed.

For example, you have a painful shoulder in circuit and you have used specific muscle mode to locate a muscle that is involved in this shoulder imbalance and entered that into circuit. If holding

more mode at this point gives an indicator change, this suggests that there is another muscle that needs to be identified to increase the effectiveness of the balance. Following an indicator change with more mode, you may then hold specific muscle again and be directed to another muscle that is involved with the shoulder imbalance. If more mode is held once more and there is no indicator change, it indicates that you have all the information needed at this time to perform an effective balance.

To continue this example, you have a painful shoulder and specific muscle mode has indicated that you have to locate a muscle and enter it into circuit. Checking more mode gives an indicator change, suggesting there is another piece of information that is needed before balancing. However, holding specific muscle mode again does not give an indicator change. This indicates that while more information is needed, it is a different type of information from that previously entered (another muscle). Instead, you may check other modes and find that emotion mode produces an indicator change, suggesting that a component of

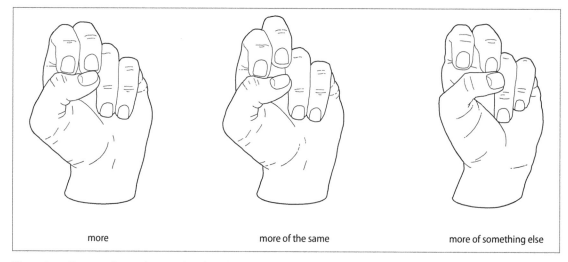

more   more of the same   more of something else

Figure 25.4 More modes. a, The more hand mode involves placing the pad of the middle finger on the edge of the thumbnail, and the pad of the index finger on the edge of the nail bed. If there is an indicator change when more mode is held, it indicates that there is additional information needed for this circuit to be fully developed. b, By lifting the middle finger while holding more mode, the mode is altered to 'more of the same'. If there is an indicator change while this mode is held, it indicates to look for imbalances within the same system you are currently working with. c, By lifting the index finger while holding more mode, the mode is altered to 'More of something else'. If there is an indicator change while this mode is held, it indicates the need to investigate other systems than the one you are currently working with for additional information.

the pain in the shoulder relates to subconscious emotions.

However, using more mode in its original form you never knew whether you needed to locate information of the same type as the original information or of a different type. In 1986, both Richard Utt in Applied Physiology and Bruce Dewe in Professional Kinesiology Practice independently had the concept that the two fingers sitting on the thumb could indicate each of these two options. Unfortunately, the assignations they made were directly opposite to each other! Utt assigned the middle finger touching the corner of the thumbnail *continue the modality*, and the index finger touching the bed of the thumbnail *locate a different modality*, while Dewe assigned the exact opposite. Because of the more prolific use of the Professional Kinesiology Practice assignations, we will use Dewe's assignation in this textbook.

Therefore when more mode gives an indicator change, the monitor need only lift the index finger or the middle finger to see which caused the indicator change. If touching the index finger on the edge of the thumbnail bed gives an indicator change, they then know to look for imbalances within the same system they are currently working with. In contrast, if touching the middle finger to the edge of the thumbnail gives an indicator change, they now know to investigate other systems than the one they are currently working with. All three more modes are shown in Figure 25.4.

However, there is another way of using more mode that is equally significant. When you have gathered all the data and located the priority technique for correcting the issue in circuit and the correction is complete, you can check more mode once again. If you get an indicator change here, it has two different meanings. First, if *more of the same* gives an indicator change, then it says that whatever technique you are doing needs to be continued; for example, neurolymphatic massage needs to be done for longer. Second, if *more of something else* gives an indicator change, then it says that the therapy you have just applied is complete; however, there is another factor that you need to locate and balance before the circuit itself is complete.

The use of circuit mode

Another concept developed by Ian Stubbings in the Stress Indicator Points System is the concept of circuit mode and extended circuit mode. An energetic circuit, particularly one created by linear stacking, is in a sense like a wire with a string hanging from it with knots or blockages along its length. The wire is the present time, and the knot attaching the string to the wire is the presenting issue, for example a muscle imbalance. Once this is pause locked and more mode shows, there is an additional factor underlying this muscle imbalance; investigation with modes and specific indicator points will identify the nature of that imbalance, that is, the next knot on the string. Because this may be repeated several times, the string hanging from the present time may have a series of knots or blockages along it, each of which is entered into circuit. In normal circumstances, this circuit would then be balanced. If the balance is effective, it will resolve the knot of the present day issue and all the related knots (blockages) identified that underlie the present issue.

In some cases, however, there may be collateral issues to one or more of the knots identified along the length of the string. For example, if it was a muscle imbalance, the first knot of the string may have been a neurolymphatic reflex point. When more mode was held, it did not give an indicator change, showing that there were no more issues on this line. However, when circuit mode is held you may get an indicator change. This indicates that the neurolymphatic imbalance just identified is associated with a collateral imbalance that is separate from the original muscle imbalance but that still may affect the original muscle imbalance via this neurolymphatic reflex. For example, there is an emotion that when active may activate this specific neurolymphatic reflex, even if it is not present at this time. When that emotion becomes active, it may very well activate that neurolymphatic reflex, recreating the muscle imbalance that was just balanced (see Figure 25.5).

This means that circuit mode allows us to include relevant collateral imbalances and information that would be hidden if we were using only more mode. Circuit mode is made by crossing the

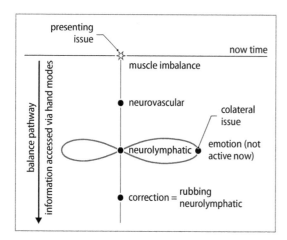

Figure 25.5 **Value of circuit mode.** The presenting issue is a muscle imbalance, and factors underlying this present-time issue were identified via a kinesiology balance using hand modes and specific indicator points. By correcting the priority issue underlying the other issues, in this case a neurolymphatic imbalance, the client may experience improvement or resolution of their muscle imbalance. Circuit mode allows us to also identify collateral issues not in the direct balance pathway but which if left unresolved may reactivate one of the factors that underlie the original muscle imbalance (e.g. the emotion underlying the initial neurolymphatic imbalance), and over time this collateral issue will recreate the original muscle imbalance.

left thumb over the top of the right thumb with the fingers extended, as shown in Figure 25.6a. If there is an indicator change when this mode is held, it indicates that there is collateral information that needs to be included in the circuit to deepen the corrections that are made.

At a later date, one of Stubbings's students in Germany suggested a modification of the circuit mode, as circuit mode just indicated that some type of collateral information was needed, with no indication of what type. So this student suggested that perhaps you could identify the domain of the imbalance by doing an *extended* circuit mode.

Extended circuit mode involves holding the original circuit mode, and if there is an indicator change, then folding all the left fingers on top of the right fingers, as shown in Figure 25.6b. A reciprocal indicator change means that you then need to identify the domain.

This is accomplished by holding first little finger over little finger, ring finger over ring finger, middle finger over middle finger, and index finger over index finger. The finger that gives a priority indicator change indicates which domain this collateral issue is in; for example, ring finger over ring finger indicates that the collateral issue is in the

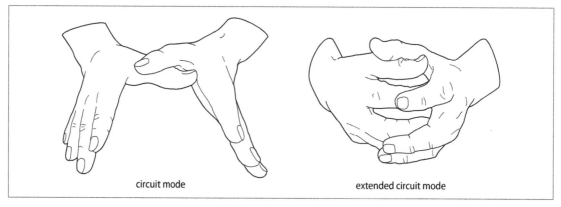

circuit mode   extended circuit mode

Figure 25.6 **Circuit modes. a, Circuit mode.** The circuit hand mode involves crossing the left thumb over the top of the right thumb with the fingers extended. If there is an indicator change when circuit mode is held, it indicates that there are collateral imbalances that need to be included in the circuit to deepen the correction(s) that are made. **b, Extended circuit mode.** This mode involves holding circuit mode then folding all the left fingers on top of the right fingers. If this mode is held after circuit mode has given an indicator change, then another indicator change means that you need to identify the domain by checking each finger one at a time. An indicator change while touching the index fingers indicates the collateral information is in the structural domain, middle fingers indicate that it is in the nutritional domain, ring fingers indicate that it is in the Emotional domain, and the little fingers indicate that it is in the electromagnetic or energetic domain.

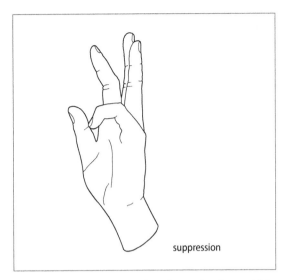

suppression

Figure 25.7 Suppression mode. The suppression hand mode involves holding the nail of the little finger to the crease of the thumb. If this mode is held, there is another indicator change; this indicates that there is information related to the issue in circuit but which is suppressed. Once this mode has been entered into circuit, then this suppressed information can now be accessed and balanced.

emotional domain. Further investigation within that domain will identify the specific collateral issue, for example emotion, flower essence or self-concept. Stubbings researched this concept and found that it did indeed work.

Uncovering suppressed information

We may suppress many things at many levels on a daily basis. We may be angry with a friend but we do not wish to hurt their feelings, so we suppress what we wanted to say. We may have the flu, so we take drugs that suppress the elimination process. We may take flower essences that in some instances could suppress an emotional reaction. We may have vaccinations that could suppress the immune system.

During a session, suppressed information can be present that relates to the imbalance in pause lock but does not give an indicator change and hence remains unknown to the monitor. How can we access this information if it has been suppressed?

The concept of suppression mode was developed by Andrew Verity, as he had done training in homeopathy and suppression is a major concept in that field. He was thinking that when we have more mode and it does not give an indicator change, does that really mean that there is no more information needed for the circuit? Or might there

be additional important information that has been suppressed and hence does not show with more mode? Andrew then discovered that when he held the nail of the little finger to the crease of the thumb, as shown in Figure 25.7, he would sometimes get an indicator change even after more mode had indicated that the circuit is complete. Because this hand mode involves the little finger, which represents the energetic–electromagnetic domain, this mode is basically representing an energetic–electromagnetic priority.

Suppression mode can be used to help identify suppressed information. This mode must always be monitored with an unlocked indicator muscle in circuit to ensure that a clear change of indicator is obtained. Suppression will often over-facilitate the indicator muscle and hence eliminate an indicator change. By starting with an unlocked muscle, you will not miss a change from locked to over-facilitated, permitting the monitor to detect any suppressed information in the circuit.

This mode can be used in a session in two ways: 1, as the last step before correction, to access any suppressed information so that it can be entered into circuit and balanced; or 2, at the end of every balance before the circuit is closed, to ascertain if the balancing has freed up any suppressed information that can now be accessed and balanced.

Chapter 26

FINDING EMOTIONS

Because over 50% of all our illnesses are said to be stress-related, it is relevant for us to know what causes the stress in our lives. Heart disease, high blood pressure, colitis, asthma, kidney disease, peptic ulcers, anxiety, depression, obesity, rheumatoid arthritis and cancer are all conditions for which stress has been implicated as a significant factor.[1] Much of the stress in our lives results from unresolved emotional issues that, even when not in our consciousness, stimulate the secretion of stress-related hormones such as cortisol and adrenaline. In fact, *Healthy People 2000*, a report from the US Department of Health and Human Services, reports that stress has a great impact on our health, with 70-80% of all visits to the doctor for stress-related and stress-induced illnesses, and stress now contributes to 50% of all illness in the United States.[2]

It would therefore appear useful for us to know how to recognize the sources of stress in our lives, and indeed how distressed we are, or stated more commonly, how stressed we are, in order to begin resolving these stressors. After all, self-awareness is one of the keys to establishing effective stress management.

Emotional stress and the brain

Because unresolved emotional stress is such a significant component of the stress in our lives, it is important to understand the nature of emotional stress. To have a conceptual understanding of emotional stress, it is necessary to know how the brain processes information, at least in broad strokes. The brain can functionally be divided into right and left brains, top and bottom brains, and front and back brains or brain regions, each with its own unique contribution to the processing of incoming sensory information and emotional response to that information.

For most people, the right cerebral hemisphere is the location of holistic gestalt lead functions, the seat of intuitive knowing. The left cerebral hemisphere in most people contains the logic lead functions, the seat of language and analytical thought. While the processing and integration of sensory information occurs at several levels in the brain, it is only in the higher cortical centers that this sensory input is interpreted and given meaning as a conscious perception.

However, there are two quite separate sensory systems that process sensory data: the conscious stream mentioned above, and the subconscious stream that assigns survival emotions to the current sensory data being processed. Because the survival emotions require only a few neural links and are thus formed rapidly, they are generated quickly, well before the more specific multistep processing in the cortex has completed its far more detailed analysis to give us a fine-grained image and all our experiential references to this current experience as a now-time conscious perception.

If the rapid subconscious processing, centered in the amygdala and related survival system, associates the current stimulus with either pain and punishment or pleasure and reward, this subconscious emotional input colors our conscious awareness developed on the basis of more in-depth cortical processing that happens after the emotional color has already been established.

Depending on the meaning assigned, emotional responses may be triggered, often out of our conscious awareness. Using sight as an example, visual images are first transferred from the retina to the primary visual cortex in the back of the brain, and then through a series of steps translated from the raw data of density patterns of light to visual perceptions (e.g. Fred's face). However, while this multistep cortical process is happening in the cortex, the amygdala has already checked out our last emotional interaction with Fred for the associated survival emotions.

So our consciousness is busy working out exactly what we are looking at and accessing referents in our long-term memory and our previous experience with similar sensory data to create a conscious perception. This perception is then integrated into our previous experience to give it meaning, and depending on how we feel about Fred, this perception could potentially elicit an emotional response, positive or negative.

The top of the brain, comprising primarily the neocortex or new cerebral cortex, is an evolutionary newcomer unique to mammals. It is most fully developed in Man and in cetaceans, porpoises, whales and their relatives. The neocortex is the seat of associative thinking (intellectual thought) and lies over the deep bottom brain as the cap of a mushroom overlays and covers its stem. The deeper bottom brain regions are composed of the brainstem: the medulla oblongata, the pons and the midbrain, below the diencephalon, the hypothalamus and the thalamus. Together, these are sometimes called the 'lizard brain' or 'reptilian brain', the seat of instinctual drives and raw emotions, for example sexual drive, thirst or rage. This is so named because these deep brain structures are found and fully developed in our reptilian ancestors.

The reptilian brain houses the survival system that controls the fight-or-flight reactions. Surrounding the reptilian brain is a band of ancient cerebral cortex, the paleocortex. The limbic system is composed of both paleocortex and parts of the reptilian brain, and is the seat of our subconscious emotions and the mediator of our survival emotions, such as fear, anger, sadness and rage. These survival emotions originate deep within our unconscious brainstem survival system and are then mediated by parts of our subconscious limbic system with regard to their social expression.

So while the brainstem survival system may elicit anger or rage to a particular situation from the *fight* of the fight-or-flight reactions, how you will express that anger or rage is largely determined by parts of the limbic system, such as the anterior cingulate gyrus, which then modulates these survival emotions relative to socially and culturally accepted norms, and the subcallosal gyrus, which overtly supresses the anger and rage. Thus, these bottom brain structures are the source of many of the feelings and emotions that reach our consciousness, albeit modified by our cultural and social norms and past associated experiences through the limbic system.

The vertical auricular line, a line drawn from one ear over the top of the head to the other ear, separates the frontal cortices from the posterior cortices. The anatomical posterior cortical regions include the parietal, occipital and temporal lobes, and are largely processing centers, where our visual, auditory and kinaesthetic inputs become fully developed into conscious perceptions of sight, hearing and touch sensations, respectively. The long-term memories associated with these senses are also stored in these same posterior cortical areas.

The rapid access to these long-term memories stored in the posterior cortical areas can be triggered by the response of the survival system to some stimuli, thus eliciting these memories. The two systems, the posterior cortical memory system and the brainstem survival system, were collectively called the *back brain* in some forms of Energetic Kinesiology. However, this totally confuses the very different roles played by these two very different brain systems.

The frontal lobes are the seat of associational thinking and working memory. Here, we analyze new incoming information in the light of our past experiences to better understand these experiences, or reanalyse past experiences to rationally understand the meaning of these past events in our lives and in our current situation. Also, working memory is the seat of our executive functions: our ability to use higher-level reasoning, analytical thinking, multitasking, decision making and problem solving. The executive functions are the source of our lateral thinking and creative problem solving. The frontal lobes also house the orbitofrontal cortices, which help direct our conscious attention, are involved in emotional conflict resolution and help us organize our behavior by providing routines for us to follow.

Much of the incoming sensory data we receive every day is quickly assessed, found to be irrelevant and dumped (e.g. the number of bricks in your garden path or the number of times your neighbour's dog has barked). A small percentage of this incoming sensory information is deemed relevant and focused on for further processing, and then if repeated often enough or of great enough relevance, is stored in posterior cortical association areas of long-term memory.

The frontal lobes are also the site where old patterns or ideas stored in the posterior cortical memory vaults can be reprocessed. Memories are brought forward from these memory areas into the frontal lobes, especially in working memory areas and the higher association areas of the prefrontal cortex. These areas can look at these past events in a dispassionate, non-judgmental and unemotional way: whatever happened, happened!

The frontal lobes then merely appraise these events in a discriminating way, using analysis and rationalization to understand why these events occurred and thus extracting life's lesson contained in them and in similar situations. Indeed, one of the most powerful aspects of having well-developed frontal lobes is the ability to learn from past mistakes and be able to alter future behaviors to prevent stressful situations from happening again, including learning from your own and other people's mistakes! However, the following quote is only too true: 'One of the most remarkable things about human beings is their ability to learn from other people's mistakes—but an even more incredible thing about human beings is their reticence to do so!' (anonymous).

For instance, you trusted someone to do a job and he or she did not do it. From this experience and the past experiences with a friend who was not particularly trustworthy, you might have developed the emotional program, largely from emotions elicited in the subconscious emotional survival centers deep within the brain, summarized as, 'Well, I can never trust anybody to do what they say again!' While this program would initially be stored in your posterior cortical memory areas, it could be brought forward into your frontal lobes in the future for analysis, which may extract the lesson, 'Well, I guess I should be more discriminating in whom I choose to trust in

the future; perhaps assess their previous track record!'

This process of re-evaluating previous emotional traumas or upsets from a non-judgmental perspective allows you to learn life's lesson contained in these events. It appears that this analysis and re-evaluation of the upsetting situation defuses the emotional stress of the situation, releasing the associated negative emotions of anger, rage or whatever has been associated with this event. This reprocessed destressed program is again sent into storage in long-term memory, but it no longer contains the stress or charge of the negative emotions previously associated with it.

As an analogy, it is the emotional juxtaposition of events that gives a joke its humorous charge. If you analyze a joke, for instance by having to explain it to someone, it ceases to be funny, as you have defused the charge by the analysis. Likewise, with emotional situations if you truly take the time to calm down and analyze the situation from a dispassionate perspective, this analysis defuses the emotional charge of the situation.

Memory and emotions

The assigning of relevance to an experience is not, however, done in an objective, emotionally neutral way. Once the perception of the event has been formed, the meaning of this perception is determined by comparison with past perceptions of similar type based on the experiential background of the person. For instance, you may be driving along in the car, when a song you have not heard in years begins to play on the radio. Suddenly, you are transported back to the first time you heard that song.

You may find yourself thinking fondly or despondently of the people in your life at that time, depending on what circumstances the song has become associated with in your memory. You are consciously aware that the reason you are thinking of X and feeling fondness or despondency was triggered by the memories associated with the song. What type of emotion the song triggers, or whether it even triggers an emotion at all, is totally dependent on the individual's past experience. Another person may have quite the opposite emotion linked to the same song or, having never heard the song before, the song may elicit no emotion whatsoever.

Both conscious and subconscious memories, however, may link emotional responses to the events in our lives. Occasionally, we are conscious of the event that is triggering the past emotional feelings we are currently experiencing (e.g. the song on the radio), but at other times, we may suddenly feel emotions (e.g. depression) for which there is no obvious conscious trigger. In these cases, the trigger is usually subconscious, with some recent event acting as a trigger that activates the emotions linked subconsciously to a similar event in our past. Thus, while we will consciously experience the emotion, we may be totally unaware of the source of this emotion.

Conscious and unconscious memories, although recording past experiences, are processed very differently. The sensory data on which conscious memories are based is first filtered by our ego, how we see ourselves and how we believe others see us. When an event happens that may reflect negatively on our ego, we may alter how we remember the event so that it was not really our fault, or the more critical statements about us may be deleted or altered so what the other person said was not so bad.

You can bet that if a man with a strongly negative opinion of women drivers observes an accident in which a woman was involved, in his memory of the accident he will find her at fault, no matter what objectively happened. Another part of his brain will also have recorded the original sensory data from his observation of the accident, but this accurate memory is recorded only in his subconscious memory. Thus, if the subconscious memory of the same event could be taped, as sometimes occurs by brain areas being activated during a brain operation, a more objective presentation of the facts may be offered in which the woman was much less at fault. There is considerable evidence that at some level within our brain there is a memory trace for every event that has ever occurred in our lives. Each of these memory traces, whether conscious or subconscious, is capable of triggering emotions associated with that memory.

There is also ever increasing evidence that much of what we remember as fact may not have happened the way we remembered it. In many cases, the brain, in the process of reassembling a previous memory, may create a new memory of considerably different content from the original memory. Or from suggestion the brain may create memory of something that never actually happened, as in the case of false memory syndrome.

The role of trigger stimuli in emotional response to memory

While the integration of processes in the right (gestalt) and left (logic) hemispheres and the top and bottom brain processes are important to the formation of emotional programs in the first place, it is the storage of these emotional programs containing emotional stress in brainstem and limbic memory areas that can be problematic in future situations in our lives. Metaphorically, our brainstem and limbic memory areas can be visualized as a huge videotape library containing tapes of every event recorded during our life, either consciously and/or subconsciously. These tapes are, however, filed in a unique way. They are filed by trigger stimulus, with the most traumatic or emotionally intense experience related to particular stimuli at the top of the stack of tapes of related experiences.

The tapes are filed in this way because traumatic, negative or emotionally intense experiences have the greatest survival value. Because the primary function of the brainstem and limbic centers is to maintain your survival, they operate by the axiom, 'Pay close attention to those events that threatened your physical or emotional ego survival the most!'

A trigger stimulus can be any sensory input from the environment that becomes associated with a particular emotion or circumstance. In phobias, for instance, the sight of a spider or snake, or even a certain color, becomes linked to the survival emotional response of irrational fear. Or, the sound or tone of someone's voice may trigger emotions related to a totally unrelated event from childhood (e.g. a parent's anger). However, the person is only consciously aware of the person who is speaking to them in that vocal tone, not the triggered anger caused by this vocal tone and its past association with their parent's anger. This occurs totally outside of their consciousness. Thus, they react with anger to the person speaking with them and blame them for making them angry, but in reality the anger was merely triggered by these childhood memories acting outside of their consciousness.

Any stimulus is potentially a trigger stimulus. The intensity and/or degree of emotion associated with the stimulus are the factors that determine whether the memory program stored in the posterior cortical areas will contain emotional stress or not. In the earlier example of hearing the old song, whether the song triggers an emotional response or not, and the type of emotional response elicited, depends entirely on the circumstances that the song had been associated with when you first encoded the memory of that event.

Only those tapes in a stimulus category that are traumatic or emotionally intense are stored on top of the pile, and thus the first ones to be replayed when similar stimuli are experienced in the future. The next time that a stimulus occurs, the brain rapidly scans the video files for the trigger stimulus category closest to the one just received. The top tape on that pile is jammed into the brain tape player. If the first message on this tape is unresolved stress, then we are switched into a reactive mode of fight-or-flight reaction, which unfortunately has only a playback function. So whatever program is on that tape, we are forced to play this program from beginning to end. However, what is on that tape is our previous reaction to another, often unrelated, emotionally stressful situation (unrelated, that is, except for sharing a similar trigger stimulus).

If, however, the emotional stress on that top tape has been resolved before this time, the brain's tape player is switched to the frontal lobes. This is the seat of *choice*, where the current event is viewed as a new event with many potential options of response, despite its association with a past traumatic situation. From a frontal lobes perspective, we look at each situation as it is now, not what associated trigger stimuli have meant in the past. We are free to choose the most appropriate

behavior or response to the current situation, including ones we have never done before.

Equally important as choice in the present, the frontal lobes also contain edit, erase and record functions, the role of introspection and analysis located in your working memories. When an emotionally stressful or traumatic tape is called up from memory, if we can stay in the frontal lobes we can employ these options and release or defuse the stressful emotions associated with these past traumas and stresses. We do this by dispassionate analysis and introspection, using the transcendent emotions accessed through the prefrontal cortex. In computer terms, the frontal lobes appear to be programmed to evaluate all events non-judgmentally, irrespective of previous emotional or traumatic content, and to extract what can be learned from a circumstance.

When the event is reprocessed in the frontal lobes, the emotions associated with it are defused and the experience is edited for life's lesson contained in the event. This life's lesson is then recorded over the previously emotionally traumatic memory of the event, and this tape is once again filed away at the top of the stack. The next time that trigger stimulus occurs, the tape on top, containing the emotionally defused memory, is now played back. We can now evaluate the current situation from the frontal lobe perspective of choice, applying life's lesson learned from the past circumstance.

When the subconscious speaks

If the source of many of our emotional stresses is subconscious, how are we to know about this stress? There are many times that emotional states just appear to take us over, with no obvious cause, and we are left in a state of anxiety, depression or tension with no idea of how to resolve it. On the other hand, there are always two different agendas active in our lives: the one we perceive consciously and the underlying subconscious emotional context. So while you may say to yourself, 'I don't have a problem with John; he's basically a nice guy. He just has a couple of irritating habits', our subconscious may have an entirely different relationship to John based on the tonal quality of his voice, which happens to trigger childhood memories of an annoyed parent. But how are we to know about our states of stress both conscious and subconscious?

One of the most direct and observable ways to know of your stress is through muscle biofeedback, which allows us to literally see and feel our stress. By monitoring a muscle at the same time as you think of a situation or an event in your life that may have been stressful, the muscle response will let you observe whether this situation or event is indeed still stressful or not, at both the conscious and the subconscious levels. If there is no stress associated with this particular situation or event, or the previous stress has been defused, then the muscle will remain locked when monitored while you think of this situation or event. If there is either conscious or subconscious stress associated with the situation or event, then the muscle will immediately unlock when monitored.

This occurs because the issue generates subconscious stress that directly alters the muscle tone controlling the load reflex; the spindle cell bag fibers become slack and the muscle unlocks. This change in muscle tone caused by emotional or mental stress is the reason that a professional golfer may miss a simple 3-foot putt needed to win the big tournament. This stress sufficiently altered their muscle tone such that they could not successfully carry out a normally easy and well-practiced action.

While we tend to think of our muscle movement as voluntary, for all but a small proportion of the time our muscle movement is actually run by the subconscious. Walking is a complex integrated muscle action requiring literally thousands of coordinated muscle movements, but how many of this cast of thousands do you actually consciously direct when you walk? Basically none; all you do consciously is give the command to walk and the subconscious deep brain nuclei (basal ganglia) and cerebellum do the rest. When you are walking down the street thinking, 'What am I going to do tonight?', who is running your feet? It is obviously not your conscious brain but rather the subconscious brain centers monitoring the millions of bits of sensory feedback required to coordinate this complex muscular activity (see Figure 26.1).

Not only does the subconscious normally control our muscular activity, but when push comes to shove it will override the conscious command. There are tension sensors in the tendons of the muscles, Golgi tendon organs, which tell the brain about how much tension is on each muscle. When tension levels reach a threshold above which mechanical damage is likely to result, the tendons may tear or muscles may rip; the subconscious sensors turn the muscles off to protect them from damage no matter what your conscious desire.

Watch any weight-lifting competition to see this principle in action. The weight lifter is consciously going for the gold and commands their body to lift the weight, and they get it to just above their head. But it just will not go any further, and the weight lifter appears to throw the weight down. What happened? While the weight lifter's conscious command was to lift, at a certain point the tension exceeded the danger threshold and the subconscious stepped in and in a sense said, 'Sorry, you have not trained long enough or hard enough to lift this amount of weight. You lose!' And it just turns off the muscles doing the lifting. It also turns on the muscles necessary to throw the bar onto the floor to release the tension as rapidly as possible.

While this was a physical example, the same thing may occur when emotional or mental stress levels get too high. In a stress-free state, these subconscious centers run our muscular movement to satisfy our conscious commands. However, should a sufficient level of emotional or mental stress enter the scene, this stress may interfere with the normally automatic subconscious processing of sensory data and alter the muscle response.

Locating stressful emotions

Because many of our emotional states originate in our subconscious, particularly our brainstem and limbic survival systems, we need a mechanism to access these subconscious emotional stressors. As previously discussed, muscle monitoring provides just such a tool.

When we have entered information into a

circuit, whether this be physical (a muscle imbalance), emotional (an issue with a parent) or mental (distressing thoughts), the underlying issue may have an emotional component. How are we to locate the relevant emotion or emotions that are part of this imbalance? By holding the emotional hand mode, it is possible to check whether an emotion is involved in the issue. When holding the emotional hand mode causes an indicator change, we know that the frequency of the imbalance in the circuit matches the emotion mode and therefore has an emotional component.

Meridian-emotion relationships

The Chinese recognized through millennia of observation that imbalances within specific organ systems, which they related to specific meridian flows, are consistently preceded or associated with specific emotional states. For instance, kidney meridian energy and kidney-related disorders are associated with the emotion of fear, while imbalances within the liver and liver meridian are associated with the emotion anger. This meridian-emotion association was well established by the time of Christ. See Table 26.1 for original Chinese psychosomatic associations.

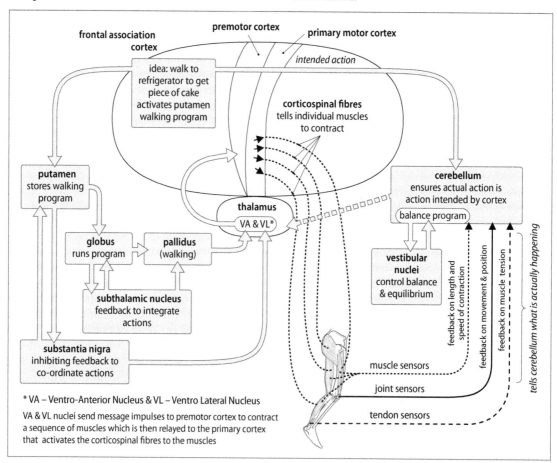

Figure 26.1 Subconscious control of movement. Note that except for the conscious initiation of the movement (i.e. 'Walk to the refrigerator'), all the centers and pathways controlling movement (the basal ganglia: putamen and globus pallidus on the lower left), its integrating and coordination centers (substantia nigra and subthalamic nuclei below left) and the cerebellum (on the right comparing intended action with actual action and sending corrective motor output when needed), including the posture and equilibrium programs (the balance program of the cerebellum and vestibular system), all the centers controlling movement are subconscious.

Table 26.1 Chinese meridian-related psychosomatic conditions

Meridian or body region	In normal function	In anomalous function
Stomach	• Outgoing • Stable sensibility	• Hesitance • Irrationality
Stomach and spleen	• Charity • Wisdom	• Greed • Deceit
Spleen	• Caring, sympathetic • Creative positive thinking • Able to accept and order life's experiences as you meet them each day, in all their variety	• Moodiness, sullenness • Worry • Unable to accept and order life's experiences as you meet them each day, in all their variety
Large intestine	• Openness, receptivity • Discrimination	• Self-opinionated, blocked • Hypercritical
Large intestine and lungs	• Forgiveness • Insight	• Pride • Misconception
Lungs	• Trusting, hopeful • Intuitive • Able to filter out the unwanted and the outgrown	• Grievous, pining, hopelessness • Closed mindedness • Unable to filter out the unwanted and the outgrown
Bladder	• All embracing, rapport • Clarity, farsightedness	• Gloominess • Introversion
Kidneys	• Confiding, giving • Concentration	• Sorrowful, needing to receive • Weak, impotent thinking
Bladder and kidneys	• Truth • Assurance • Able to evaluate life's experiences in the clear light of truth	• Fear • Isolation • Unable to evaluate life's experiences in the clear light of truth
Gall bladder	• Capable, good management • Decisiveness	• Escapist, non-committal • Indecisiveness
Gall bladder and liver	• Selflessness • Patience	• Envy • Intolerance
Liver	• Courage, fortitude • Organized thinking • Balanced mental activity • Able to regulate and manage life's experiences	• Anger, depression • Emotion rules the thinking • Too much mental activity • Unable able to regulate and manage life's experiences
Small intestine	• Listener, comforter • Intentionality	• Bitter, conniving • Poor memory, unreliability
Small intestine and heart	• Compassion • Love	• Hate • Deprivation
Heart	• Joyful, loving • Judge of what is best • Autonomous self-identity • Self is equal to others	• Resentful, insatiably desirous • Self-destructor • Savior seeking • Inferior to others

These original meridian-emotion associations were added to Applied Kinesiology and the Energetic Kinesiology modalities that followed by using muscle biofeedback to determine more specific meridian-emotion relationships. Once you have access to direct muscle biofeedback and the alarm points of Chinese medicine, which meridian becomes active or is affected by a specific emotion can be directly determined. Thus, a number of kinesiology modalities developed meridian-emotion charts that can now be used to locate specific emotions via their meridian relationship.

The first associations were those taken from the Chinese with respect to the primary emotions associated with each meridian. However, with advent of muscle monitoring once emotion mode is entered into circuit, the nature of the emotion can be easily located by circuit-localization of the alarm points for each meridian. This is possible because each emotion has a primary frequency signature related to a particular meridian.

As other Energetic Kinesiology modalities developed, this meridian–emotion relationship was elaborated, with additional emotions assigned to a meridian relationship. One of the first Energetic Kinesiology modalities was Biokinesiology, developed by John Barton. One of the core features of this kinesiology was the relationship of the organs, and hence meridians, with a number of very specific positive and negative emotions. Barton ran summer camps while he was developing these meridian–emotion relationships. He and his colleagues would test a large number of individuals and see which meridian alarm point was related to a specific emotion, by having the person state that emotion and monitoring the alarm point. He would consider the meridian–emotion relationship valid only when a thousand muscle tests had confirmed this relationship.

Kinesiologists working in other Energetic Kinesiology modalities used muscle monitoring to develop emotional charts based on other models, rather than just the meridian–emotion relationship. There are a large number of these charts now available, such as the Behavioral Barometer in Three In One Concepts and the Kinergetics Emotions Chart developed by Philip Rafferty. It is useful to have a large selection of emotional trigger words available to scan when working with clients, so that the client's emotional state can more specifically match their issue.

Scan mode and information gathering

While one of the more esoteric methods used in Energetic Kinesiology, scan mode has proven to be one of the most powerful tools in identifying specific emotions as well as other information. Developed by Richard Utt, scan mode is accessed by holding the thumb pad over the proximal knuckle of the index finger, as shown in Figure 26.2. Scan mode selects the frequency interference pattern held in circuit to match against other potential frequencies, such as various emotions or acupoints.

Currently, the exact mechanism by which scan mode actually works, besides frequency matching,

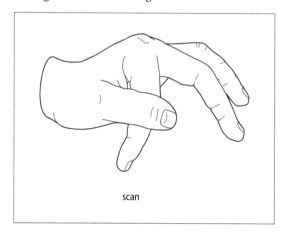

scan

Figure 26.2 Scan mode. The scan hand mode involves holding the thumb pad over the proximal knuckle of the index finger. If scan mode is held while a list or diagram is scanned, then an indicator change will identify the item in that list or diagram that is relevant to the issue in circuit.

remains unknown. However, it has consistently proven to provide accurate information relative to the imbalance held in circuit and is especially useful in identifying emotions that are relevant. Once emotion mode has indicated that emotions are a component of the imbalance, and this has been entered into circuit, then with scan mode it is possible to scan a list of emotions that may be relevant to the issue in circuit. This allows you to identify the specific emotion that is indicated by the more general emotion mode.

Scan mode is an information mode, and it therefore does not cause an indicator change when held by the monitor but rather provides a context to identify information, such that when you hold scan mode there is no indicator change, but when emotion mode has been entered into circuit and you then scan a list of emotions while holding scan mode, the relevant emotion will now give an indicator change. This allows the monitor to identify the emotion relevant to the frequency interference pattern held in circuit, out of an endless list of possible emotions.

Krebs, coming from his analytical chemistry background, initially found scan mode a challenging concept, particularly as there was no cogent mechanism by which it might work. However, based on his consistent observations over the past 25 years, scan mode appears to work exceedingly well and produce results that defy statistical probability. For example, Krebs was working with a man at Richard Utt's center in Tuscon, Arizona, and emotion mode came up as a frequency match for the back problem being held in circuit. But it did not match any of the numerous lists of emotions that he had at hand. So he held scan mode and scanned the books in the room and a specific book then gave an indicator change. Within this book it then indicated a specific aphorism labelled *solitude*. Initially, Krebs felt very reticent to even say this word to the man, because it

seemed so implausible, but then when he had the man state 'solitude', the man said 'That's exactly my issue! I just can't get any solitude in my life!'

Because Krebs was having great difficulty consistently getting an indicator with this client, when Utt returned Krebs asked him to investigate the problem. Utt took the man into his office, put the back problem into circuit and emotion mode came up. Again, none of the normal lists of emotions were relevant, and so Utt held scan mode and scanned the books in his office. A specific book was indicated, and Utt located a specific page and then scanned the page. Low and behold: the word indicated was *solitude*. Because there are probably 10 million words in all the books in those two separate rooms, the probability of scan mode twice selecting the word *solitude* in the context of the man's back problem is statistically improbable. So, we may not yet understand the mechanism by which scan mode works, but we know it does work!

Scan mode has now become an important tool in finding emotional information, as it allows the rapid assessment of even long lists of potential emotions to locate the specific emotion involved in the issue held in pause lock.

A conceptual model could be analogous to the barcode scanners used in supermarket checkouts. The employee scanning your groceries merely passes an item over the scanner and it goes, 'Green beans, $2.39'. However, the scanner did not actually say anything; it just detected white bar, black bar, white bar, black bar ... which was the programmed code for 'Green beans, $2.39'. In a similar way, written words have pre-programmed energetic patterns that have been assigned by billions of minds. Therefore when the monitor is holding scan mode as it passes over a specific emotional word, there can be a frequency match, giving an indicator change. This indicates that this word has a frequency match with the imbalance in circuit.

References

1. Selyes, H 1976, *The Stress of Life*, McGraw-Hill, New York, pp. 171–227.
2. US Department of Health and Human Services 2000, *Healthy People 2000 Final Review* [online] Available at: http://www.cdc.gov/nchs/data/hp2000/hp2k01.pdf

Chapter 27

AGE RECESSION

The exact origins of age recession in kinesiology remain unclear at this time, but it has proved to be an important technique for gathering essential information for resolution of stress in circuits and is now used in a wide variety of Energetic Kinesiology modalities. In psychological literature, this technique was called *age regression* and has been used since Freud's time. This technique involves the concept of going back into a person's history, often into their childhood years, using various techniques, such as hypnosis, trance state work or guided imagery. The intent is to seek the underlying events related to their current emotional state or trauma.

The psychological concept of age regression was renamed *age recession* by the founders of Three In One Concepts, Gordon Stokes, Daniel Whiteside and Candace Callaway, and this term is now generally used in Energetic Kinesiology. While the person clearly remains consciously in the present, they are now accessing memories of events that happened in their past that are relevant to the information in circuit. Indeed, one of the things that often create stress for us in the present has its origins in our early childhood, as many of our basal emotional programs are set between the ages of 18 months and five years.

The brain's memory systems

Why this critical age period? This results from the development of the nervous system, especially myelination of the hippocampus, the short-term memory center. It is only possible to store things in long-term memory that have first been held in short-term memory long enough to be transferred to long-term memory by the process of consolidation. Thus, before the hippocampus is fully myelinated, which is not complete until approximately age three, a child's short-term memory is indeed short term and it is difficult for them to lay down

long-term memories. Hence, you start the trip to Grandma's and two minutes down the road you are asked, 'Are we there yet?', and five minutes later the child asks again, 'Are we there yet?', with no memory of having just asked it five minutes before!

Freud noticed that people seldom have personal memories of even very traumatic events and situations that took place in their lives before the age of three. While they remember being told about these events or situations, they do not have actual personal memories of them. Freud termed this *infantile amnesia*, but it is not really amnesia, rather just the lack of myelination of the hippocampus supporting the creation of long-term memories. If you had asked the child about this event shortly after it had happened, they would have been able to tell you about it from their personal memory; however, because they could not hold this information in their short-term memory long enough to consolidate the memory, no conscious long-term memory is laid down.

We have two quite separate memory systems. The one that we are most aware of is our conscious memory or declarative memory, which means that you are able to consciously tell (or *declare*) what you remember. One of the most frustrating parts of declarative memory is that we often forget things we did know or remembered previously. It is suggested that this is caused by memory interference, that is, that newer memories tend to push older memories further and further back in our memory vaults, making them less and less retrievable in the present. One major component of declarative memory is that we often forget things we have learned or experienced in the past. The further it is in the past, the less likely we are to remember it in the present moment.

The second type of memory is subconscious or non-declarative memory, which means that you do not have conscious access to this information. This is the primary memory of the survival systems of the brain stem and limbic system. One of the major differences between subconscious and conscious memory is that subconscious memory is complete, that is, you do not forget what you have experienced. However, the recording of subconscious memory is dependent on the survival relevance of the event and the associated survival emotion. It must be understood that the subconscious survival system does not think, does not reason and is not rational; it is only associative.

The subconscious associates an event with a particular survival emotion and then believes this association. Therefore it can make associations that are totally illogical, and indeed not even correct, but that nevertheless fire the same survival emotions whenever an event triggers this memory. For instance, as a child you were eating spaghetti and you happened to have a stomach virus that caused you to vomit. This created a most unpleasant feeling, and unfortunately the spaghetti happened to come out of your nose! From that day, you have never been able to eat spaghetti again, even though it had absolutely nothing to do with you being sick. It has become guilty by association.

So the subconscious memory system not only activates the survival emotions but all the surrounding context as well, even factors that were uninvolved in the generation of that survival emotion. This is the basis of phobias. A neutral stimulus happened to be present at the same time that a strong survival emotion was generated, and it becomes linked to that survival emotion. In the case of phobias, the survival emotion is fear and has become linked to a particular stimulus.

For example, you are a young child on the floor and this really interesting animal, which happens to be a spider, is walking across the floor toward you. To you, it is only a furry object of interest, which you are curious about. However, at that moment your mother enters the room, grabs a book and shrieks as she slams it down on the spider. Now while you were not afraid before, you are afraid now! The fear comes from both your surprise and the noise of the book slamming down and your mother's reaction, and perhaps even her vocal tone in the shriek. So now, for you, spiders and fear have become permanently linked in your subconscious memory, and the mere presence of a spider elicits extreme fear, which then controls your behavior.

As an adult with considerable experience and knowledge, you know that a daddy longlegs is a harmless spider-like creature and presents absolutely no threat to you, particularly if it is on the wall several meters away. However, if you have a spider phobia, the instant your eyes register 'spider' all this rational knowledge is shut down and you react as if it is a deathly threat and you must leave the room. This is because the subconscious survival system must inhibit thinking in order for you to physically survive.

In our evolutionary past, those people who thought first and initiated a survival reaction second did not survive to leave many offspring! The people who reacted to survive first and then thought about it are our ancestors! For physical survival, it is often fractions of a second that determine life and death, and so there is no time for the slower process of thinking. For instance, you are stepping off the curb and in your peripheral vision you detect a car approaching rapidly. Without thinking, you jump back just in time to prevent being hit by the car. Had you first thought, 'What kind of car is it?', it would have been your last thought!

Therefore there is a powerful brain mechanism, finely honed by evolution, called the *fight-or-flight reaction*, which provides you with the necessary reflex reactions to keep you alive in life-threatening circumstances. In order for this reaction to work unimpeded, the subconscious survival system must shut down the frontal cortex so that you do not think. This is easily accomplished by output from the survival center, the amygdala, to reduce blood flow to the frontal lobe areas, effectively turning them off.

This has significant consequences for accessing memories of traumatic experiences during childhood, because while the conscious memory of these traumatic experiences was never properly laid down, and at best is incomplete, the subconscious emotional memories of these experiences were fully formed and encoded in the subconscious survival memory system.

Because we must survive between birth and the age of three, we thus rely on our subconscious survival memories. It is indeed these subconscious survival memories that form to keep us alive and out of harm's way. However, they are based on association, not rational thought or understanding, and may be accurate to the events that happened or distortions of what actually happened because of our lack of experience and understanding. And like all survival emotions, they are retrieved not by conscious recall but by an associated trigger stimulus. Therefore events that were traumatic in this critical period often lay down triggered patterns of behavior that persist well into our adulthood, affecting our behavior and emotional states.

For example, you are two years old and it is necessary for you to have a minor operation. Because you are not able to rationally reason or understand, your parents cannot explain to you why it is necessary for you to go to hospital, be separated from them and, from your perspective, be accosted by strangers who may even hurt you. For you, this is a terribly traumatic experience activating a powerful survival program: hospitals and/or doctors are dangerous. This makes it traumatic for you to go to hospital or seek medical attention, even as an adult.

Another fact that must be understood is that when we are talking of trauma, we are talking about trauma from a child's perspective rather than from the rational perspective of an adult. Indeed, childhood trauma is not only the cause of many psychoemotional issues later in life but is also usually the basis of learning problems. An example of this that demonstrates the role of the child's perspective of trauma is a case Krebs had of a nine-year-old boy who could not spell. This was caused by the lack of brain integration, in which the functions necessary for making pictures in his head had been shut off as a mechanism for surviving a trauma with which he could not cope.

When the lack of brain integration was entered into circuit, emotion mode gave an indicator change and scanning of an emotion list and age recession indicated that he was angry at his mother at the age of 2½. His mother then did the mental mathematics and said, 'Oh, I know exactly what

the issue was. This would be just before Christmas and I always make Christmas cookies the week before. I had just pulled a tray of cookies out of the oven when Johnny came into the room. Of course he said "Cookie, cookie, cookie", to which I replied, "No, you can't have the cookies until next week because they're Christmas cookies." At which point, he put on such a performance: crying, throwing himself on the floor in a tantrum—that I still remember it today."

What this illustrates is the difference in perspective of the rational adult mother and the non-rational 2½-year-old child. While for her it was a question of cookies next week, just not now; for him, who lives only in now time, with no appreciation of the future, it was, 'I'm never going to get a cookie!' Remember: children under the age of 3–5 have no sense of time but live in the eternal now, and it is either 'now' or 'not now', and next week is a 'not now' time so far into the future that it equals 'never'.

In addition, while he does not have rational thought, the subconscious survival system is making important associations for his psychoemotional survival. One of these associations is objects that represent approval and love. He had made a very definite association that when he is a good boy, his mother gives him a cookie, demonstrating her approval and love of him. So for him cookie equals mother's approval and love; denial of a cookie equals mother's approval and love withheld, which is tantamount to annihilation to the two-year-old ego. So while the mother was hearing, 'You can have a cookie next week', Johnny was thinking, 'I'm never going to have your love and approval again!' This is a situation he did not know how to cope with psychoemotionally, leading to the emotional outburst and tantrum the mother observed.

So this one traumatic incident from Johnny's point of view resulted in a learning problem, his inability to learn to spell, but was rooted in a 2½-year-old's subconscious emotional program.

The process of age recession

How did Krebs determine that Johnny's stress was at 2½ years of age? By using the process of age recession with muscle monitoring, Johnny's subconscious was able to indicate the exact time in the past when the psychoemotional program blocking the functions needed to spell originated, because the subconscious never forgets.

There is extensive evidence that non-declarative memory is basically complete, that is, it does not forget any survival related experience—for obvious reasons. This is the basis of much of our early learning involving interactions with our environment. Mum says to her two-year-old child, 'Don't touch the stove; it's hot and you'll burn yourself.' Now while the child knows what 'Don't touch' means, they do not yet know what 'burn yourself' means, so most often they touch the hot stove. The intense burning sensation and pain makes a very strong association between 'hot stove' and 'Don't touch' in their survival system. The child does not need to burn their hand monthly because they forget that hot stoves burn, as this association is indelibly recorded in the subconscious memory. And furthermore, this reaction is generalized to any object that might be a 'hot stove' and might burn.

Once an issue has been identified as having an emotional component, it is useful to challenge whether age recession is appropriate or not. As you will recall, to challenge is to make a statement and then observe the indicator muscle response. So if there is an indicator change when the monitor states 'age recession', it indicates that it is important to locate the time of an antecedent issue that is the basis for the current emotional context. Alternatively, you could have the client state 'present', 'future' or 'past' and monitor after each statement. The statement giving an indicator change indicates what you should do.

If 'present' gives an indicator change, then just continue working with the circuit as it is a present time issue. If there is an indicator change on 'future', this indicates that the stress at the present time has its origins in something that is yet to happen. For instance, if you are told that next week you will be talking in front of 500 people, you might become overtly stressed now, even though the event is not until next week. If stating 'past' gives an indicator change, it indicates that the issue in

circuit at the present time has an antecedent cause that occurred sometime in the past, but when in the past?

The process of identifying the time of the antecedent issue is then quite straightforward. You start with the client's current age, for example 36, then you would say out loud '36 to present day' and monitor the indicator muscle. If there is no indicator change, then state '36 to 30', '30 to 20', '20 to 10', '10 to 5', '5 to birth', 'birth to conception' and 'preconception', while monitoring the indicator muscle after each age range is stated. When an indicator change occurs, you then need to locate the exact year and month in that time period. For example, if birth to 5 causes an indicator change, then you would check 'birth to 1', '1 to 2', etc. If the indicator changed at '4 to 5', then you would check '4 to 4½' and/or '4½ to 5'. If the indicator changes at 4½ to 5, you would then state '4 years, 6 months', '4 years, 7 months', etc. until an indicator change occurs. This year and month would then be the time of the issue underlying the present day psychoemotional stress. The final step is to have the client state that age out loud while you pause lock the indicator change.

It would seem strange to many people that times before birth could be related to their adult psychoemotional states. But this is not surprising if you understand that the amygdala and the brain stem survival system are fully functional by seven months in the womb. And therefore psychoemotional events that may occur with your mother may become part of your psychoemotional subconscious memories. Thus, associations with events such as noises, vocal tones and physical and psychoemotional traumas experienced by your mother are still encoded in your subconscious memory. This is sometimes the reason that people cannot make any conscious connection between a psychoemotional state and the events that triggered these states.

What does it mean when 'preconception' gives an indicator change? Directly, it is indicating that the source of the stress associated with the present issue originated before your conception. How this is interpreted is based on your personal and philosophical beliefs and those of your client. This is something the monitor needs to investigate before proceeding with the age recession. As previously discussed, the client's religious and philosophical beliefs must be respected, and preconception needs to be put into a context that is acceptable to them.

Why do we so often age recess to the ages 18 months to 6 years?

There is extensive work done by Dr. Laibow in investigating the amount of time that you spend in different brainwave states, as measured by electroencephalograms (EEGs) at different ages. Both adults and children display EEG variations that range from low-frequency delta waves to high-frequency beta waves. However, researchers have noted that EEG activity in children reveals the predominance of specific brainwaves at each developmental stage.

The slowest brainwaves are *delta* waves (0.5–4 hertz) and indicative of deep sleep. *Theta* waves (4–8 hertz) are indicative of light sleep. *Alpha* waves (8–16 hertz) indicate the transitory state between sleeping and waving and are characteristic of calm wakefulness. Low *beta* waves (16–24 hertz) are the normal waking state when you are actively processing sensory information. High *beta* waves (24–32 hertz) are generally indicative of heightened anxiety and tension.

Between birth and two years of age, children's brains spend most of their time in delta, although they may exhibit short bursts of higher EEG activity. Children then begin to spend more time at higher levels of EEG activity, characterized as theta and alpha, between 2 and 6 years of age, and have more extended periods of both low and high beta. It should be noted that the hypnogonic state, the state entered when you are under hypnosis, is characterized by the dominance of alpha–theta brainwaves. Children aged 2–6 spend much of their day in this highly programmable state.

This probably has an evolutionary origin, in that children have so much to learn, about their physical environment and even more about their social environment, including the rules and mores of their social group. Therefore this property of being programmable and being able to take in data, particularly into the subconscious survival systems, allows you to rapidly store the essential data you will need for day-to-day life.

There is a downside to this though. If your mother, in a moment of frustration after you have spilled the milk for the fourth time today, says to you, 'You're so stupid! How many times do I have to tell you to be careful with the milk!' and you happen to be in theta–alpha at that time, this becomes a programmed statement of you and how you are: 'I am stupid.' However, this program is totally outside your consciousness, and consciously you would have forgotten this comment within the hour. Unfortunately, the subconscious survival system never forgets, and acts as if this comment is true. How many people do you know who make a simple error and hit themselves on the forehead and say, 'I'm so stupid', when they are actually very intelligent?

Therefore, fundamental behaviors, beliefs and attitudes that we observe in our parents can become hardwired in our subconscious minds. Once programmed into the subconscious, they then control our behavior and beliefs, as they become our truths that unconsciously shape not only our behavior but also our perception of our potential and can last a lifetime.[1]

This is perhaps why in age recession the ages 18 months to 6 years of age are most commonly involved with core issues underlying much of our adult emotional reactions. Indeed, when an adult is acting like a 2- or 3-year-old, it is because they are running a program that was encoded at 2 or 3 years of age; in a sense, they *are* acting their age!

Reference

1. Lipton, BH 2005, *The Biology of Belief*, Mountain of Love Productions, Santa Cruz, pp. 162–165.

Chapter 28

IDENTIFYING ANCILLARY FACTORS INVOLVED

Once an emotion mode has been entered into pause lock and the relevant time identified via age recession, it is then important to know what other factors are involved with the issue. One of the most important factors to determine is whether there is another person involved or another relevant circumstance or event.

Identifying person(s) involved

To determine if a person is involved in this emotional context, you may circuit locate acupoints to know whether the person involved was male or female or the client themselves. This is easily accomplished by circuit-localization of the acupoints kidney 27 or Central Vessel 22. If kidney 27 on the right gives an indicator change, it says that the person involved is male. If kidney 27 on the left gives an indicator change, this indicates that the person involved is female. Should the acupoint Central Vessel 22 give an indicator change, it indicates that the issue relates to the client themselves.

Further, if the point kidney 27 right or left shows only in combination with Central Vessel 22, it states that the issue is with the yang or masculine aspect of the client themselves (kidney 27 right) or the yin or feminine aspect of themselves (kidney 27 left). However, if both kidney 27 right and left should show, especially if you have age recessed to early childhood, this almost always refers to the person's parents.

This is how Krebs knew that the issue with Johnny and spelling was an issue of anger at his mother. The anger was identified by an indicator change when he circuit located the liver alarm point. Then an indicator change on the left kidney 27 acupoint indicated that the anger was with a woman. When you are 2 years old, the most important woman in your life is usually your mother. When Johnny stated 'Mum', this gave an indicator change, confirming that the woman involved was indeed his mother. But if it were not the client's mother, then you would just challenge other relevant females in their life, for example sister, grandmother, aunt or teacher.

Identifying circumstances or events involved

When the issue is not associated with another person, it may then relate to the client and a particular circumstance or event. The amount of information that you need to effectively defuse this emotional context in the client's life varies considerably with the issue. If more information is necessary, this can be identified by using muscle monitoring and challenging different statements, such as the context of the emotional issue, for example 'at home' or 'at work', until the necessary context is identified by an indicator change. Once this context has been identified, a more specific component may then need to be identified. For instance, if the context is work, is it the client's boss or a colleague or a difficult customer? This questioning is repeated until all the information necessary to resolve this emotional issue has been entered into the 'biocomputer'.

How much information do you need before you can begin the correction process? This can be determined by the more modes and the circuit modes. After each new piece of data has been identified and entered into the biocomputer, you can use circuit modes to identify any collateral information related to that particular piece of data. Then more modes can be used to see if there is any additional information required in order to effectively balance this circuit.

Chapter 29

ACCESSING THE AMYGDALA AND SUBCONSCIOUS SURVIVAL EMOTIONS

The amygdala, an almond-shaped nucleus in the medial temporal lobe, just lateral to the hippocampus, the short-term memory center, is the sentinel of the periventricular survival system, consisting of the periventricular and periaqueductal gray matter making up the very core of the brainstem. The amygdala receives all sensory input before it has been processed in the cortex, and hence before it becomes a conscious perception. Based on only a few neural links, the amygdala makes a coarse-grained image of this sensory experience and then errs on the side of caution, asking only 'Could this stimulus be dangerous?' And if it could be dangerous, the amygdala treats it as if it is dangerous and then fires the fight-or-flight system of the periventricular survival system.

The amygdala also plays an important role in reward and punishment, associated with learning, and maintaining brain integration. In fact, reward and punishment are the very mechanism of learning, because only if a stimulus is associated with reward or punishment can it be remembered and thus learned! Therefore the recently discovered role of the amygdala in emotional learning and memory needs to be discussed.

Research over the past couple of decades has revealed a startling fact: the brain has two perceptual and memory systems that provide the basis for survival and learning. These two systems are normally seamlessly joined in our mental processing. One is cortical, which creates the fine detail and nuance of our conscious experience. The other is subcortical, providing only a coarse-grained view of our world but ever vigilant for threat and danger; this system creates the subconscious emotional context of our lives. These two perceptual and memory systems are derived from parallel transmission of visual, auditory and probably other sensory information to the brain.

These two parallel perceptual–memory systems generate two different types of learning from life's experiences. One is via sensory input to the thalamus, which is then relayed to the primary sensory cortex interpreting that type of sensory information. For instance, visual and auditory inputs go to the lateral and medial geniculate nuclei of the thalamus and are then relayed to the primary visual and auditory cortices, respectively. Similar pathways are probably followed by the other senses for conscious perception (see Figure 29.1).

Visual and auditory information is then processed with reference to previous information of the same type held in association memory areas of the cortex, and intricate interpretation of the information is fully developed into conscious perceptions about our environment and about objects and events in that environment. The hippocampus appears to be instrumental in laying down memories about these events and objects, recording them as facts that are then generally consciously accessible (at least for a time). The hippocampus also mediates the retrieval of these memories, as it is only the information currently being processed in the hippocampus that you are consciously aware of. This hippocampal mediated memory is called declarative memory and involves explicit, consciously accessible information about objects and their identity as well as spatial memory (e.g. the relationship of the object or event to its environment).

While an understanding of the dynamics of declarative memory has progressed rapidly over the past 50 years, the existence of the other perceptual–memory system has begun to emerge only over the past two decades. This other perceptual–memory system is subcortically based and relies on the amygdala as its central processing unit for memory storage and retrieval.

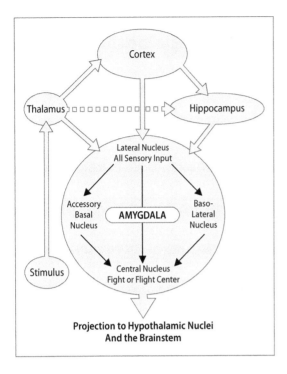

Figure 29.1 Sensory input to the amygdala and output pathways of the amygdala. The lateral nucleus receives sensory information directly from the sensory nuclei of the thalamus and relays this sensory data either directly or indirectly via the basolateral and accessory basal nuclei to the central nucleus of the amygdala. Central nucleus rapidly assesses this sensory information for potential threat or danger, and then activates the periventricular survival system: the periventricular hypothalamic gray matter. Then it initiates hard-wired behavioral reactions associated with the fight or flight within the periventricular gray matter (of the thalamus), and the periaqueductal grey matter of the midbrain.

In this subcortical system, sensory data is also relayed via the sensory thalamus and then directly to the amygdala without the multistep cortical processing of conscious perception. Only a crude perception of the external world is generated in the amygdala, but it relies on largely hard-wired brainstem processing that requires only a few neural links, and thus this subconscious perception is formed far faster. This coarse-grained perception in the amygdala is not used to understand our environment and the objects or events in it, but rather to act as an early warning system for potential threat and danger. The amygdala then lays down memory of these perceptions of threat or danger, creating emotional memory, which is subcortical and subconscious, having never involved any conscious areas of the brain. Note that the amygdaloid subcortical system does not appear to have any working memory or means by which you can introspect on the emotions you are experiencing, or retrospect, meaning literally to look back on these emotions and experiences.

Thus, while the cortical conscious memory of the hippocampus–cortex system is declarative, with objects and events perceived only as cold facts, the amygdala–subcortical system generates feelings about the objects and events crudely perceived, largely based on two things. First is 'Are these objects or events threatening?', in which case emotions based in fear are elicited and withdrawal behavior initiated. Second is, 'Are these objects or events nurturing or supportive of my existence?', in which case dopamine and endorphins (brain opiates) appear to be released into other subcortical areas, such as the nucleus accumbens, acting as reward and creating positive pleasant feelings and emotions: pleasure.

The emotional memory generated by fear-based learning is, however, stored and retrieved differently from the emotional memory creating pleasure or reward-based learning. Current evidence suggests that fear-based emotional memory is stored and retrieved subcortically outside our consciousness and is relatively permanent. Once that object or event has been associated with fear subconsciously, it is extremely hard to extinguish the behavioral response elicited from these fear-based memories. This is clearly illustrated by phobias, which although consciously irrational responses to neutral stimuli are extremely hard to extinguish. Somehow, these neutral stimuli activated an amygdala reaction and were incorrectly assigned a potentially dangerous label and then stored in the fear-based emotional memory. Once established, these fear-based behaviors persist, even when the conscious mind knows this behavior to be totally irrational and often quite consciously inconvenient, for example not being able to use an elevator in a tall building.

Pleasure or reward-based memories, on the other hand, appear to be created subcortically via output of the amygdala to other subcortical areas, such as the nucleus accumbens, but are then stored cortically. When an animal has been conditioned to respond to a specific sensory stimulus, sound or light to gain a reward, removal of the areas of the cortex storing this particular type of sensory input, and/or the hippocampus, results in loss of the reward-based memory. In contrast, removal of the cortical areas storing the stimulus that generated fear-based memory does not affect this memory or the behavior it elicits.

The thalamic–amygdala pathways are therefore critical to survival, as they provide rapid response to potentially, although not fully identified, threatening stimuli. Eliciting fear, triggering fight-or-flight reactions, in response to benign stimuli is less costly than taking the time to consciously analyze and positively identify stimuli that may prove dangerous. This tendency for the brain to err on the side of caution is also seen when two stimuli (objects or events) are presented simultaneously, one with fear-based aversion and the other with pleasure-based reward; the subconscious fear-based memory wins out every time! The object is avoided and the behavioral response is one of fear, not pleasure.[1]

The amygdala and emotional stress

The above discussion highlights the amygdala's critical role in generating fear-based emotional learning and memory that override our conscious desire and often create subconscious states creating anxiety, leading to loss of the ability to think clearly and problem solve. A single fear-based memory linked to a particular type of situation may be enough to produce a lifelong loss of brain integration whenever confronted with that situation, or even stimuli reminding us of that original situation. Likewise, anxiety resulting from the subconscious emotional context of fear-based memory related to any situation may also result in loss of an ability to respond effectively.

However, because these fear-based memories are encoded in protected subconscious circuits related to our survival, they are difficult to access or bring up on the 'biocomputer' for balancing. Yet as long as they persist in the subconscious, they hold the potential to disrupt our brain function and behavior whenever activated. These fear-based memories appear permanent, being difficult to extinguish through conscious means, and generally do not show as an indicator change when balancing. However, recent research has demonstrated that the amygdala can mediate both the acquisition and extinction of emotional learning and memory.[2] Figure 29.2 graphically demonstrates these points.

When the eyes see an object, the visual information takes two separate pathways, one subcortical and subconscious, and the other cortical ending in conscious perception. Visual information goes straight to the amygdala via the visual thalamus as well as branches of the optic nerve (as in Figure 29.2). The amygdala forms only a coarse-grained image based on rapid processing involving only a few neural links, and then immediately references subcortical memory of similar objects, with special emphasis on potentially dangerous objects of similar shape. The amygdala sees a twisted object on the ground (B), references 'possibly a snake' (i.e. danger) and sends signals to the hypothalamus to initiate the fight-or-flight response. Signals are then sent to the adrenal glands (C) to release adrenaline, increasing heart rate, blood pressure and the power of muscle contraction, and you may jump back to avoid the object.

At the same time, visual information is also

Figure 29.2 Dual visual and memory systems in the brain. When the eyes see an object, the visual information takes two separate pathways: one subcortical and subconscious, and the other cortical and ending with conscious perception. **a, Visual information goes straight to the visual thalamus and is relayed to the amygdala.** The amygdala forms only a coarse-grained image based on only a few neural links but immediately references any subcortical memory of similar objects, with emphasis on potentially dangerous objects of similar shape. **b, The amygdala references 'Snake: danger'.** It then signals the hypothalamus to initiate the fight-or-flight response. **c, The fight-or-flight response.** The adrenals are activated to release adrenaline, increasing heart rate, blood pressure, and the power of muscle contraction, and you jump back to avoid the object. **d, At the**

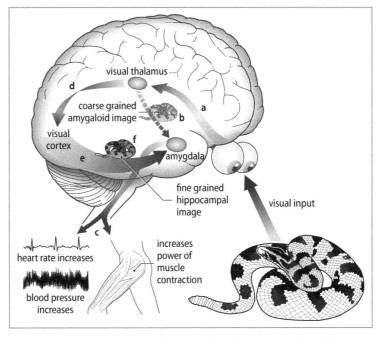

same time, visual information is also traveling back to the primary visual cortex. The information travels via the optic tracts and optic radiations from the visual thalamus to the primary visual cortex. **e, Further processing.** The visual information then undergoes multistep and multilevel processing involving many neural links. **f, The resulting fine-grained image of the object is then sent to the hippocampus and other cortical memory areas.** This creates a conscious visual perception. After Le Doux, JE 1994, Emotion, memory and the brain, *Scientific American*, Vol. 270, No. 6, p. 38.

travelling back to the primary visual cortex via the optic tracts (A) and optic radiations (D) from the visual thalamus. Once at the primary visual cortex, this information then undergoes multistep and multilevel processing involving many neural links to form a fine-grained image of the object (E), which is then sent through the hippocampus to other cortical memory areas for final identification at the level of consciousness.

Two outcomes are possible following this conscious image formation, which occurred well after the amygdaloid image had caused the fear reaction: 1, the fine-grained image is a snake, in which case the fear reaction and avoidance are continued; or 2, the fine-grained image is a twisted bit of vine, in which case the amygdaloid fear reaction is turned off and you walk calmly past the twisted vine, as your heart rate and blood pressure decrease once again to normal.

Formatting for the amygdala circuit

Therefore the trick is *how* to access the fear-based emotional memories blocking or affecting critical brain functions? Formatting for the amygdaloid circuits controlling the survival responses was adapted from Richard Utt's original amygdala formatting by Dr Charles Krebs, and it opens the door to deeper, more permanent corrections of many issues than possible before. Research at Melbourne Applied Physiology, Ballarat, has developed the following formatting to access and balance these fear-based emotional memories via the amygdala.

While the effects of amygdala activation of survival emotions underlie many of the indicator changes in most circuits containing psychoemotional stress, often the amygdala reactions linked to these issues remain unknown. Without resolution of these amygdala reactions, the issue may persist over a period of time and be recalcitrant to change. Only when you directly access the amygdala survival circuits can you fully resolve these issues. Therefore formatting for the amygdala is extremely important any time fear, sadness, grief, anger or reward and punishment are overtly involved in the issue. But how do you access these deep amygdaloid issues that appear so important to their effective resolution?

In order to access the amygdala, we first have to access the limbic system, of which the amygdala is only one component. Using the limbic acupressure format (anatomy mode × gland mode × Central Vessel 23 × Central Vessel 24) gives you access to the whole limbic system and normally does not give an indicator change unless a number of components of this complex system are under stress. Remember, an indicator change is a 51% phenomenon and would require more than 50% of all the limbic components to be overtly stressed.

Once you are in the limbic system, then it requires additional acupressure formatting to specifically access the amygdala (+ Central Vessel 14). Further formatting is then necessary to access specific functions of the amygdala (+ physiology mode + Central Vessel 12–16), the fight-or-flight responses of the central nucleus of the amygdala.

Note that in Figure 29.3, when the amygdala has been formatted for and then physiology mode + Central Vessel 16 gives an indicator change, it does not indicate that you are having too much pleasure and reward but rather that the issue in circuit blocks your access to pleasure and reward. In contrast, when physiology mode + Central Vessel 14 gives an indicator change it does indicate that some kind of aversive emotion, panic, pain or punishment is associated with the issue in the circuit.

From our previous discussion on emotions, in chapter 26, it is clear that when the amygdala associates an aversion emotion with a particular stimulus and this activation reaches a critical threshold value, it then shuts down the thinking and reasoning in the frontal lobes and results in loss of coherent thinking and behavior. So you are no longer *responding* to the situation but now only *reacting*.

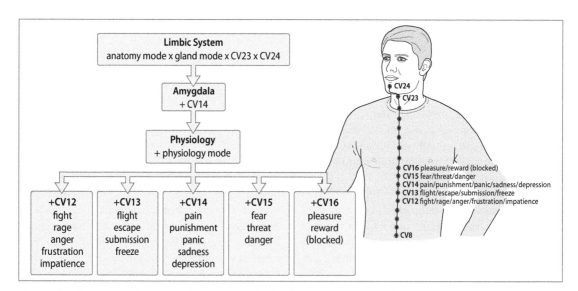

Figure 29.3 Acupressure formatting for the amygdala circuit. Procedure to format for the fight-or-flight responses of the central nucleus of the amygdala. 1, Pause lock the limbic acupressure format: anatomy mode × gland mode × Central Vessel (CV) 23 × CV 24. 2, Pause lock acupressure format to specifically access the amygdala: + CV 14. 3, Pause lock format to access the functions of the amygdala: + physiology mode. 4, Circuit locate acupoints for amygdala survival emotions: + CV 12–16.

References

1. Sah, P & Westbrook RF 2008, Behavioural neuroscience: the circuit of fear, *Nature*, Vol. 454(7204), pp. 589–590.
2. Likhtik, E, Popa, D, Apergis-Schoute, J, Fidacaro, GA & Paré, D 2008, Amygdala intercalated neurons are required for expression of fear extinction, *Nature*, Vol. 454(7204), pp. 642–645.

SECTION VII

Core correction techniques

The correction phase of a kinesiology balance follows the set-up phase. As discussed in chapter 48 under *The role of the healer or kinesiologist*, the purpose of the correcting phase of a balance is to provide the information or energy flow necessary to help the client's systems re-establish equilibrium closer to homeostasis. In the words of William Tiller, 'The correction(s) applied appear to initiate a flow of organizing energy and it is this transfer of "organizing" energy that constitutes or initiates the healing process within the client.'

This correction section is intended not as an encyclopedic collection of all the techniques used in Energetic Kinesiology but as an introduction and guide for those practitioners and/or students who wish to learn a general approach to Energetic Kinesiology. The correction techniques we have chosen from the plethora of possible correction techniques in the many and varied Energetic Kinesiology modalities are not meant to be comprehensive. Indeed, some of these correction techniques may not be used in all modalities of Energetic Kinesiology, and likewise, we may have omitted some widely used correction techniques. The techniques we present were chosen on the basis of historical precedent and commonality of use in most foundation Energetic Kinesiology programs in colleges and other professional trainings.

These fundamental correction techniques are presented as generic templates that may have been embellished with many 'bells and whistles' in different training programs. Therefore the presentation is not a 'how to' manual approach but rather a description of the common principles employed in their use and the factors that need to be addressed in their application. Wherever details of application are given, it is to illustrate a basic principle or is a necessary consideration for their application.

Chapter 30

APPLYING CORRECTION TECHNIQUES

Determining the techniques to apply

Muscle biofeedback provides an extremely effective tool to locate and identify imbalances in many different domains of our multidimensional body. As discussed above, this tool is very useful for locating stressors within the body and even informing the monitor when they have completely collected all the information necessary to balance the issue in circuit.

One of the amazing aspects of kinesiology is that the same techniques used to gather information about the client's issue are also used in the resolution of this issue. Through the use of hand modes, specific indicator points, challenges, verbal questioning and other techniques, there are many possibilities of how to correct the information we have gathered into a circuit. So how do we locate the most effective techniques and apply these techniques to correct the imbalances in circuit? By the very same hand modes, specific indicator points, challenges, verbal questioning, etc. that you have used to identify the issues that are now in circuit.

The difference is the mental context. In the information-gathering phase, the mental context is what factors relate to the imbalance in circuit and are necessary for its resolution. In contrast, in the correction phase you will now interpret indicator changes from the hand modes, specific indicator points, challenges, verbal questioning, etc. as specifying possible correction modalities.

Once all the relevant information has been identified, you will then be looking for a correction technique to apply to bring the person back into or nearer to homeostasis. Indeed, this is the mental context with which you now hold a hand mode, circuit locate an acupoint or ask a question. An indicator change at this point, for example emotion mode, now indicates that you need to select an effective emotionally based correction technique to balance the information in circuit.

For instance, when gathering information your mental context is 'What factors are related to this particular imbalance?' So if emotion mode gives an indicator change, in this context it indicates that you need to locate a specific emotion and enter this information into circuit. Entering the emotion into circuit actually changes the overall energy interference pattern of that circuit. Another type of information, for example specific muscle, may now have a frequency resonance with the new interference pattern created by the emotion. Therefore the identification of the emotion permitted you to gather more information, that is, take the next step and identify the specific muscle and its state of imbalance, which then creates a new interference pattern.

In contrast, once you have entered the correction phase you now have the mental context of 'What technique is needed to balance this circuit?' Now if emotion mode gives an indicator change, in this context you would then be seeking a type of Emotional Stress Defusion technique to resolve the emotions that generated the issue in the first place. In both circumstances, emotion mode is identified as the priority component of the circuit, but how you interpret its meaning is dependent on the phase of balancing that you are in.

Once the monitor is in correction mode, what they need is a system to identify the most effective correction technique from the many different techniques known to them. In this textbook, we have included a series of what we are terming *core techniques*, and these techniques are accessed via the use of hand modes, specific indicator points and acupressure formatting, with a more sparing use of verbal challenge and asking questions.

Stack or correct?

The use of verbal challenge can also be a very important technique for determining which type of therapy to apply. One of the areas in which verbal challenge is most useful is when you have reached the correcting phase. Do you go straight to correction or do you need to seek additional information of a similar nature to be entered into circuit before correction?

For instance, a person presents with a series of muscle imbalances and you have entered the priority muscle into circuit and reached a point where more circuit and suppression modes no longer give an indicator change. Therefore you then have all the information in circuit that you need to balance that muscle. However, should you proceed to balance this specific muscle? Or is it more appropriate to enter the next priority muscle into circuit and go through the process of gathering information until no more, circuit or suppression modes show for that second muscle? Here, the response to the verbal challenge of 'Stack?' or 'Correct?' will inform the monitor as to how best to proceed. Depending on which of these verbal challenges gives a priority indicator change, you would then enter the second muscle into circuit if *stack* were the priority, or proceed straight to the correcting phase if *correct* were the priority.

What would determine the outcome of the challenge 'Stack?' or 'Correct?' In the example above,

it is the nature of the issue(s) underlying these two muscle imbalances. If the primary issue underlying the first muscle imbalance is unrelated to the primary issue underlying the second muscle imbalance, then the challenge would indicate 'correct'. However, if the primary issues underlying both muscle imbalances are related, for example they share the same emotional issue, then the challenge would indicate 'stack'. This is because addressing the common issue would resolve both muscle imbalances, as they have the same origin.

Determining the time of application

One of the most important considerations in applying many different types of corrections is how long should this therapy be applied. For example, if you were to apply acupressure therapy, light therapy or sound therapy, the length of time you apply that technique may be a very important factor in its effectiveness. But how are you to know the length of time to apply this technique? The monitor may simply use time mode and pineal tap to establish the optimum time for application.

Time mode is the tip of the fingers curled into

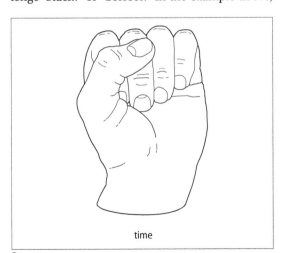

time

a

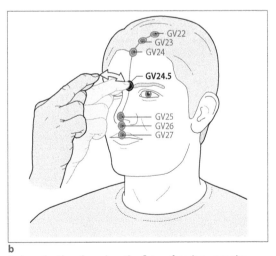

b

Figure 30.1 a, Time mode. Curl all the fingers into the palm and place the thumb pad on the flat surface between the second and third joints of the middle finger. **b, Pineal tap.** Gently tap on the acupoint Governing Vessel (GV) 24.5. When holding time mode, each tap on the pineal point can be assigned a time unit (one second, one minute, etc.). An indicator change then indicates how many units of time are required for the type of correction that is to be employed (e.g. acupoint stimulation).

the palm with the thumb pad on the flat surface between the second and third joints of the middle finger, as shown in Figure 30.1a. Pineal tap, shown in Figure 30.1b, is a technique developed in Applied Kinesiology for bringing both conscious and subconscious awareness to what is being addressed in circuit at that moment. Pineal tap consists of gently tapping the acupoint Governing Vessel 24.5 at the same time as holding time mode and monitoring an indicator muscle. So each tap on the pineal point can each be assigned a particular time unit, for example 10 seconds or 1 minute, that is relevant to the type of correction to be employed.

For instance, if tuning forks are the priority correction to be applied to a particular acupoint the monitor then needs to know for how long. Or the monitor may need to know the amount of time to apply acupressure to a particular acupoint. To determine the amount of time, the correction technique first needs to be activated, for example ding the forks once or briefly stimulate the acupoint and then enter this response into pause lock. This is important, as it provides a context for the time component of the technique you are now about to apply. When monitoring the indicator muscle while holding time mode and tapping the pineal point, the monitor states various time intervals. The indicator change then indicates the optimum amount of time to perform this technique.

The amount of time indicated to apply the technique may also provide other information. For example, if an acupoint point is blocked or frozen and you pineal tap for the amount of time to stimulate the acupoint, it may be in minutes rather than seconds, which is far more common for acupoint stimulation. The longer the treatment time, the more blocked the acupoint is. In this case, rather than treating the acupoint you would enter this acupoint imbalance into circuit and find the reason for the blockage. That is, an extraordinarily large amount of time to apply any technique would suggest there is a factor compromising the effectiveness of this technique and that factor should be identified and resolved before applying the original correction technique identified.

Chapter 31

NEUROLYMPHATIC REFLEXES

Development of the neurolymphatic reflexes[1]

In the early 1960s, Dr George Goodheart began using manual muscle testing in his chiropractic clinic. His early work with muscle monitoring was to test the effectiveness of his spinal manipulations. He would test a series of muscles before and after spinal adjustment to see if a previously unlocking muscle subsequently locked. This gave him valuable feedback on the effectiveness of a manipulation for the condition he was treating.

In common with other chiropractors, he experienced great frustration in the inability of some of these manipulations to hold when the patients went about their normal lives. In these cases, the muscle spasms would return with the associated pain or stiffness. This led Goodheart to look further into the nature of muscle spasm, using muscle monitoring as his investigative tool.

It was while working on a man with considerable lower back pain and a consistently unlocking upper leg muscle (tensor fascia lata), that Goodheart discovered a revolutionary technique for correcting muscle imbalances. The pain became far more severe when the man would sit or lie down for a period of time, but it disappeared when he walked. This type of condition indicated lymphatic involvement.

The lymphatic system

The lymphatic system is a network of fine capillaries, throughout the whole of the body, leading to larger lymph vessels. It drains fluid from the spaces between cells and is the body's primary pathway for removing metabolic waste. The lymph is a clear fluid propelled primarily by compression of the lymphatic vessels from movements such as breathing, walking, intestinal activity and muscle action. Lymph is prevented from flowing backward by a series of one-way valves in the bigger lymph vessels.

There is no primary pump for the lymphatic system, such as the heart for the cardiovascular system, so lack of movement can soon exacerbate any lymphatic drainage problems. Along the lymph vessels are lymph nodes ranging in size from 1 to 25 millimeters, which filter the lymph fluid and remove then destroy foreign substances such as bacteria. Thus, the lymphatic system is also an essential part of the immune system.

Lack of lymph drainage results in localized build-up of toxic material in the tissue, fluid retention, swelling and even infection (see Figure 31.1).

Chapman's reflexes

In an attempt to encourage lymphatic drainage, Goodheart massaged the painful site (around the sacroiliac joint) looking for swollen lymph nodes, which he could not find. Out of frustration, he finally briskly massaged the offending muscle. The man's pain disappeared and the muscle locked for the first time. Subsequently, he tried massaging other unlocking muscles but without success.

Still holding to his earlier reasoning, Goodheart concluded that he had somehow worked on a reflex associated with lymphatic drainage in the muscle. He turned his attention to the work, done in the 1930s, of osteopath Frank Chapman and described in the book by Charles Owen entitled *An Endocrine Interpretation of Chapman's Reflexes*, written in 1937.[2] In this work, reflexes are described that can be used to consistently improve lymphatic drainage in organs and tissues related to this reflex. When active, these reflexes consist of localized tissue changes at particular points often quite distant from the organs they affect.

Because lymph drainage is extremely important in the removal of toxic materials as well as the delivery of important nutrients, Chapman believed that most disease is caused by inadequate

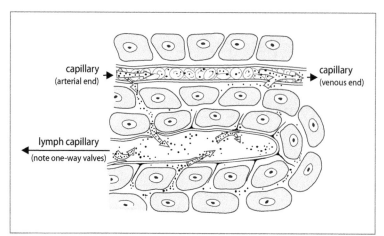

Figure 31.1 a, Lymph capillaries.
Because of increased hydrostatic pressure in the capillaries, proteins, fats and other large molecules are pushed out of blood capillaries into the interstitial spaces. These large molecules cannot return to the blood capillaries and are returned to the circulatory system via lymph capillaries draining into bigger ducts with one-way valves, as the lymph flow is driven by muscular activity.

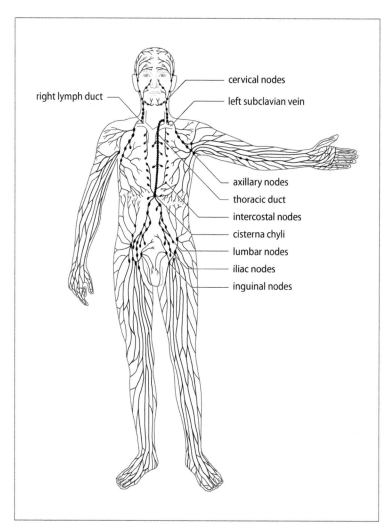

b The lymphatic system. Lymphatic vessels drain the entire body, penetrating most of the tissues and carrying fluid from the intercellular spaces back to the bloodstream. The primary left thoracic duct, which arises at the cisterna chyli in the abdomen, drains the legs, abdomen, left side of the head and left arm, emptying into the left subclavian vein. The right lymph duct drains the heart, the lungs, part of the diaphragm, the right upper part of the body and the right side of the head and neck, emptying into the right subclavian vein. Lymph nodes interspersed along the vessels trap foreign matter, including bacteria and viruses, as well as clearing toxins from the interstitial fluids. After Walther DS, 1988, *Applied Kinesiology: Synopsis, Second Edition*, Systems DC, Pueblo (a) and Guyton, AC 1991, *Textbook of Medical Physiology, Eighth Edition*, WB Saunders, Philadelphia (b).

lymphatic drainage. By trial and error, he correlated various organ and gland dysfunctions with these reflex points (see Figure 31.2). He found that the conditions improved when lymphatic drainage was increased. This was done by stimulating these points via deep massage.

Goodheart experimented with the Chapman reflexes looking for nodulation in the suggested areas for those patients who showed symptoms of imbalance in the related organs or glands. In addition, he monitored various muscles throughout the body to find which muscles were unlocking. On deeply massaging these often tender areas, certain muscles would now lock firmly. By trial and error, Goodheart related specific muscles to reflex points. Finally, by discovering nodulation in areas that Chapman had not discussed, he was able to link most of the muscles with these reflex points, which he then called *neurolymphatic reflexes.*

Working through the relationships: muscle « neurolymphatic (connections he had discovered) + organ/gland « neurolymphatic (connections of Chapman), it was readily apparent that muscles could be related directly to organs or glands. In addition, the state of muscle imbalance was able to give a direct readout on the state of imbalance of the related organ and/or gland. It finally started to explain why there was frequently a sudden and dramatic improvement in health when the muscle imbalance was corrected. The muscle response did not show that pathological changes had taken place in the organ or gland, but it indicated that they were improperly functioning.

Sometimes the effect of neurolymphatic reflex stimulation is only temporary, in which case a deeper cause would need to be found and corrected. Other things that can affect lymph drainage are, for example, lack of exercise, poor diet, toxic overload, or many of the other types of imbalances that can be identified by kinesiology techniques.

In many cases, however, the correction is quite long lasting. Goodheart proposed that the neurolymphatic reflex is a type of circuit breaker that needs to be reset by stimulation. Frequently, he would have corrected a spinal subluxation at the same level as the neurolymphatic reflex, but the muscle failed to be corrected until the neurolymphatic reflex was also massaged.

Physiological explanation of the neurolymphatic reflexes

To understand this circuit breaker concept better, we turn back to look at the mechanics of the lymphatic system again. In fact, the lymphatic system does have another system of pumping that, if not functioning adequately, leaves us very dependent on movement for lymph drainage. The larger lymph vessels have smooth muscle fibers that contract when the pressure in the lymphatic system exceeds a certain threshold. This propels the lymph fluid through the one-way valves to its final destination in the large veins of the neck region. Smooth (involuntary) muscle contraction is mediated through local factors, reactions to hormones and the autonomic nervous system from control centers in the brain (limbic and hypothalamic centers), whose responses are based on sensory feedback from the body.

Because the neurolymphatic reflexes are frequently at quite a distance from the organs or glands they affect, it would appear that the action of the neurolymphatic reflex is to reset these brain control mechanisms to more appropriate levels (in relationship to the feedback they are getting from the body sensors). These brain control mechanisms include the levels of facilitation to the related muscles and the contraction of tissue at the neurolymphatic reflex, and all these typically have nerve pathways that are entering or exiting at the same spinal level. Therefore when an organ's lymphatic drainage is lowered, the related muscle is also

Figure 31.2 Chapman's neurolymphatic reflex points. The neurolymphatic reflexes discovered by Chapman are found on both the front and the back of the body, with sets of usually bilateral reflex points on the front of the body, generally along the midline of the body, and another set on the back that are usually paired paravertebral points along the spine. When the points are associated with acute conditions, they are usually soft or doughy, but with chronic conditions the tissues become hard and painful when massaged. After Walther DS, 1988, *Applied Kinesiology: Synopsis, Second Edition*, Systems DC, Pueblo.

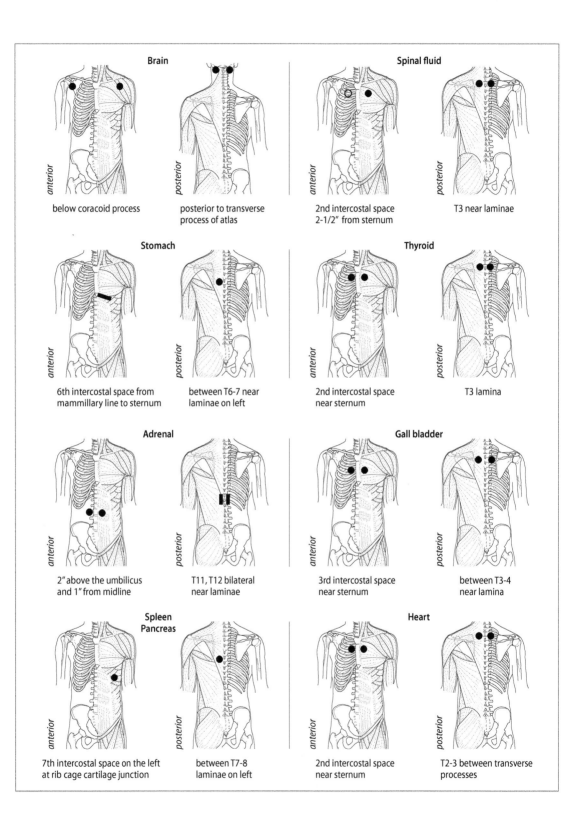

Brain

anterior — below coracoid process

posterior — posterior to transverse process of atlas

Spinal fluid

anterior — 2nd intercostal space 2-1/2" from sternum

posterior — T3 near laminae

Stomach

anterior — 6th intercostal space from mammillary line to sternum

posterior — between T6-7 near laminae on left

Thyroid

anterior — 2nd intercostal space near sternum

posterior — T3 lamina

Adrenal

anterior — 2" above the umbilicus and 1" from midline

posterior — T11, T12 bilateral near laminae

Gall bladder

anterior — 3rd intercostal space near sternum

posterior — between T3-4 near lamina

Spleen Pancreas

anterior — 7th intercostal space on the left at rib cage cartilage junction

posterior — between T7-8 laminae on left

Heart

anterior — 2nd intercostal space near sternum

posterior — T2-3 between transverse processes

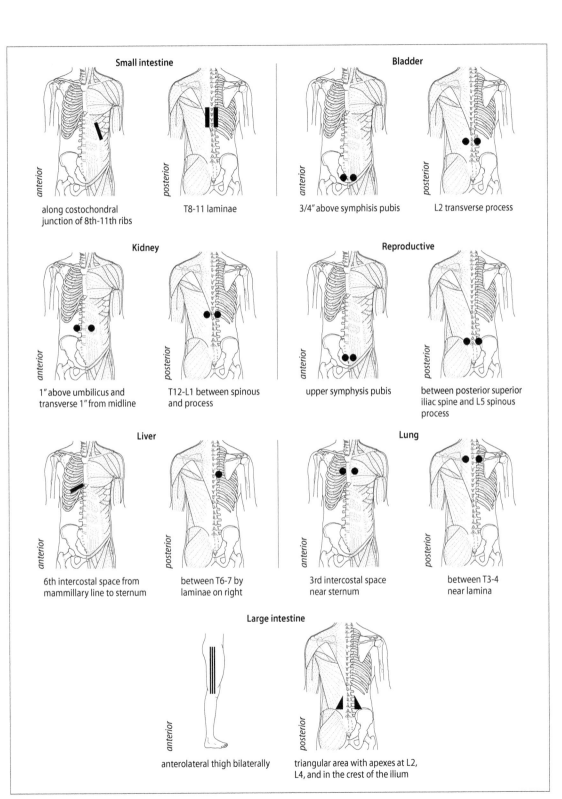

Small intestine

anterior — along costochondral junction of 8th-11th ribs

posterior — T8-11 laminae

Bladder

anterior — 3/4" above symphisis pubis

posterior — L2 transverse process

Kidney

anterior — 1" above umbilicus and transverse 1" from midline

posterior — T12-L1 between spinous and process

Reproductive

anterior — upper symphysis pubis

posterior — between posterior superior iliac spine and L5 spinous process

Liver

anterior — 6th intercostal space from mammillary line to sternum

posterior — between T6-7 by laminae on right

Lung

anterior — 3rd intercostal space near sternum

posterior — between T3-4 near lamina

Large intestine

anterior — anterolateral thigh bilaterally

posterior — triangular area with apexes at L2, L4, and in the crest of the ilium improperly facilitated, and the tissue of the neuro-lymphatic reflex swells then eventually contracts.

One model suggests that the muscle tissue surrounding the neurolymphatic reflex is initially under-facilitated (like the unlocking associated muscle) and becomes over-facilitated and hard (like muscle spasm) as the associated muscle also becomes over-facilitated.

Working backward, when the neurolymphatic reflex is corrected by stimulation, the brain control centre is reset, which in turn resets the muscle facilitation to appropriate levels and increases the lymphatic drainage of the associated organ or gland.

The neurolymphatic reflexes are mainly located between the ribs close to the sternum (breast-bone), along the spinal column and on the front

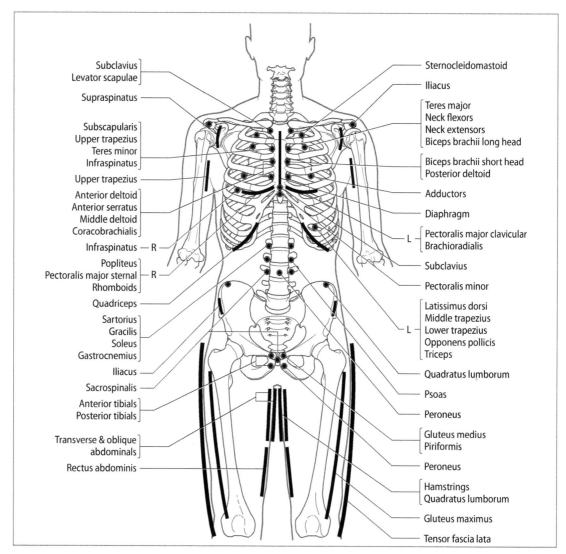

Figure 31.3 Neurolymphatic reflex point muscle chart. Using Chapman's original reflex points, Goodheart researched which muscles were related to which points he now called *neurolymphatic reflex points*. Note how a number of muscles all share a common set of reflex points. Interestingly, muscles sharing the same neurolymphatic reflex point also are associated with the same acupuncture meridian, representing a physical expression of the muscle–organ/gland–meridian matrix.

of the abdomen, with some reflexes on the arms and legs (see Figure 31.3).

The degree of contraction of the tissue of the reflex area increases with time. Originally, it will be puffy, with a dough-like feeling over the entire area of the reflex (typically about 3 centimeters in diameter). With time, the doughiness contracts down into globules the size of small lima beans and finally to numerous hard little beads like shotgun pellets. The tenderness increases with the degree of contraction, the hard little beads being extremely painful to touch.

The reflexes on the front of the body are usually far more tender than those on the back of the body and tend to contract down into beads or pellets far more. The reflexes on the lower parts of the body are much larger and feel like stringy masses of knotty plaques when active.

Correction of the neurolymphatic reflexes is with manual pressure working to the point of pain, and gradually increasing pressure as it can be tolerated. This can take anything from some seconds to several minutes, depending on the severity of the neurolymphatic reflex imbalance. The treatment should continue until the tenderness has gone and/or until the related muscle locks.

Application of the neurolymphatic reflexes

When the specific indicator point for all neurolymphatic reflexes, stomach 35 (see Figure 31.4), has given priority indicator change, then by circuit locating each alarm point the meridian-related muscle of the neurolymphatic reflex can be quickly located. These neurolymphatic reflex reflexes (see Figure 31.3) are then firmly massaged by the monitor to the level of their client's pain tolerance. It must be noted that chronic neurolymphatic reflexes can be extremely painful when massaged, and so care must be taken to stay within the client's pain tolerances. It is recommended that you start with very gentle pressure and gradually increase this pressure as the pain or tenderness subsides. You should continue massaging with increasing pressure until the point is no longer tender. This may take only 20 to 30 seconds or a number of minutes, depending on how chronic the neurolymphatic reflex imbalance has become. People often report a warming or even energy-moving sensations after application of this technique.

The presenting issue is then re-entered into circuit once more and is reassessed for imbalance by circuit locating stomach 35. If there is no indicator change, this suggests there is no longer any neurolymphatic reflex imbalance present. As a final check, the neurolymphatic reflex treated should be circuit located while monitoring an indicator muscle to confirm that the correction is complete.

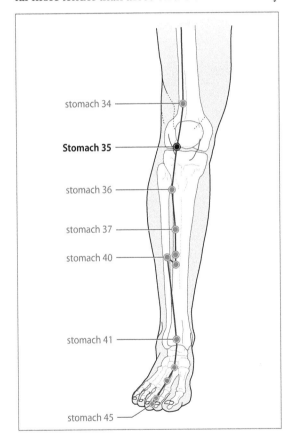

Figure 31.4 Neurolymphatic reflexes specific indicator point: stomach 35. When the knee is flexed, stomach 35 is in the center of the depression slightly below and lateral to the patellar ligament. An indicator change when stomach 35 is circuit located indicates either that a neurolymphatic reflex imbalance is involved with the issue in circuit or that neurolymphatic reflex stimulation is the correction for this issue.

References

1. Dickson, GJ 1990, *What is Kinesiology?*, IHK Publishing, Melbourne.
   Goodheart, GJ *You'll Be Better: The Story of Applied Kinesiology*, AK Printing, Geneva.
   Walther, DS 1976, *Applied Kinesiology: The Advanced Approach in Chiropractic*, Systems DC, Pueblo.
   Walther, DS 1981, *Applied Kinesiology, Volume I: Basic Procedure and Muscle Testing*, Systems DC, Pueblo.
   Walther, DS 1988, *Applied Kinesiology: Synopsis*, System DC, Pueblo.
   Guyton, AC 1991, *Textbook of Medical Physiology, Eighth Edition*, WB Saunders, Philadelphia.
2. Owens, C 1937, *An Endocrine Interpretation of Chapman's Reflexes*, Academy for Applied Osteopathy, Carmel.

Chapter 32

NEUROVASCULAR REFLEXES

Development of the neurovascular reflexes[1]

In the mid-1960s, while working on a boy with severe asthma, Dr George Goodheart discovered another important technique for correcting muscle imbalances. Frequently, an asthma attack is directly related to lack of adrenal hormone production, and Goodheart was working on an unlocking sartorius muscle, which is related to the adrenals.

Having exhausted his usual repertoire of correction techniques, Goodheart attempted a cranial bone manipulation, trying to free the parietal bones along the top of the head. Although the correction did not produce the desired result, Goodheart noticed a faint but insistent pulse under the two fingers that were resting on the boy's posterior fontanel (the indentation close to the back of the head).

He compared it with the boy's pulse rate and respiration rate, and then Goodheart held his own fingers up against the wall to see that it was not in fact his own finger pulses that he was feeling. None of these matched the 72 beats per minute he again felt when he reapplied his fingers. The pulsation kept increasing in strength and became more rhythmic and regular until the boy's breathing eased. The sartorius muscle was now locked firmly.

Shortly after this observation, Goodheart had a woman come to his practice complaining of a headache she had had continuously for 29 years. The only thing that varied was the intensity. Once again, he found that it was a cranial imbalance, and he applied his fingers to the parietal bones to make a cranial adjustment. Again he noticed this strange pulsation under the tips of his index fingers. When he removed his fingers the pulsation ceased, and when he put them back it reappeared and was a consistent pulse between 72 and 74 beats per minute.

Instead of making the cranial adjustment, he held his fingers on the parietal eminences and with slight traction waited until the pulse became stronger and synchronized on both sides. Reassessment of the original cranial imbalance showed that it was now absent, and within a few minutes the women exclaimed, 'Oh my God, my headache is gone! It's gone!' To which Goodheart replied, 'Of course it is; that's why you came here.'

Realizing that he had discovered another important muscle-balancing technique, Goodheart turned to the literature to find out more about these neurovascular reflexes. In the early 1930s, a chiropractor named Dr Terrence Bennett developed a technique that related certain points on the head and the front of the body with blood flow to specific organs or glands, and which influenced particular body functions (see Figure 32.1).

By means of a radio-opaque dye and a fluoroscope, Bennett observed that when these points were held with gentle finger pressure and slightly tugged to create traction, the X-ray showed blood flow increasing in specific glands and organs. In addition, pulsation would appear under the holding fingers at a rate of typically 70–74 beats per minute, regardless of the pulse rate or heartbeat.

Using Bennett's organ or gland « neurovascular reflex, and his own organ/gland « muscle correlations, Goodheart was able to find which neurovascular reflex related to which muscle. Although a specific muscle would be corrected by only one of the neurovascular reflexes, most of the reflexes influenced more than one muscle.

Although Bennett had numerous reflex points on the head, trunk and legs, Goodheart used only the Bennett reflex points on the head, with very few exceptions. Bennett also had various approaches to manipulate the points, whereas again Goodheart used only the approach that suits the points on the head. Goodheart called

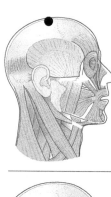

Heart   Sub-scapularis
Gall bladder   Anterior deltoid
Lung   Middle deltoid
Lung   Diaphragm
Brain central   Supraspinatus

Bregma: junction of coronal and sagittal suture (anterior fontane - baby's soft spot). Measure from the bridge of your nose with the heel of your hand and the middle finger is on the Bregma.

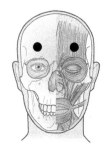

Stomach   PMC
Bladder   Anterior tibialis
Bladder   Sacrospinalis
Liver   Rhomboids

Bilateral frontal eminences are the bumps on the forehead halfway between the eyebrows and hairline.

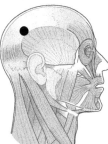

Small intestine   Quadriceps
Large intestine   Tensor fascia lata
Large intestine   Quadratus lumborum
Pericardium   Gluteus medius

Parietal eminence posterior aspect is the widest aspect of the head; above and behind the ears.

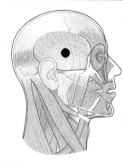

Th - Thyroid   Teres minor
Spinal fluid -   Teres major
  governing

1" below the pterion on the temple at the hairline; slightly above and in front of the ear, and at the junction of the 1st rib, clavicle, and sternum.

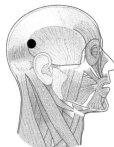

Spleen/Pancreas   Latissimus dorsi

Superior to temporat bone on line slightly posterior to the external auditory meatus.

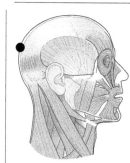

Spleen/Spleen   Middle trapezius

1" above lambda.

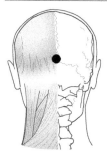

TH - Adrenals   Sartorius

Lambada - posterior fontanel where the lamboid and sagittal sutures meet.

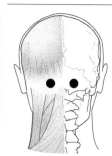

Kidney   Psoas

1/2" lateral to external occipital protuberance.

Figure 32.1 Bennett's neurovascular reflex points. Goodheart selected Bennett reflex points primarily on the head and then researched which organ–meridian matched each reflex point, and further then determined which meridian-related muscles were associated with each specific neurovascular reflex. After Walther DS, 1988, *Applied Kinesiology: Synopsis, Second Edition*, Systems DC, Pueblo.

these Bennett reflex points *neurovascular reflexes* to signify their effect on the microcirculation of the tissues in the body.

Physiological explanation of the neurovascular reflexes

The location of skin receptors that can influence blood flow to specific organs appears to stem from embryological development, during which skin and nervous tissue originate from a common area.

Increased blood flow, brought about by the neurovascular reflexes, provides additional nutrition (including oxygen) to the related organs or tissues it affects. Without adequate nutrition, the cells begin to under-function and eventually die. Adequate blood flow is also responsible for flushing and removing other products of metabolism, such as dissolved carbon dioxide, toxins and the proteins (such as hormones, enzymes and antibodies) that the cells produce.

The 74 beats per minute pulsation that is unrelated to pulse rate or heartbeat appears to result from capillary pulsation of the microcirculation in the tissues. Arteries connect with veins via a capillary network that has a large number of branching and interconnecting pathways: artery to arteriole to capillary bed to venule to vein.

At the junction of the arteriole and the capillary (known as the vasomotor plexus) is a muscular sphincter known as a precapillary sphincter. Blood flow to the capillary bed is being continually monitored and adjusted according to the needs of the tissue it feeds, for example muscle tissue will have high needs when the person is active and low needs when they are resting. The adjustments are achieved by the muscular coat of the arteriole, primarily at the precapillary sphincter. These smooth (involuntary) muscles are controlled by the sympathetic branch of the autonomic nervous system.

Control of this action comes from the vasomotor center in the brainstem, which in turn can be modified by higher brain centers. The arterioles can be constricted by facilitating impulses into the vasoconstriction area, or dilated by inhibitory impulses into this area. The vasoconstrictor area fires impulses at a rate that corresponds to the 74 beats per minute rate and causes a continuous partial contraction of the blood vessels known as vasomotor tone.

It is hypothesized that the pulsing felt at the neurovascular reflexes is from the tonic pulses of the vasoconstriction area of the brain that also transmits impulses to the arterioles resulting in capillary bed pulsations. If the brainstem centers are inappropriately set, this could lead to deficiencies in the function of these arterioles and result in local blood flow deficiencies.

Working backward, stimulating the neurovascular reflexes by touch normalizes this action via brainstem centers and so increases microcirculation to specific organs or glands. The fact that this has been successful is indicated by the proper tonic impulses also being fed back to the corresponding neurovascular reflex, creating the regular even pulsing. These brainstem centers may have related control over the blood flow in the muscle that monitors unlocking when the neurovascular reflex is active. Therefore if the muscle itself is similarly deprived of oxygenated blood, lactic acid builds up faster than it can be removed, leading to muscle weakness and pain.

The fact that the neurovascular reflexes are controlled by the vasomotor centers of the medulla, which is in turn innervated by various outputs from the hypothalamus and brainstem areas involved with survival, is one of the reasons that muscles unlock when these reflexes become imbalanced. These same vasomotor centers are involved in blood flow changes in reaction to fight or flight. Therefore subconscious emotional factors may be associated with or underlie neurovascular imbalances. This may be why the Bennett reflex points related to stomach muscles, found just under the frontal eminences and on the temples, were labeled *emotional points* by Bennett. Indeed, emotional issues are often felt in our stomach, a gut reaction.

Interestingly, almost all the Bennett points on the head are also specific acupoints, for instance the Bennett emotion points gall bladder 14, just under the frontal eminences and just above triple heater 23 at the end of the eyebrows on the temples. While only these two points were labeled emotional points by Bennett, all the neurovascular reflex points are probably similarly affected by the subconscious emotions altering vasomotor centers in the brainstem.

Furthermore, there is anecdotal evidence that these emotional points of Bennett not only change blood flow in their associated muscles and organs or glands but also in the brain. The premise of these points affecting emotions and being the primary points held during Emotional Stress Release and Emotional Stress Defusion is that holding these points also brings blood flow back into the frontal cortex when it has been inhibited by output from the survival centers in the amygdala and brainstem as a result of activation of the fight-or-flight reaction. Thus, holding the emotional neurovascular points brings blood flow back into the frontal cortex, the centers that are involved in accessing a higher perspective than our ego-controlled limbic and brainstem survival systems. This brings back online our rational analytical thinking, problem solving, and access to retrospection and introspection of past events related to the current emotional issues. This permits these now accessible resources to be used to resolve the associated emotional issue.

Application of the neurovascular reflexes

When circuit location of the specific indicator for neurovascular reflexes, triple heater 10 (see Figure 32.2), gives an indicator change, it confirms that neurovascular reflexes are the priority imbalance to be entered into circuit or the priority correction. The monitor then need only circuit locate the alarm points to find the meridian-related muscle and its associated neurovascular reflex point (see Figure 32.3). Gentle pressure, approximately the amount of pressure you can apply to the closed eyelids, is then applied to the active neurovascular reflex points. Slight traction is applied, and the monitor then holds these points until a pulse is felt beneath the fingertips. At first these pulses may be erratic, first on one side and then the other, and even come and go, but in time the pulses synchronize. Once

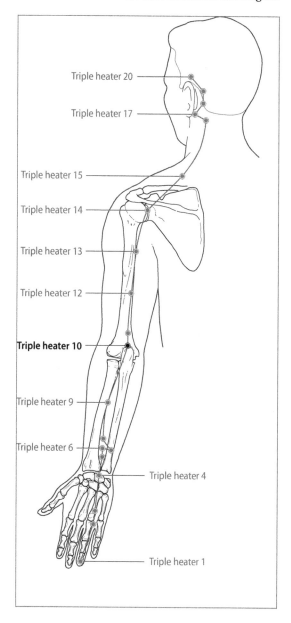

Triple heater 20
Triple heater 17
Triple heater 15
Triple heater 14
Triple heater 13
Triple heater 12
Triple heater 10
Triple heater 9
Triple heater 6
Triple heater 4
Triple heater 1

Figure 32.2 Neurovascular reflex specific indicator point: triple heater 10. When the elbow is flexed, triple heater 10 is on the lateral aspect of the arm, in the depression 1 cm directly above the tip of the elbow. An indicator change when triple heater 10 is circuit located indicates either that a neurovascular reflex imbalance is involved with the issue in circuit or that neurovascular reflex stimulation is the correction for this issue.

the pulsation in the neurovascular reflex points is synchronous and continuous, the neurovascular reflex correction is complete.

The circuit is then closed, and the presenting issue is re-entered and reassessed by circuit locating triple heater 10. If there is no indicator change, this suggests there are no longer any neurovascular reflex imbalances present. As a final check, the neurovascular reflex point treated should be circuit located while monitoring an indicator muscle to confirm that the correction is complete.

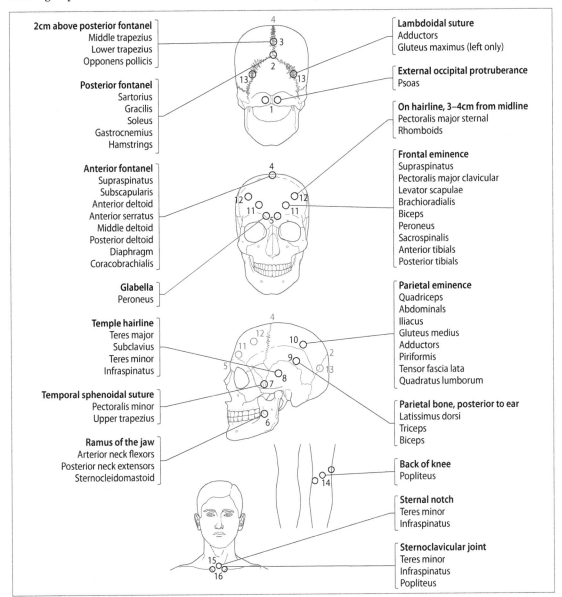

2cm above posterior fontanel
Middle trapezius
Lower trapezius
Opponens pollicis

Posterior fontanel
Sartorius
Gracilis
Soleus
Gastrocnemius
Hamstrings

Anterior fontanel
Supraspinatus
Subscapularis
Anterior deltoid
Anterior serratus
Middle deltoid
Posterior deltoid
Diaphragm
Coracobrachialis

Glabella
Peroneus

Temple hairline
Teres major
Subclavius
Teres minor
Infraspinatus

Temporal sphenoidal suture
Pectoralis minor
Upper trapezius

Ramus of the jaw
Arterior neck flexors
Posterior neck extensors
Sternocleidomastoid

Lambdoidal suture
Adductors
Gluteus maximus (left only)

External occipital protruberance
Psoas

On hairline, 3–4cm from midline
Pectoralis major sternal
Rhomboids

Frontal eminence
Supraspinatus
Pectoralis major clavicular
Levator scapulae
Brachioradialis
Biceps
Peroneus
Sacrospinalis
Anterior tibials
Posterior tibials

Parietal eminence
Quadriceps
Abdominals
Iliacus
Gluteus medius
Adductors
Piriformis
Tensor fascia lata
Quadratus lumborum

Parietal bone, posterior to ear
Latissimus dorsi
Triceps
Biceps

Back of knee
Popliteus

Sternal notch
Teres minor
Infraspinatus

Sternoclavicular joint
Teres minor
Infraspinatus
Popliteus

Figure 32.3 Neurovascular reflex points: muscle chart. When the specific indicator point for the neurovascular reflexes (triple heater 10) has indicated a neurovascular imbalance, using the alarm points the meridian-related muscle with a neurovascular imbalance can be quickly located, and inspection of the neurovascular muscle chart will provide the neurovascular points to hold for correction.

References

1. Dickson, GJ 1990, *What is Kinesiology?*, IHK Publishing, Melbourne.
Goodheart, GJ *You'll Be Better: The Story of Applied Kinesiology*, AK Printing, Geneva.
Walther, DS 1976, *Applied Kinesiology: The Advanced Approach in Chiropractic*, Systems DC, Pueblo.

Walther, DS 1981, *Applied Kinesiology, Volume I: Basic Procedure and Muscle Testing*, Systems DC, Pueblo.
Walther, DS 1988, *Applied Kinesiology: Synopsis*, System DC, Pueblo.

Chapter 33

MUSCLE BALANCING

Development of the muscle–organ/gland–meridian matrix

One of the core concepts of Energetic Kinesiology, developed by Dr George Goodheart and his colleagues in Applied Kinesiology, is the essential relationship between specific muscles of the body and specific meridians and their associated organs or glands. This became known as the *muscle–organ/gland–meridian matrix*. Energy imbalances within specific meridians would be expressed as various types of imbalances within the meridian-related muscle.

So how did Dr Goodheart realize this relationship existed? You remember in the discussion on neurolymphatic reflexes and neurovascular reflexes that Dr Goodheart utilized Chapman and Bennett points. The way he identified the organ–reflex point relationship was by observing which muscles showed imbalance when he was dealing with specific organ-related problems. For instance, when there were issues related to the stomach organ, the pectoralis major clavicular (PMC) muscle would consistently show imbalance.

Chapman and Bennett both assigned their reflex points on the basis of organ relationships. For instance, Chapman would say that stomach problems originated from poor lymphatic drainage of the stomach organ and could be rectified by firm massage to the fifth intercostal space on the left side until the tenderness and pain disappeared. In a similar fashion, Bennett's model was that organ dysfunction related to poor microcirculation within that organ, and that holding the Bennett point specific to that organ would increase its blood flow and restore the organ function. In the case of imbalances within the stomach organ, Goodheart would hold his emotional points just beneath the frontal eminences.

With this information at hand, Goodheart simply noted when he had a stomach-related problem, if the stomach-related Chapman and Bennett points were also active and according to the state of balance or imbalance within muscles he had identified as being related to stomach function. If he had a patient with a stomach-related issue, he would first test the PMC and other stomach-related muscles for their state of balance. Then he would assess the Chapman neurolymphatic points and/or the Bennett neurovascular points and look for correlations in these stomach-related systems.

For example, he might find that PMC was under-facilitated, and that the Bennett point was not active but the Chapman neurolymphatic reflex was active, as indicated by an indicator change when it was circuit located. Then he would treat the active point, Bennett or Chapman, until that point was in balance. He would then remonitor PMC for its state of imbalance. He found a very strong correlation between the activity of the organ-related reflex points and the state of balance of the PMC. He could now use this muscle–organ relationship to both identify organ imbalances and then measure the efficacy of the treatments he applied by remonitoring the muscle and observing changes in its state of balance.

Following President Nixon's trip to China in 1972, this closed society with its knowledge of acupuncture and acupressure suddenly became accessible to the West. Goodheart was an extremely eclectic reader, and he began to read information about the Chinese acupuncture meridian system and how it worked. With his genius for synthesis, he suddenly realized he had organ-related reflex points, muscle-related organ reactions and a whole system of Chinese medicine linked to organ functions through the meridian energy flows. With his ability to integrate different systems, Goodheart linked the meridians to the muscles via their common organ associations, which then in turn linked them to the organ-related reflexes. Thus was born the concept of the muscle–organ/gland–meridian matrix.

For example, if the meridian were under-energy the meridian-related muscle would monitor under-facilitated. Similarly, if the meridian were over-energy the meridian-related muscle would monitor over-facilitated. Likewise, imbalances within the meridian-related organ or gland would also be represented as imbalances within the meridian-related muscle.

In the Chinese system, every meridian is not only linked to an organ but also directly to acupoints on that meridian, acupoints on other meridians that affect its function, an emotional state, a sense and even a color. This discovery by Goodheart extended the use of muscle monitoring from identifying purely physical muscle-related imbalances to indicating imbalances within other domains from the physical through to the emotional, mental and even energetic.

Goodheart even found that in certain cases of organ imbalance, tracing the pathway of the meridian with his hand just above the body would often eliminate the organ problem and restore that meridian-related muscle to balance. Thus, the muscle–meridian relationship opened up access to our multidimensional being, with all dimensions now accessible through this powerful tool of muscle monitoring. While there can be purely physical factors causing muscle imbalance, often the muscle response reflects the state of energy flow in its associated meridian. So any factor that alters the balance of energy in any particular meridian will result in a reciprocal imbalance in the function of the meridian-related muscles.

Applying muscle-balancing techniques

Muscles make up approximately 80% of the physical mass of the human body and are the primary mechanism by which we interact with our physical world. They also provide the 'keys to the kingdom' for kinesiologists, as it is by muscle biofeedback that we unlock the door to our unconscious and subconscious imbalances, which affect not only our muscles, emotions and mind but also indeed the quality of our lives.

Indicator muscles

In kinesiology, the concept of an indicator muscle has assumed pre-eminence, because a generalized indicator muscle provides a very effective biofeedback tool with broad application. There are two types of indicator muscles: 1, a general indicator muscle (e.g. anterior deltoid or PMC), which can indicate stresses within the physical, etheric, emotional, mental and spiritual systems of the body; and 2, specific indicator muscles that have direct meridian-related associations (e.g. PMC when it is used as an indicator of stomach meridian and/or organ imbalances).

When using a generalized indicator muscle, the muscle circuit is indirectly linked to the source of imbalance that it is indicating. Therefore to be a reliable indicator a muscle such as the anterior deltoid must be in perfect homeostasis within its own circuitry, as previously discussed. Then when the anterior deltoid is monitored at the same time as an alarm point is circuit located, if that meridian has over-energy the homeostatic anterior deltoid will now give an indicator change or even perhaps become over-facilitated, reflecting the state of imbalance within that meridian. While a generalized indicator muscle can indicate that there is stress within a system, it does not indicate the specific nature or location of that stress.

Likewise, a homeostatic indicator muscle may suddenly go into a state of under-facilitation when a particular emotion or attitude has been entered into circuit, again reflecting that there is stress generated by this emotion or attitude. The specific nature of this emotion or attitude then has to be determined by using hand modes, specific indicator points, challenges, verbal questioning or other techniques, and may indeed indicate stress in a meridian that is different from the meridian associated with the indicator muscle being used. For instance, anterior deltoid is a lung meridian–related muscle, but as a generalized indicator it may indicate an imbalance in the bladder meridian.

In contrast, when a muscle is used specifically

as an indicator for the meridian energy to which it is directly linked, it is now specifically indicating the stressors only within this muscle–organ/gland–meridian matrix. In addition, the meridian-related muscle has the strongest frequency resonance, with imbalances within that specific meridian–organ/gland matrix such that the exact nature of an imbalance in the meridian, organ or gland will be accurately reflected in the state of the meridian-related muscle. For example, if the stomach meridian should become under-energy, the PMC will always monitor under-facilitated. Likewise, if the stomach organ should have an inflammatory condition, for example an ulcer, the PMC will become over-facilitated because inflammation in the Chinese system equals over-energy.

While any muscle in the body may be used as a generalized indicator muscle, the most commonly used muscles are the anterior deltoid, PMC and brachioradialis. Both PMC and anterior deltoid are easily accessible; are relatively sensitive, because of the fact that they have a relatively long lever arm; and are usually stable in terms of maintaining homeostasis over time. However, when you are going to do repetitive monitoring, the long lever arm means that they may fatigue rather quickly. For this reason, many kinesiologists switch to the brachioradialis when they are doing repetitive monitoring, which is often the case in the information-gathering phase. The brachioradialis is the muscle that lifts the lower arm vertically while the upper arm rests on the table, providing a shorter lever arm and support against gravity.

Types of muscle balancing

Muscle balancing can be of three different types: 1, general meridian-related muscle balancing; 2, using a combination of a meridian-related muscle and a generalized indicator muscle to assess specific and/or deeper states of imbalance; and 3, Holographic 14-Position Muscle Balancing.

The first type is a meridian-wide muscle balancing in which a meridian-related muscle is used to indicate the overall balance of its associated meridian and organ. For instance, in the Touch for Health system, 14 primary meridian-related indicator muscles are assessed for their state of balance. Each meridian-related muscle represents the balance of the meridian itself and all its related functions. Using biofeedback from the 14 meridian-related muscles, each meridian is returned to a generalized state of balance and the body is now in overall homeostasis. So while the more overt imbalances have been resolved, the more highly compensated states of balanced or imbalance may still persist.

The second type of muscle balancing addresses more specific physiological, physical, energetic and/or psychoemotional imbalances in specific systems, for example the immune system, organ systems, hormonal systems and even neurological systems. This approach to muscle balancing uses a combination of both specific meridian-related muscles and generalized indicator muscles.

For instance, the set-up to assess stress within the immune system could be an acupressure format of organ mode × anatomy mode × circuit-localization of the spleen alarm point + gland mode × circuit-localization of Central Vessel 18 (thymus gland). The middle trapezius muscle of the Chinese spleen–pancreas meridian has a stronger frequency match with the spleen component of this two-phase meridian. Therefore the balance of the middle trapezius muscle indicates the state of balance within the immune system. If after entering the acupressure format for the immune system, the middle trapezius shows any state of imbalance, it indicates that there are stresses affecting the immune system. This imbalance can then be entered into pause lock. At this point, the monitor normally changes to a generalized indicator muscle, for example brachioradialis, to gather more information about the specific nature of the imbalances within the immune system and the causal factors underlying these imbalances.

The third type of muscle balancing is Holographic 14-Position Muscle Balancing. In this type of muscle balancing, the object meridian is assessed in relation to one or more of the 14 reference positions on both sides of the body. The object meridian may be chosen because of its direct relationship with a specific organ that demonstrates a state of imbalance, or it may be chosen because muscle hologram was indicated as the priority correction. This technique will be discussed in detail later, in chapter 40.

For example, a person may present with a specific organ-related issue such as tachycardia. This is clearly a heart-centered issue but involves feedback from a number of other meridian and physiological systems. In this case, the object meridian would be heart and the heart meridian–related muscles would be used to assess the specific stresses in all 14 positions. The imbalances in each position may then be balanced individually using a generalized indicator muscle to first locate the anatomical, physiological and/or psychoemotional stresses underlying each imbalance, and second, to find the appropriate techniques to correct these imbalances.

General meridian-related muscle balancing

The primary example of meridian-related muscle balancing would be Touch for Health, created by Dr John Thie. What Thie had recognized from Goodheart's work with meridians and muscles is that the state of balance of meridian-related muscles directly reflects imbalances within the related meridian. The Chinese clearly state that when all the meridians in the body are in balance this sustains health and well-being.

Indeed, in the ancient Chinese medical system a traditional Chinese medical practitioner was paid a small sum every day that a person in the village was well. As soon as they became ill, they stopped paying. It was then the traditional Chinese medicine practitioner's job to employ their skills at balancing the body's energy. They traditionally used herbs, acupuncture, moxibustion and other techniques to restore the meridian balance of the body–mind–spirit. Therefore a good doctor could keep a large number of people well and receive a reasonable sum for his efforts, while a poor doctor spent most of his time trying to get his patients well and would therefore make very little!

Following in this tradition, Thie developed the system he called Touch for Health so that individuals could maintain the health of their family and friends with simple meridian-related muscle-balancing techniques. The concept was prevention of disease by maintaining meridian balance. This was accomplished by regular 14 Muscle Balancing, in which each of the 14 meridians is represented by a muscle related specifically to that meridian. This gave individuals the opportunity to maintain health with techniques that anyone could learn in a relatively short time. Indeed, Thie said, 'I see Touch for Health as a candle lighting for others the way to better health and living. And I believe each of us holds such a candle—perhaps as yet unlit—that can serve to guide those we cherish safely toward a more abundant life.'[1]

This muscle balancing can be done in both general and specific contexts. For instance, you may do a 14 Muscle Balance 'in the clear', with no particular issue in circuit. This may show imbalances caused by the current stresses in the person's life. Following the 14 Muscle Balance, perhaps involving corrections using neurolymphatics, neurovasculars and even Emotional Stress Release, all the meridians would now be in balance. However, if you now should have that same person address a specific issue in their life by, say, focusing on a physical pain or a distressing psychoemotional issue and then recheck the 14 meridian-related muscles, you may now find a number of muscle imbalances. Correcting these imbalances is now not correcting generalized meridian flow, as in the first instance, but rather the imbalances in that flow created by the specific issue being addressed. The result, however, is a deeper, longer lasting balance.

Reference

1. Thie, JF 1979, *Touch for Health*, De Voross, Marina del Rey, CA.

Chapter 34

REACTIVITY

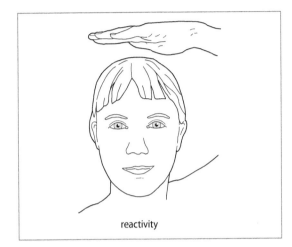

reactivity

Figure 34.1 **Reactivity mode.** The reactivity hand mode involves placing the hand over the top of the client's head. If this mode is held, then an indicator change indicates that there is reactivity involved in the imbalance being investigated. Reactive imbalances can take the form of either physical muscular reactions or energetic reactions.

Reactivity is the term used when one component of a system directly causes a reaction in another component of the same or another system. Energetically, this normally takes the form of a component of one system going over-energy, which then creates under-energy in a component of the same or another system. In the muscular system, as discussed earlier, the over-facilitation of a meridian-related muscle is the physical representation of over-energy in the associated meridian. Therefore reactivity can take the form of either physical muscular reactions or energetic reactions.

All reactivity has two components: the reactor and the reactive(s). When the reactor is activated, it will instantaneously cause a reaction in the reactive(s) such that the reactive component that was in balance before the reactor's activation suddenly displays imbalance. For example, in muscle reactivity when an over-facilitated muscle is activated this will often result in the inhibition

of another muscle some place in the body. The reactive muscle pair may be related by physical position (such as overlapping muscles or muscles sharing a common origin or insertion), by sharing a common meridian association, or by being involved in the same action(s) and thus active at the same time.

However, the reactivity may appear to be totally spurious. For example, the reactive muscle (the muscle inhibited) may be located in a totally different part of the body from the reactor causing this inhibition, with no apparent functional relationship between them. For instance, the reactor muscle may be a muscle in your wrist and the reactive muscle may be a muscle in your back, such that activation of the wrist causes inhibition and muscle weakness of one or more of the back muscles. This is why treatment of a sore back may be ineffective, because the actual origin of the problem may not be in the back and is therefore never addressed.

A real world example of the power of muscle reactivity is highlighted in the case of a man who presented with osteoarthritis of his left wrist and chronic lower back pain. On investigation, a muscle reactivity was revealed between his wrist supinator and his quadratus lumborum, the strongest muscle in the lower back. Activation of his wrist would cause instantaneous inhibition and hence weakness of his lower back muscles, creating pain and soreness. When asked what he did for a job, he replied that he built the hydraulic systems on heavy equipment. Indeed, one of the actions he performed almost every day was to take a heavy hydraulic piston and hold it vertically with his right hand while supporting it in his left palm, then twisting while inserting it into the hydraulic unit. All the while, he was bent over at an angle.

He had been to see several health care practitioners for treatment of his problems, and indeed was on anti-inflammatory medication for the osteoarthritis in his wrist and receiving chiropractic and massage treatment for the pain in his lower back. Superficially, these two problems would appear to be, and were treated as, two unrelated clinical conditions. While the treatment had been ongoing, the anti-inflammatory medication had proved to be only palliative, with the pain returning as soon as the medication was stopped. In addition, the chronic back pain persisted despite regular treatments.

Kinesiological investigation quickly revealed a muscle reactivity between the left wrist supinator, which twists the wrist, turning the palm upwards, and the quadratus lumborum of both sides of the lower back. This unlikely reactive pair was discovered through direct muscle biofeedback and was represented energetically by a meridian over-energy and a meridian under-energy. Application of the Law of Five Elements to rebalance the meridian energies resulted in almost immediate relief from the osteoarthritis of the wrist and the lower back pain. Relief from these symptoms was ongoing for at least six months.

This example highlights the difference between treating the symptoms of an imbalance, the osteoarthritis of the wrist and the lower back pain, rather than treating the cause of the problem, that is, the over-facilitation of the wrist muscle, which then caused a concomitant inhibition of the lower back muscles. Even though the muscles involved two totally different pathologies (osteoarthritis and lower back pain), they were both involved in the same action the man did repeatedly in his work.

Types of reactivity
Muscular reactivity

Muscular reactivity is one of the primary causes of muscle imbalance and musculoskeletal pain within the body. Muscle reactivity may result from over-facilitation of a muscle, and hence over-energy, caused by repetitive use activating a tendon or ligament guard reflex, inhibiting another muscle or muscles. Likewise, when the muscles are activated in an unexpected order, for example slipping on a banana peel or missing a step, it may also create a muscle reactivity resulting in inhibition of one or more muscles in the body.

Repetitive use of a specific muscle often leads to muscle fatigue and recruitment of its synergists. Continued use at this point often drives the synergist muscles into over-facilitation, that is, borrowing energy from other meridians in order to maintain their function. This may result from switching to alternative biochemical pathways because of low oxygen levels in the muscle and/or the building up of lactic acid in the muscle itself.

The Golgi tendon organs (GTOs) and the Golgi ligament organs (GLOs) both have thresholds for reflex inhibition of the muscles that they are attached to (GTOs) or the muscles of the joint in which they are located (GLOs). They prevent excessive tension from causing mechanical damage and/or injury. Unexpected muscle actions may cause the threshold for reflex inhibition to become unset, thus creating an over-facilitated muscle because of the tendon or ligament guard reflex. The tendon or ligament guard reflex is the automatic alteration of the threshold of reflex inhibition caused by injury.

Every action creates proprioceptive flow to the cerebellum. When these proprioceptive signals are received within a specific time window, to be discussed in detail below, related to the successful completion of each action, it informs the cerebellum that 'All is in order'. However, should various proprioceptive signals arrive outside this time window, it indicates that an action other than the intended action has occurred. If the reception of the signal exceeds the threshold for that time window, it is normally associated with the potential for mechanical damage to the associated tendon or ligament or damage to associated soft tissues.

Therefore to prevent damage to tendons, ligaments or soft tissues and allow for recovery and healing of these tissues should damage occur, the GTOs and GLOs reset the threshold of inhibition. This reduces the mechanical stress on these tissues by initiating reflex inhibition sooner than normal. These inhibited muscles then monitor unlocked to reinforce this 'Do not use now, I'm healing', and there is normally coactivation of the nociceptors (pain receptors). This restricted range of motion caused by muscle inhibition and pain limits the range of motion of that muscle. This resetting of the threshold for reflex inhibition of the tendon or ligament is termed the tendon or ligament guard reflex, as it guards against further injury and allows healing to proceed unhindered by excessive mechanical stress.

For instance, you are walking down the stairs and miss the last step. The unusual pattern of proprioceptive input elicited by this action causes the cerebellum to misinterpret these signals as indication of potential injury. To protect the body, it activates the tendon or ligament guard reflexes in a belief that it is protecting the injured muscles. If these reflexes are activated and the thresholds reset but there is no actual injury, these aberrant thresholds persist, often over long periods of time.

Other types of reactivity

Reactivity is normally a component of one system, for instance a muscle, causing inhibition of another component of the same system, for instance another muscle; this is a muscle reactivity. However, in other situations a muscular imbalance may create a reaction in another system other than muscles. For instance, an over-facilitated muscle that is reflected energetically as an over-energy meridian may cause an under-energy in another meridian, which in turn can have physiological, glandular or physical effects such as pain. Physical pain is always represented energetically as over-energy, and dissipation of this over-energy results in resolution of the pain.

For completeness, we need to note that there are other types of reactivities that do not involve muscles but may involve other physical components of your body (e.g. organ reactivity), physiological components (e.g. gland reactivity) or energetic reactivity (e.g. chakra and meridian reactivity). There may even be mixed reactivity, in which an inhibited muscle may result from an emotional state. It is possible to have an over-energy emotional state, which via the output of the limbic and amygdaloid connections to our reticulospinal tracts unset the spindle cell bag fiber output, rapidly decreasing the muscle tone, which is observed as an unlocking muscle. So every time this psychoemotional state is activated, in reaction specific muscles become inhibited.

Neurophysiology of muscle reactivity

To understand the origin of muscle reactivity, we have to delve more deeply into muscle proprioception and proprioceptive processing in the brain. There are two primary tracts that carry unconscious information about muscle, tendon and joint proprioception to the cerebellum. Because there are no tracts from the cerebellum directly to the cortex with regard to this proprioceptive input, this input remains totally subconscious. However, it is this proprioceptive input to the cerebellum that sets the tendon and ligament guard reflexes that control reflex inhibition to protect muscles, tendons and ligaments from damage. Also, when damage has occurred it protects the injured tissues by resetting the threshold to limit the range of motion while the tissue heals.

Indeed, to ensure that you do not further damage the injured tissue, the resetting of the tendon and ligament guard reflexes causes muscle inhibition well before any significant physical stress is applied to the tendons or ligaments. It does this by activating the nociceptors or pain receptors to enforce this limited range of motion while you are healing. When the tissue is healed, the cerebellum should reset the tendon and ligament guard reflexes to their original length, thus permitting a full range of motion while at the same time protecting the muscle or tendon from injury in the future. However, as anyone who has broken a bone and had their limb immobilized for an extended period knows, this automatic reset of the guard reflexes may need to be assisted by forceful physical stretching, which can be quite painful.

The ascending pathways from the spinal cord into the brain carry both conscious and subconscious information. The subconscious information is carried largely by the dorsal and ventral spinocerebellar tracts from the spinal segments innervating each muscle to the cerebellum. The ventral spinocerebellar tract carries information from the GTOs and GLOs to the cerebellum via type 1b myelinated sensory fibers, which carry information on tension and changes of tension in the tendons and ligaments.

These signals are relatively fast, but not as fast as signals carried by the type 1a highly myelinated sensory fibers carrying information from the annulospiral endings of the bag fibers in the muscle spindle cells. These fibers carry information about the changes in length and rate of change of changes in length to the cerebellum via the dorsal spinocerebellar tracts. Additional proprioceptive information on muscle stretch and length are sent to the cerebellum via the type 2 less myelinated sensory fibers of the dorsal spinocerebellar tracts. Additional skin stretch information is likewise carried to the cerebellum via type 2 sensory fibers in the spinocerebellar tracts.

The degree of myelination determines the speed of conduction, so muscle spindle bag fiber signals traveling along the type 1a fibers reach the cerebellum before the length signals from the flower spray endings traveling along type 2 fibers. The tendon stretch and tension receptor signals travel along type 1b fibers and are initiated at the same time as the muscle stretch signals, but they travel slightly slower and therefore arrive after the bag fiber output. Information from skin stretch receptors traveling along type 2 fibers is usually elicited later than the spindle cell and GTO or GLO signals. Furthermore, the GLO signals of the joint ligaments have a higher threshold before the reflex inhibition is initiated and therefore arrive later than the signals from the GTOs. To provide an idea of the relative speeds of these tracts and their order of arrival in the cerebellum, Table 34.1 shows the speed of transmission for the different tracts and types of proprioceptors.

Table 34.1 Spinocerebellar tracts: rates of transmission of nerve impulses and types of proprioceptors

Tract	Fiber	Rate of transmission (milliseconds)	Proprioceptor
Ventral spinocerebellar tracts	Type 1b	~ 4	GTOs and GLOs*
Dorsal spinocerebellar tracts	Type 1b	~ 4	GTOs
	Type 1b	~ 6	GLOs
	Type 1a	~ 2.5	Spindle bag fibers
	Type 2	18–25	Spindle chain fibers

*GLO = Golgi ligament organ; GTO = Golgi tendon organ.

Therefore we have a variety of signals from various proprioceptors arriving at the cerebellum at different time intervals. Each of these carries information about a specific component of muscle and joint function. The cerebellum basically sets up a window of response times in which these signals should arrive (see upper panel of Figure 34.2). Because the intended plan for every action you do is recorded in the cerebellum before you act, it compares the proprioceptive signals carrying the *actual* action with the *plan* of the intended action. If these do not match, the cerebellum sends

out corrective motor output so that the intended action becomes the actual action.

When these signals from different proprioceptors do not arrive within the intended window of response times (see lower panel of Figure 34.2), the cerebellum may perceive this as evidence of potential injury. The cerebellum will then reset the threshold for GTOs, GLOs and spindle inhibitory reflexes to protect this 'injured' tissue. Normally, this will result from actual injury, such as a tendon strain, and is indeed necessary to allow the injured tissue to heal, at which time the threshold will be reset to allow the normal range of muscle motion once more. However, should the signals arrive at the cerebellum in an unexpected order because of an unintended action, such as missing a step, this will often be misinterpreted by the cerebellum as actual injury. In response to this perceived injury, the cerebellum will reset the threshold via the guard reflex, creating an 'over-protected' state of muscle function, which is reflected physiologically as over-facilitation.

The reset procedure should occur automatically with the healing of the injured tissue; however, because there was no actual injury, this over-protected state may persist for an extended period of time, even years.

Muscle reactivity: the cause of many musculoskeletal problems

Many musculoskeletal problems are represented by complex patterns of over-facilitated and under-facilitated muscles. Some of these over-facilitated muscles may become reactor muscles in a muscle reactivity. An initial muscle reactivity may generate a complex pattern of compensatory reactivities over time but often begin with a single incident, perhaps trying to lift something too heavy or at a wrong angle, missing a step, slipping and falling or repetitive activation of muscles that leads to

fatigue. However, once this initial reactivity has been established, it may lead to a series of inter-connected muscle reactivities over time because of compensation.

The creation of an over-facilitated muscle will often result in the establishment of a muscle reactivity such that activation of the over-facilitated muscle will actually inhibit another muscle that may otherwise be in homeostasis. This inhibition of the homeostatic muscle now leads to a secondary muscular imbalance, which then must be compensated for.

Each muscle is a prime mover in a particular action in which its orientation and position give it the maximum mechanical advantage for that action. For instance, the biceps muscle fibers are oriented from the shoulder to the elbow and cross the elbow joint to insert on the lower arm close to the elbow joint. When the biceps contracts with the palm facing up, it lifts the lower arm upward and has the maximum mechanical advantage to perform this action. When you attempt to lift a considerable load, the beta efferents of the biceps will automatically recruit its synergists, the brachialis and brachioradialis muscles, to assist it.

When the biceps is reactive to another muscle, the reactor, it will be overtly inhibited every time that reactor is activated, preventing it from developing its full power. The consequence is that when performing actions in which biceps is a prime

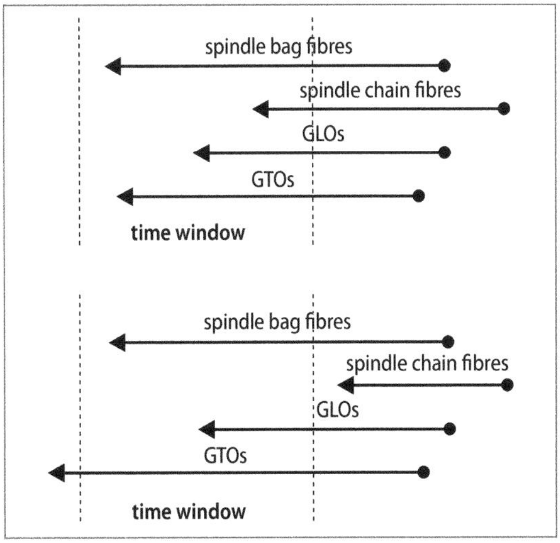

Figure 34.2 Cerebellar time windows. Subconscious proprioceptive signals arrive at the cerebellum via several different types of spinocerebellar tracts of varying myelination and therefore speed. Thus, the cerebellum sets an expected time window for each, and if all inputs arrive within this time window (top), all is well. If these sensory inputs arrive outside their expected time window, this normally indicates injury to the muscle, tendon or joint (bottom).

Note: GLO = Golgi ligament organ; GTO = Golgi tendon organ.

mover, it will need to recruit its synergists much sooner and they will do more of the work as a compensation for the weakened (inhibited) biceps. However, the synergists do not have optimal mechanical advantage to perform this action and therefore now have to work much harder than normal to assist the designated prime mover, the biceps.

Of course, one of the primary ways of producing muscle over-facilitation is to repetitively over work a muscle, particularly when working at reduced mechanical advantage. An example would be you carrying a bucket of sand directly at your side versus holding your arm out horizontally to the side; which would you find harder? Clearly, you will find holding the bucket out horizontally to the side much more effort, and your muscles will fatigue much more rapidly. If this action is repeated a number of times, it may create over-facilitation of the synergists trying to assist the inhibited prime mover created by the original muscle reactivity. This newly created over-facilitated muscle may in turn initiate a new muscle reactivity, inhibiting yet another prime mover in another part of the body.

In this way, the original muscle reactivity may result in a chain of muscle reactivities with each later reactivity being the result of compensation for the reactivity preceding it. Therefore, over time the muscle soreness and dysfunction may become far removed from the original cause. This is one of the reasons why long-term musculoskeletal problems are often difficult to resolve. Treating the most recent painful over-facilitated muscles and dysfunction has only palliative effects, as these are often only treating compensations and therefore the original cause of the muscle reactivity is not addressed.

This demonstrates the importance of two things: 1, locating the original muscle reactivity; and 2, addressing the factors causing the original muscle reactivity, which are not necessarily only mechanical or physical in origin. Remember the earlier discussion regarding the emotional control of muscle response. Emotions can cause muscle over-facilitation which can trigger muscle reactivity. Unless the causative factors, emotional in this case, are addressed, these musculoskeletal problems may remain unresolved.

The significance of muscle reactivity

While muscle reactivities may indeed be local phenomenon, for example the reactor overlaps or is contiguous with the reactive muscle, it is possible for the reactor and its reactive to be widely separate from each other in the body, and for them to be ipsilateral (on the same side) or contralateral (on opposite sides) or both to a single reactor. In the example given earlier, the man's left wrist supinator was the reactor that inhibited both sides of his lower back muscles, quadratus lumborum.

So how can it be that muscles so widely separated from each other physically on the body can interact so strongly? Indeed, it is possible for a muscle on the face to inhibit a muscle in the foot! Neurologically, this is totally plausible, as one-third of all the fibers in the spinal cord are called propriospinal fibers.[1] Propriospinal fibers connect one spinal segment to the one above or below it, two above or below it, three above or below it, etc., between the cervical spine and the lumbar spine. The muscles of the shoulders are activated by the motor neurons in the cervical enlargement, and hip, leg and foot muscles are activated by motor neurons in the lumbar enlargement. As these two spinal areas are directly connected by propriospinal fibers, an over-facilitated shoulder muscle could easily be a reactor inhibiting an ankle or a foot muscle.

Much of our normal movement and muscular activity is coordinated by a series of subconscious reflexes. Reflexes are spinal arcs in which the coordination of one muscle is programmed to coordinate with the activation or inhibition of another muscle. There are many types of these reflexes, from the simple monosynaptic reflex arc of the muscle load reflex to complex cross-extensor withdrawal reflexes. Thus, when a muscle reactivity inappropriately inhibits one of the muscles in a reflex arc, it has the potential to disorganize the function of this automatic reflex. This then results in loss of coordination, and considerably more effort is now required to perform normal actions or movements.

For instance, there are a major set of reflexes called the righting reflexes that are largely responsible for the coordination of postural muscles to keep you in an upright position. This happens completely outside your consciousness, as these reflexes are all subconscious in origin. If a reactor muscle should inhibit a key postural muscle in one of the righting reflexes, every time the reactor is activated you will suffer postural distortion caused by inhibition of the reactive postural muscle. This in turn may produce compensated patterns of muscle function that further distort your posture, creating additional compensatory muscle reactivities.

Another major set of reflexes are the gait reflexes that automatically organize the contralateral muscles needed to walk and run. When these reflexes are disturbed by muscle reactivity, there is always a loss of coordination in contralateral activities.

Clearly, muscle reactivity is a major player in musculoskeletal problems, and unless muscular reactivity is addressed these problems are unlikely to be resolved even with normally effective treatments.

Reference

1. Williams, PL, Bannister, LH, Berry, MM, Collins, P, Dyson, M, Dussek, JE & Ferguson, MWJ, eds 1995, *Gray's Anatomy. The Anatomical Basis of Medicine and Surgery*, Churchill Livingstone, Edinburgh, pp. 1003–1004.

Chapter 35

CENTERING

What is centering?

Centering is a set of interactive reflexes built on patterns of integration of even simpler spinal reflexes that coordinate our equilibrium and posture when standing and sitting, as well as coordinate our walking, running and other complex movements. The cloacal or righting reflexes begin developing in the womb and are the basis of our primitive reflexes, which are brainstem reflexes that provide coordinated body movement before the full development of our integrated postural and gait reflexes by about the age of three years. By this time, the cortex is sufficiently myelinated to take over control of these movements.

The most basal of these reflexes are the cloacal reflexes, an integrated set of basic spinal reflexes that act as our earliest form of righting reflexes. These then become integrated with higher-level brain areas to form the adult postural righting reflexes. These are called *cloacal* reflexes because they begin development when the fetus has a cloaca, that is, before the separation of the urinary and genital systems. *Cloaca* comes from Latin and means 'common sewer'. In tetrapods, these cloacal reflexes are not only involved in maintaining upright posture, the reason they become integrated with the other righting reflexes, but are also very important for mating. During mating, they control the hip–body alignment and movement necessary for successful intercourse when you cannot see what is happening 'down there'.

The primitive cloacal reflexes are first integrated with the labyrinthine (vestibular) and visual righting reflexes with development of the vestibular ocular reflexes, and then with the neck-righting reflexes as the cortex gains more direct control of head and neck posture, as the child lifts their head to look around. Other primitive reflexes begin *in utero* and reflexively organize early movement patterns. For instance, the asymmetric tonic neck reflex coordinates head movement with arm and leg movement; turning the head activates ipsilateral extension on the side to which the face is turned and ipsilateral withdrawal on the occipital side. This reflex begins *in utero* and is important to assist the birth process and then after birth to help the child to roll over.

Most of these specific primitive reflexes should be integrated into more mature postural reflexes within the first year of birth, and all of them should be well integrated into the postural reflexes by the age of three years. In the past, it was often said that these primitive reflexes were extinguished by the age of three years, but they are not extinguished but rather integrated into more mature coordinated movement patterns. When, for whatever reason, the primitive reflexes do not become fully integrated in the higher cortical postural reflexes, various motor coordination and even cognitive problems may develop, including learning difficulties.

As the cortex continues to myelinate, the control of arm, leg and body movements is progressively transferred from the brainstem-controlled primitive reflexes into the mature cortically activated 'higher' postural righting reflexes to coordinate our standing posture and equilibrium. By about 7–9 months after birth, the cloacal and the neck-righting and visual righting reflexes have been integrated into the more mature postural reflexes, permitting the child to now sit unaided and begin to stand on their own (although often holding onto something). Then, by about 12 months, the development of our gait reflexes begin to coordinate specific contralateral (opposite side) shoulder–arm and hip–leg muscles to organize our walking and running movements.

To recapitulate, as the primitive reflexes become progressively integrated with our cloacal, labyrinthine, neck- and visual righting reflexes, we develop our postural reflexes controlling static posture and equilibrium, and then the gait reflexes begin to organize the cross-lateral movement patterns of walking and running.

To provide a stable visual horizontal, which is so important for our equilibrium, requires an effective feedback mechanism for the location of the head in space. While the vestibular apparatus provides one point of reference for head position, and horizontal visual cues in our environment provide another, the tension and relative length of the neck muscles provide a third input for comparison, completing the *equilibrium triad*. One of the reasons for this redundancy is the same reason all airplanes have not one but three gyroscopes. If one gyroscope is malfunctioning and you only have two, how do you know which one is in error? But if you have three, then you go with the two that agree!

This third reference point for equilibrium is provided by the sensory feedback of the hyoid bone. The balance of the hyoid bone becomes a major feedback control input because of its unique location and structure. The hyoid bone is suspended halfway between the head and the chest on the stylohyoid ligament from the tip of the styloid process of the temporal bone to the greater *cornu* or 'horn' of the hyoid by eight pairs of muscles: four suprahyoid muscles and four infrahyoid muscles. Because of this unique free-floating arrangement, the hyoid acts like a gyroscope for the position of the head in space relative to the body. Changes in length of any of these muscles thus moves the hyoid, changing the proprioceptive output to the cerebellum, informing the brain of a change in position of the head relative to the body or the body relative to the head.

So when this hyoid position is combined with vestibular and visual input, it creates a unified view of the position of the head in space relative to the body. These combined vestibular, visual and hyoid inputs are then integrated by the vestibulocerebellum to provide a point of reference for alignment of the head, and for the proprioceptive input to the spinocerebellar vermal zone to then align the body relative to the head position. To maintain

coherent visual function, the vestibular input is linked to the visual input via the vestibulo-ocular reflex, which allows you to maintain a visual horizontal of the head, independent of body movement, and then use this visual horizontal as a reference point for position of the body. This is why when you enter the fun house at the circus, with mirrors that distort your visual horizontal, you have so much trouble with equilibrium and posture. You find yourself twisting your body to match the distorted visual horizontal, even though your proprioceptors of your neck muscles, including hyoid input and vestibular input, are screaming, 'No, this is *not* horizontal!'

The cloacal and other righting reflexes are an integrated set of crossed and uncrossed (contralateral and ipsilateral) extensor–flexor reflexes primarily of the axial muscles along the spine and neck, as well as groups of proximal shoulder and hip postural muscles required to maintain the position of the head and body in space against the force of gravity. The labyrinthine or vestibular apparatus of the membranous labyrinth in the mastoid bone coordinates these reflexes by direct output to the vestibular nuclei of the pons via the medial and lateral vestibulospinal tracts to the body, secondarily via output of the vestibulocerebellum and spinocerebellum vermal zone, and also by activation of the same medial and lateral vestibulospinal tracts (see Figure 35.1).

The hyoid reflexes integrate the position of the head relative to the body in relation to the vestibular input and vestibulo-ocular reflex visual horizontal. This integrated input and feedback from the righting and hyoid reflexes about where your head is in space, and the alignment of your body beneath your head, allows you to maintain two things: 1, static posture, that is, standing and sitting upright; and 2, coordinated movement, such as walking and running.

However, walking and running require another reflex system to become fully integrated: the gait mechanism. The gait mechanism is again a coordinated system integrating crossed extensor–withdrawal spinal reflexes, which coordinate the movement of specific contralateral muscles of the shoulders and hips to facilitate and inhibit reciprocal pairs of contralateral muscles to keep the arms and legs aligned during walking and running.

Unlike the contralateral righting reflexes that control groups of postural muscles of the shoulders and hips, the gait mechanism activates and coordinates specific individual proximal flexor and extensor muscles of the shoulders with the opposite side specific flexor and extensor muscles of the hips. Thus, as the right anterior deltoid is activated, it inhibits the left anterior deltoid and is coactivated with the contralateral (left) rectus femoris, which when activated automatically inhibits the right

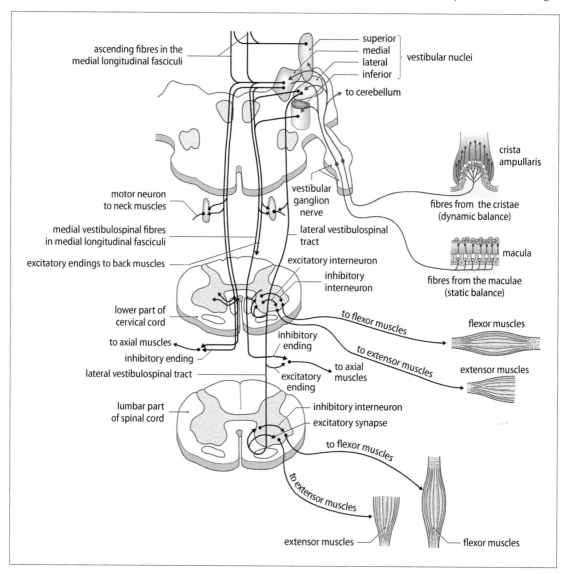

Figure 35.1 Vestibular apparatus and vestibular system. The vestibular apparatus consists of the cristae of the semicircular canals of the membranous labyrinth that detect the angular rotation of the head, and the maculae of the saccule and utricle that detect the static position of the head. The vestibular system consists of the output from the cristae and maculae to the vestibulocerebellum and the vestibular nuclei of the pons. The vestibulocerebellum and vestibular nuclei then integrate this input to provide the location of your head in space, the reference point for all actions, and they activate and inhibit the postural muscles via the medial and lateral vestibulospinal tracts to maintain your posture and equilibrium.

rectus femoris. Likewise, as the pectoralis major clavicular is activated, it inhibits the opposite side pectoralis major clavicular and is coactivated with the contralateral psoas, which when it is activated inhibits the psoas of the opposite side. The end result is smooth, coordinated, alternating movement of the specific muscles guiding contralateral arms and legs so that they move in alignment with the body to maintain coordination while walking or running.

However, standing, as well as walking and running, needs additional feedback about *how* your foot is contacting the ground; this is the role of footpad pressure sensors (FPSs). Likewise, when you are sitting you need feedback about *how* your ischial tuberosities, the blunt ends of your ischial bones, which you sit on, are contacting the surface you are sitting on; this is the role of your ischial or buttock pressure sensors (BPSs). Both the FPSs and the BPSs have the same structure and differ only in their location. FPSs are located on the pad of each toe, along the ball of the foot, along the outside edge of the foot and across the heel, with a subset in the arch of the foot, while the BPSs are located across the ischial tuberosities.

The FPSs and BPSs are specialized corpuscles of groups of Ruffini end organs and Pacinian corpuscles, which provide sensory feedback on the instantaneous pressure and changes in pressure (the Pacinian corpuscles) on the skin and instantaneous direction of movement of the skin (the Ruffini end organs). The output of these sensors goes to spinal segments controlling the antigravity postural muscles initiating reflex correction of postural muscle tensions to compensate automatically for changes in pressure on the foot or buttock. Changes in pressure on the foot or buttock result from variations in the surface on which you are standing or sitting, and these need to be compensated for to maintain upright posture (see Figure 35.2).

For example, you are standing with your right foot on a flat surface while your left foot is placed on a sloping surface to the left. Clearly, there will be an increase in pressure on the left FPS along the side of your left foot and a decrease in pressure on the FPS on the upslope side heel and ball of the foot. The FPS along the side of the foot on the downhill sloping side will therefore fire more rapidly, initiating both centering and spinal reflexes activating the extensor muscles on the downslope side of the body and inhibiting extensors on the upslope side of the body, while facilitating flexors on the upslope side and inhibiting the flexors on the downslope side to maintain your body in an upright position. If you continue to stand in this position, the steady state output of the Ruffini end organs will maintain this postural stance.

The basal ganglia do *not* store a motor program for every surface you might walk on; rather, they store a basic motor program for standing on a flat horizontal surface and then let the FPS output

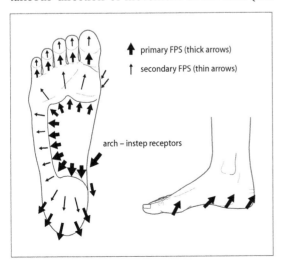

↑ primary FPS (thick arrows)

↑ secondary FPS (thin arrows)

arch – instep receptors

Figure 35.2 **Foot pad pressure sensors (FPSs).** The primary FPSs (large arrows) are located along the posterior edge of the ball of each toe, along the posterior border of the ball of the foot, along the medial border of the lateral side of the foot, and across the posterior border of the heel, with a set of sensors at the lower, posterior arch, where it joins the heel. Secondary sensors (small arrows) provide output to fine-tune the output to the spinal segments and reflexes, activating postural muscles to maintain posture.

modify this standing-up program in real time via the centering and spinal reflexes. The same is true of your sitting posture, with BPS feedback compensating for variations in the surface your buttocks are sitting on. Of course, this FPS and BPS input to the central nervous system also provides proprioceptive feedback to the vestibulo-cerebellum and spinocerebellum vermal zone. This then adjusts your final posture, in conjunction with vestibular output via the reticulospinal and vestibulospinal tracts, direct output to the ventrolateral thalamic nuclei and the motor cortex, and then output via the extrapyramidal tracts controlling the proximal shoulder and hip muscles and the axial muscles along the spine. Further discrete direct output to specific spinal segments from the fastigial nuclei via the fastigio-spinal tracts fine-tunes your new posture (see Figure 35.1).

So in a sense you have default standing and sitting programs for regular flat surfaces, and these default programs are then modified by FPS and BPS output for variations in these surfaces. Clearly, this FPS and BPS output needs to be taken into consideration when you are balancing the centering reflexes, as they strongly interact with these spinal reflexes.

Development of the centering techniques

Dr George Goodheart discovered the gait mechanism from a kinesiology perspective by analysis of the muscles involved in walking. He tested the muscles in different patterns and observed the patterns of inhibition and facilitation of these gait muscles. For instance, when you step forward with your right foot, the same side anterior deltoid and opposite side rectus femoris muscles are inhibited, while the right side rectus femoris and opposite side anterior deltoid are facilitated. When a person stands upright on both feet with their right foot in front of their left foot and the weight evenly distributed between the two feet, if anterior deltoid muscles are monitored, both will be locked. But as soon as the person leans forward on to the ball of

their right foot, the same side anterior deltoid is suddenly inhibited and the opposite side anterior deltoid is facilitated because of activation of the gait reflexes.

Goodheart also discovered the hyoid reflexes by noting postural deviations when testing postural muscles as he moved the hyoid into different positions. He discovered that under-facilitated muscles related to this postural deviation would suddenly disappear when the hyoid was pushed into the direction of the distortion. Goodheart also noticed that muscles tested differently when a patient's eyes are oriented in different directions, according to the postural distortion he observed in the patient. This is apparently because of an adaptation of the oculomotor muscles to the individual's distorted posture. In patients who have adapted to their condition, numerous unlocked muscles may appear when the eyes are put into the direction of distortion, termed *eyes into distortion*. When the eyes are held in this position, it takes away the adaptation the extrinsic eye muscles have made to the distorted posture, but movement of the hyoid into the direction of distortion caused the same muscles to lock again.

Dr Alan Beardall discovered the cloacal reflexes from both a mechanical and an energetic perspective. The mechanics of the cloacal reflexes are rooted in the primitive reflexes, which become integrated into the righting reflexes as you mature. These righting reflexes have both ipsilateral and contralateral components and are an integrated set of spinal and brainstem–run reflexes. The brainstem components are the vestibular righting reflexes and the vestibular–cerebellar controlled vestibulo-ocular reflex, while the primary spinal components are the ipsilateral extensor and flexor reflexes and the crossed extensor–flexor withdrawal reflexes.

Because Beardall was also a sensitive who could see body energies, he noticed energy flows that were persistent from person to person. He observed flows of energy from just lateral to the pubic symphysis (stomach 30), ipsilateral to the supra-orbital foramen (an extrameridianal acupoint) on both sides of the body, and from the right stomach 30 to the opposite side supraorbital foramen, as

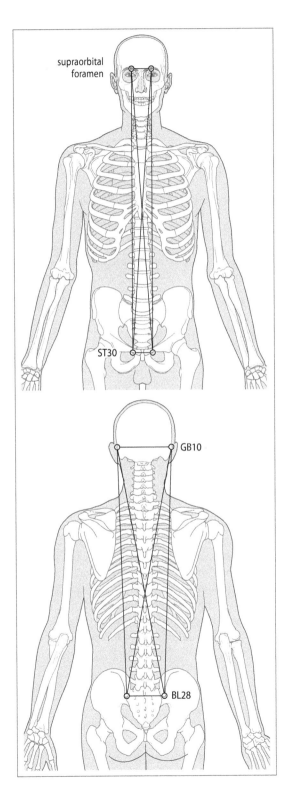

Figure 35.3 **Centering energy flows.** BL = bladder; GB = gall bladder; ST = stomach.

well as the same flows on the left side of the body. Together, the flows created a figure 8 energy pattern on the front of the body.

On the back of the body, Beardall observed a similar pattern of flows, with energy exiting from between the fourth and fifth sacral tubercles (bladder 28) of the right side of the back and flowing ipsilateral to the temporal–parietal junction just behind the mastoid process of the temporal bone (gall bladder 10). Again, as on the front of the body, he observed another flow from between the right sacral tubercles across the back to the opposite side mastoid process, with the reverse flows on the left side of the back. Together, the flows on the back created a figure 8 energy pattern as on the front of the body (see Figure 35.3).

Beardall observed that when these energy flows were out of balance or unequal, people commonly had cloacal and righting reflexes that were also out of balance, and when the righting reflexes were balanced, the energy flows were also balanced and even. Beardall associated the following righting and cloacal reflexes with each of the points he observed, as shown in Table 35.1.

Beardall then researched what he termed the *righting and cloacal reflex indicator points* to locate each of these reflexes. When the indicator point was circuit located and there was an indicator change, this indicated that there was an active imbalance in this particular reflex (see Figure 35.4).

These cloacal and righting reflexes were introduced into Applied Kinesiology, and the standard correction became strong manual or finger stimulation on the associated cloacal points which were also acupoints. For instance, if the right supraorbital foramen gave an indicator change when circuit located, then this cloacal point was *active*. Correction involved firm pressure on this cloacal point until there was no longer an indicator change when this point was circuit located. While usually effective, this Applied Kinesiology technique was often very painful!

In a similar way, the gait reflexes had a series of gait indicator points on the feet. When there was

Table 35.1 Righting reflexes and their specific indicator points

Righting reflex(es)	Specific indicator point(s)
Labyrinthine righting reflexes	Inner ear to mastoid torque (finger in ear, thumb to mastoid process and torque)
Vestibulo-ocular reflex	Supraorbital foramen to mastoid process (R to R, L to L, R « L and L « R)
Neck-righting reflexes:	
Labyrinthine	Therapy localization axis to R or L mastoid processes and to R or L supraorbital foramen
Visual	
Labyrinthine	Therapy localization third thoracic vertebrae to R or L mastoid processes and to R or L supraorbital foramen
Visual	
Visual righting reflexes:	
Front	Supraorbital foramen
Back	R temporal bone behind ear
Cloacal righting reflexes:	
Front	Superior ramus of pubis either side of pubic symphysis
Back	Fourth and fifth transverse tubercles of sacrum and lateral margins of coccyx or ischial tuberosities

L = left; R = right.

a gait imbalance, one or more of these gait points became active. The standard Applied Kinesiology correction for gait imbalance was to use firm pressure on the gait indicator points until no further indicator change occurred on challenge. Again, this could be extremely painful.

Likewise, in Applied Kinesiology centering, hyoid imbalances could be found by moving the hyoid bone into different positions while monitoring the indicator muscle, stretching each of the suprahyoidal and infrahyoidal muscles in turn. An indicator change indicated that the muscle or muscles stretched was *over-facilitated* or *hypertonic* in old Applied Kinesiology terms. So the standard Applied Kinesiology correction was to spindle off the over-facilitated muscle and then move the hyoid around to release the over-facilitated state of the hyoid muscles.

Richard Utt revolutionized these Applied Kinesiology centering imbalances by researching the relationship between each of the centering reflexes and the Law of Five Elements Command Points. This not only made locating these centering imbalances easier, it also allowed for more precise correction. Not only that, it linked these centering reflex imbalances to specific muscle positions, acupoints and even emotions and attitudes. This provides deeper, longer-lasting corrections to correct these important reflexes that are not painful.

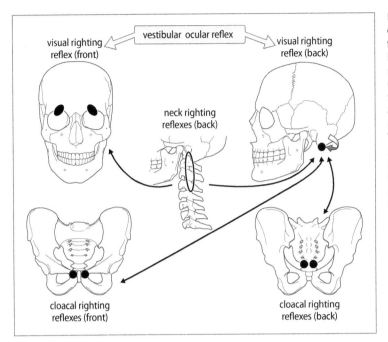

Figure 35.4 Righting reflex or cloacal indicator points for the front and back of the body. The indicator points for the front righting reflexes are the supraorbital foramen (the dent in the superior orbit above the pupil of the eye) and the acupoint stomach 30 (the inguinal crease lateral to the pubic symphysis). The indicator points for the back righting reflexes are the acupoint gall bladder 10 (the dent at juncture of the mastoid and parietal bones) and the acupoint bladder 28 (between the fourth and fifth sacral tubercles).

Chapter 36

EMOTIONAL STRESS DEFUSION

Emotional Stress Defusion techniques

Most of what we find stressful in our lives results from the triggering of old emotional patterns by often apparently unrelated stimuli. As previously discussed, stress activates the fight-or-flight mechanism, which immediately reduces blood flow to our frontal cortex, the site of all processing of new information and the reprocessing of old patterns. We are then left acting out of our survival system and memories activated by our survival emotional reactions. For evolutionary survival purposes, these brainstem–limbic reactions are programmed to just rerun previous emotional and behavioral patterns because they had survival value. These reactions are not responses chosen by your consciousness. There is no choice involved, as brainstem–limbic processing is both subconscious and reactive to trigger stimuli. In the words of Joseph LeDoux, one of the premier researchers of the amygdala, you have just experienced an 'amygdala hijack!'[1]

Once the trigger stimulus has been called forth by an associated memory with enough stress to shift us into survival–limbic processing, your action then becomes merely a subconscious reaction to the emotions evoked by the trigger stimulus. Have you ever observed yourself running an old emotional program, sometimes childish and inappropriate to the situation at hand, yet not been able to stop it? You may have even said to yourself afterward, 'I can't believe I acted that way!' That was the emotional survival system in full control.

To relieve the stress and emotionally defuse the situation, all you have to do is get your frontal cortex turned on, providing the opportunity to act differently to the trigger stimulus based on rational consideration of the total circumstances: a choice to act, not subconsciously react. The problem is how to get back into the frontal cortex for analysis after being confronted with a trigger stimulus that

drops you into brainstem–limbic reaction, for example someone who sounds like your father raising their voice to you. Fortunately, there are several acupressure points that may be held by yourself or another person that will switch on frontal cortical function and get you out of the survival system's reactive programming. This then allows you to now assess the current situation free of your reactions to past trauma associated with this particular type of stimulus.

Two of these acupoints are gall bladder 14, located just below the broad bumps on your forehead called the frontal eminences (which simply means the 'front bumps' in Latin), and gall bladder 20, located on bumps either side of the base of the skull called the occipital protuberances. These points may be held either separately or together, with one hand on the forehead and the other holding the base of the skull; this is called *Frontal–Occipital Holding*. Or the fingertips of each hand may be applied only to the frontal eminences, which is called *Emotional Stress Release*. The pressure applied to the frontal eminences during Emotional Stress Release or during Frontal–Occipital Holding is similar to the pressure that you can comfortably apply to the eyelid of the closed eye.

What this acupressure holding does is stimulate blood flow to return to the frontal cortex, despite the fact that you are now involved in an emotional reaction to a previous trauma. Once the frontal cortex is turned on, it does what it is programmed to do, that is, resolve emotional stress by turning on your problem solving and rational processing of the actual situation.

However, it actually does far more than just permit you to access rational reasoning, as the prefrontal cortex also provides access to our transcendent emotions. We call these *transcendent* emotions because to access them you have to transcend your personality ego self. The ego can see events only from its egocentric perspective: what is good for 'me' or what has been done to 'me'. Thus, the ego can never forgive and always wants to get even.

When blood flow returns to the prefrontal cortex, we can now access our higher self, which allows us to access and express the transcendent emotions of compassion, empathy, unconditional love, forgiveness and altruism. From this higher transcendent perspective, we can understand why another person slighted us, lied to us or treated us badly, and through heartfelt unconditional love truly forgive them. Forgiveness sets us free, because as long as you hold onto anger, jealousy, revenge, etc., you are locked into an ego-driven reaction that controls your emotional states and behaviors; you are not truly free.

There are other acupoints that affect the blood flow patterns in the brain. In Terrence Bennett's original research with neurovascular points, he found that when the temple is held above both triple heater 23 acupoints, just below and behind the outside end of the eyebrow in a small hollow on the skull, this reflect point affects emotional processing. It is hypothesized that by holding these points blood flow to the deeper brainstem areas is increased. While people generally experience no conscious images or content when these points are held, they often experience a variety of body and energetic sensations, such as tensions in the viscera, coldness in different body regions, and flows of energies down or around the body.

How does this switch on the frontal cortex? Brain researchers have shown that whenever a specific area of the brain is neurologically active, for example processing information, the blood flow to that area is greatly increased, while those areas with low blood flow show little neurological activity. Indeed, this is exactly what you see when you become stressed, as the blood flow to the deep brainstem–limbic survival system is greatly increased and the blood flow to the frontal cortex is greatly decreased. Thus, the areas of the brain receiving increased blood flow are activated, or 'turned on', and doing the processing, while the other brain areas are put on hold or 'standby'. Both of these acupressure holding Emotional Stress Defusion (ESD) techniques stimulate increased blood flow to the frontal cortex, in effect, turning it on.

Applying the Emotional Stress Defusion techniques

Although these stress release techniques seem too simple to be useful, they can be very powerful. Simply doing Emotional Stress Release by holding the frontal eminences or performing Frontal Occipital Holding is enough to pull a person out of the limbic survival system reaction to life's situations. Once they are viewing life's stressful situations from a new, less emotional perspective, they are now free to choose the most appropriate response to the current situation. So if a present situation stresses you, simply think about it while doing ESD, going through each detail in your mind.

How do you know when you have defused the situation? Generally, you will feel pulses appear under your fingertips after a few seconds to a few minutes (these are much like your wrist pulse), and when they become synchronized, beating together on both sides of the forehead at the same time, the ESD is complete. Just think once again of the previously stressful situation. Normally, you will find the emotional charge or tightened gut has been eliminated and you can just think of it as something that has happened.

To test this technique, think about something that has happened to you within the past few days that has caused you either annoyance or irritation. Perhaps it was an argument you had with a friend or disagreement in the workplace. As you think about it, get a sense of what you really felt and where in your body you feel it. You will often find that you have tightness in the stomach or chest, your jaw may clench and you may feel mental tension and/or a specific emotion. While continuing to think about this event, apply the acupressure techniques described above and be sure to breathe slowly and deeply. Once the pulses have appeared, or a minute or two has passed, then think again about the same event and notice how you feel about it now. Most often, you will find you just cannot contact those feelings again. The tightness in the stomach has disappeared and the mental tension has vanished.

Emotional defusion points

Below, we present the significance of the different types of emotional defusion points that may be used in ESD and what they are hypothesized to do. These ESD holding points are shown in Figure 36.1.

Frontal Holding

Holding gall bladder 14 right/left, an emotional neurovascular point of Bennett, can release stress resulting from a present-time issue or event. Holding these points brings blood flow to the frontal cortex for now-time processing of the past stressful issue from the perspective of the higher self, via access to the transcendent emotions, such as unconditional love and forgiveness. This is often accompanied by vivid visual processing of the events. The previously emotionally charged issue is now seen as life's lesson to be learned. From analyzing and understanding what happened, you can now learn from these experiences and deal with them more effectively and with far less stress in the future.

Frontal–Occipital Holding

Holding gall bladder 14 right/left and gall bladder 20 right/left, emotional neurovascular points of Bennett and neurovascular points for kidney (fear), can release stress in the present, which is usually related to a past issue or event. Holding these points brings blood flow to the frontal and occipital lobes to maintain the stressful situation in memory, while now-time processing of the issue occurs in the frontal lobes from the viewpoint of the higher self. This is often accompanied by vivid visual processing of past events and how you felt at that time.

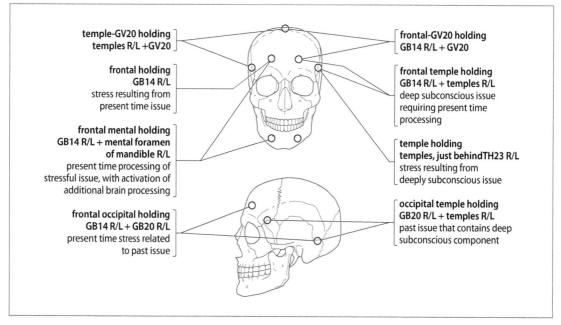

Figure 36.1 The different types of emotional holding points. Each of the primary sets of acupoints that when held with light finger or thumb pressure bring blood flow back into the frontal, temporal or occipital cortical areas are shown. Each combination of acupoints appears to activate different patterns of cortical and subcortical brain areas, and through this simultaneous activation emotional issues are reprocessed, and the stress, the 'emotional charge', held is released or defused in a process termed *Emotional Stress Defusion*. GB = gall bladder; GV = governing vessel; L = left; R = right; TH = triple heater.

Temple Holding

Holding just above triple heater 23 right/left, another emotional neurovascular point of Bennett, appears to give similar results and be related to deeply subconscious issues or events. Holding these points appears to bring blood flow into the deep subconscious brainstem areas and limbic centers for processing of past emotional experience, with a strong subconscious component related to the survival system. This results in resetting or inhibiting the underlying autonomic physiological reactions creating fear; anger and rage; panic, grief and depression; or frustration and affective rage. Considerable overt processing may occur, such as rapid eye movement, deep breathing and tension in viscera. However, there is almost always no conscious content, just very strong body feelings, like waves of anxiety flowing down the body or tightness in the stomach, which subside when the defusion is complete.

Frontal–Temple Holding

Holding gall bladder 14 right/left simultaneously with points just above triple heater 23 right/left is beneficial when deep subconscious brainstem and limbic issues or events require processing in the frontal lobes for conscious awareness to be brought to the issue or event. This not only defuses past deep subconscious issues but brings a higher perspective and greater consciousness into the defusion process.

Occipital–Temple Holding

Holding gall bladder 20 right/left (occiput) and triple heater 23 right/left (temple) is beneficial when past issues or events contain a significant deep subconscious component that requires blood flow into both memory areas of the cortex and deep brainstem and limbic areas simultaneously for effective defusion.

Frontal–Mental Holding

Holding gall bladder 14 right/left simultaneously with the mental foramen of the mandible brings blood flow to the frontal lobes for now-time processing of the stressful issue or event. This type of ESD was developed by Carl Ferreri in his Neural Organization Technique program. This activates other brain processing to defuse the issue or event. Although the exact type of processing is not known, muscle monitoring will often show this to be the priority type of holding for effective defusion.

Frontal–Governing Vessel 20 Holding

Holding gall bladder 14 right/left simultaneously with Governing Vessel 20 (Spirit Gate), on top of the head between the ears, brings blood flow to the frontal lobes for now-time processing of the stressful issue or event. It also activates Governing Vessel 20, initiating access to your higher self or soul. This type of ESD shows the priority points to hold less often than other ESD points but can be very effective when it is needed. It indicates that a spiritual level is required to resolve this issue.

Temple–Governing Vessel 20 Holding

Holding triple heater 23 right/left simultaneously with Governing Vessel 20 (Spirit Gate), on top of the head between the ears, brings blood flow to the brainstem–frontal system for now-time processing of the stressful survival–brainstem–limbic issue or event. It also activates Governing Vessel 20, initiating access to your higher self or soul. This type of ESD shows the priority points to hold less often than other ESD points but can be very effective when it is needed. It indicates that a spiritual level is required to resolve this issue.

Reference

1. LeDoux, J 1996, *The Emotional Brain*, Touchstone, New York.

Chapter 37

ESSENCES

Development of flower essences

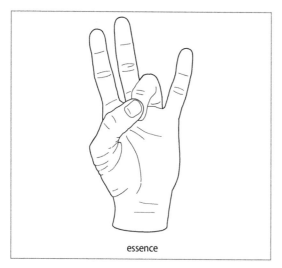

Figure 37.1 **Essence mode.** The essence hand mode involves placing the thumb pad on the nail of the ring finger, using light touch. If this mode is held, then an indicator change indicates that an essence correction should be applied.

Bach Flower Remedies

Dr Edward Bach developed the Bach Flower Remedies, powerful healers from the plant kingdom. Flower essences can be considered homeopathics for the emotions and spirit. Unlike true homeopathics, however, with flower essences there is no *proving*, that is, taking large doses of an essence will not produce a negative emotional state. Dr Bach did, however, do a form of psychic proving by inducing within himself a particular negative emotional state and then locating the flower in whose presence the state would dissipate.

In the preparation of flower essences, the water is potentized with vibrational qualities from the sun and the flower or devic kingdom. These vibrational patterns affect the higher vibrational energies of the astral, mental and spiritual bodies of the human aura. Introducing the flower essence vibrations into the body creates a resonance that reinforces the vibrational pattern of particular positive emotions, thoughts and spiritual attitudes. But how did Dr Bach discover these vibrational remedies?

Dr Bach was both a medical doctor and a homeopath. While working in a hospital, he would make a note of the mental and emotional states of his patients on his morning and afternoon rounds. He began to notice that sometimes the moods or emotional or mental states of his patients would show a marked improvement between the morning and afternoon rounds. These changes in state were very often accompanied by improvement in their clinical condition.

He noted that a common pattern accompanying these changes in mental or emotional state appeared to correlate with flowers being brought into the room during the day. He then hypothesized that the presence of the flowers was in some way associated with the change in the patient's mood and clinical condition. Thus, he began to systematically and experimentally investigate this potential relationship.

Dr Bach was also an empath and had the unique ability to put himself into specific emotional states, for example anger, grief or anxiety. He would enter one of these empathic states and then wander around the Oxfordshire countryside until he felt a sudden shift in his emotional state. He would then collect all the flowers present in that locality and take them back to his laboratory. At his laboratory, he would develop the emotional empathic state once more and have his assistant bring each flower collected one at a time into the laboratory and sit them in front of him. When he suddenly felt a shift toward normalizing or eliminating that emotional state, and this was observed on several occasions, he then attributed this change in state to the presence of that specific flower. Dr Bach, like other sensitives, was able to 'bring through' or 'realize' the emotional and spiritual qualities to which each flower essence resonated for each of the essences he developed.

Dr Bach developed a technique to prepare a type of homeopathic, energetic preparation of each flower he had associated with a specific emotional state or mood. He discovered that by placing the freshly cut flowers into a crystal bowl with natural springwater and placing the bowl in direct sunlight for several hours, the frequency resonance of the flower appeared to be transferred to this water. He would then preserve this frequency resonance of the flower by taking some of this 'stock' water and putting it into a 60% brandy solution. This greatly increased the polarity of the solution and stabilized the structure of the water holding the resonance frequency of the flower.

To test his flower remedies, Dr Bach would once again establish a specific emotional state and check that the water with the flower resonance would result in the same change of emotional state as being presented with the actual flowers. He found that these flower remedies did indeed work the same as the actual flowers. What Dr Bach's investigations had found is that when a person is experiencing or feeling a specific negative emotional state, the flower essence that resonates with the opposing positive emotional state will entrain these positive vibrations into the aura, eliminating the negative emotions.

Flower essences therefore work at the highest vibrational levels of emotions (astral body), thoughts (mental body) and attitude (spiritual body). As stated in Richard Gerber's book *Vibrational Medicine*, 'Healing from the highest vibrational state is the most powerful type of healing,' as the higher vibrational energies are capable of changing the vibrational pattern of energies at any lower state.[1] This is in accordance with the laws of physics, in which more coherent vibrational patterns will always entrain and hence bring greater coherence to less coherent vibrational patterns. The vibrational pattern of flower essences represents highly coherent states and can therefore entrain and eliminate the less coherent patterns of negative emotional, mental or attitudinal states.

Other types of essences

For several decades, Bach Flower Remedies were the only widely used flower essences. Recent decades have witnessed an exponential increase in the number of different flower essences available: North American Flower Essences, Australian Bush Flower Essences, Desert Alchemy Flower Essences and Saskia's Flower Essences, to name but a few, with newer sets of flower essences being added every year.

Once Dr Bach established a method to make flower essences, many other gifted and intuitive people began to develop not only other types of flower essences but also a number of different types of essences, from gem and crystal essences to even sound essences. Any of these essences can be used in vibrational healing, and muscle biofeedback provides a useful tool to determine the type of essence and the means by which is can be best administered to the client.

Applying flower essences in treatment

With all the different essences available today, how do you locate or identify the appropriate essence for the specific issue the person is experiencing? Historically, the practitioner would take a history of the client's complaints and then on the basis of the symptoms presented, experience and intuitive feeling, would match this clinical and intuitive picture to the appropriate essence. Often the matching procedure may involve various methods of 'tuning in' to the person's state via intuition alone or dowsing with a pendulum to confirm the match of the essence to the condition.

In recent years, kinesiology has been adapted to identify the appropriate essence for therapeutic use via a frequency match of the vibrational pattern of the client's condition to the vibrational pattern of the essence, indicated by a change in muscle response. Muscle biofeedback can be used in two ways: 1, to confirm the choice of an intuitively sensitive practitioner; and 2, to access the client's 'biocomputer' to indicate via muscle monitoring the appropriate essence to match the client's specific issue.

Locating essences

Whether muscle monitoring is to be used in either the first way, to confirm intuitive knowledge, or in the second way, to select the relevant essence to match the issue in pause lock, it is a very powerful adjunct to any balancing procedure. When you arrive at a point in the balance where you either need more information to continue or you need to define the exact nature of the problem to be balanced, accessing essences can add another dimension to your balancing techniques.

For instance, you have now aged recessed to the causal age and are going to balance the circuit, but first it is useful to establish what emotions or attitudes are associated with this issue in the person's subconscious. So at this point it is useful to go through the hand modes, checking both emotion and essence modes for an indicator change that will indicate which type of emotion or which attitude is involved with the issue in circuit. Essences usually represent the attitude behind our thinking and emotions, while emotions represent an expression of our feeling about the issue.

The attitude is our more broadly held beliefs about our perception of the reality of the issue based on our sensory input from the world. For example, you look into your cup and receive visual sensory input reporting that the cup is half filled with fluid. If you have an attitude of lack of abundance, you may then express an emotion on seeing the half cup of liquid: 'Oh, my God, it's almost gone; there's never enough for me!' This may then generate a whole series of feelings resulting in you expressing the emotion of sadness or fear. On the other hand, if you have an attitude of abundance, you will look at the same amount left to drink and express an entirely different set of feelings and emotions: 'Great, there is still half a cup left to drink; I'm going to enjoy every last drop!' This may very well result in an entirely different set of emotions of joy, gratitude and happiness.

Essence affirmations and the essence frequencies reflect the underlying attitudes that then generate our many and varied emotions. So when we arrive at the point of balancing and there is an indicator change when essence mode is held, you then need to locate which essence frequency matches the issue. One of the most direct ways to do so is to simply monitor an indicator muscle and scan each type of essence to locate the type of essence involved.

Once you have located the relevant type of essence, then by scanning each essence in this series, either from the list of essences in the book or by touching the cap of each bottle of essence, an indicator change indicates which essence matches the frequency of the attitude associated with the issue in circuit. You may then place this essence on the navel to enter this energetic pattern in circuit and then read, or have the client read, the attitude or emotion statement associated with this essence.

It is usually best to test whether the monitor should read the issue to the client, they should read it out loud or they should read it to themselves. Each way activates different neurological circuitry in their brains, retrieving information from different components of the associated survival and memory systems. If you read it only to yourself, only visual pathways and processing centers are activated, while hearing someone else read it to you activates only auditory pathways and processing centers. Reading it out loud obviously activates both auditory and visual pathways and centers. However, hearing someone else's voice may be a stronger trigger eliciting more emotions than hearing your own voice, or vice versa.

Then while the person reads, hears and/or says the essence information, the practitioner holds continuous recording mode to record all reactions both conscious and subconscious, and then enters all this into pause lock. While again holding continuous recording mode, the monitor may ask the person how they think or feel the essence information relates to their life or issues in their life.

Determining use of flower essences

Once a specific flower essence to be employed in a balance has been found, then the monitor needs to know three things: 1, where to apply the essence; 2, how many drops of essence to use in the balance; and 3, whether a dosage bottle of the essence is required for ongoing treatment, the number of drops per dose and the length of time to continue the essence therapy.

While the most common place to apply the essence is orally under the tongue, there are a number of other possibilities. The essence may be applied to an acupoint (or acupoints) or to an area of the skin, for example the back of the hands. The essence may need to be applied in the cone of a chakra or more often the *kshetram*, the entry point of the chakra into the physical body, which is almost always an acupoint. On occasion, it may even need to be placed in a spray bottle and applied to the aura. Once the location at which to apply the essence has been established, then the number of drops needed can be determined using muscle biofeedback and time mode.

Following completion of the treatment, the essence bottle can be placed on the navel and the client challenge for 'home reinforcement'. If there is no indicator change, the client needed the essence only as a component of or a correction for the treatment. However, an indicator change indicates that the client needs to take the essence for a period of time. To do so, you need to determine the number of drops from the essence stock to add to a dosage bottle. The dosage bottle is then filled with 30% alcohol solution, for example brandy, and succussed a number of times to transfer the energetic pattern of the stock essence into the dosage solution. Next, the dosage bottle is placed on the navel, and using time mode and pineal tap you determine: 1, the number of drops per dose needed; 2 the number of times per day the dose should be taken; and 3, the number of days or weeks this dosage should be taken to complete the therapy.

One of Krebs's most interesting experiences with flower essences was with a young client for whom flower essence had been indicated for the correction for a rather long, multicomponent set-up. Muscle biofeedback had indicated that three drops of the Desert Alchemy Flower Essence Creosote Bush was to be dropped from about 90 centimeters above her body through the heart chakra. The negative emotional state associated with creosote bush is intense inner desolation, feeling forever alone and cut off, and sadness. Indeed, this young girl was extremely introverted,

sad (for no apparent reason) and isolated, and she had no friends, something that had bothered her mother for several years.

As the first drop dropped through the auric layers of her heart chakra, the girl began to cry, with tears streaming down her face, and Krebs had never felt such deep sadness and desolation within himself! After the session, the mother reported she had also felt the same deep sadness herself. As the second drop passed through the heart chakra, the girl's whole countenance changed and her tears stopped. As the third drop passed through the chakra, her whole being brightened and she lost her normally morose appearance.

The next week, her mother called to tell Krebs that her daughter was now a totally different person. She had made three new friends in school and was openly expressing her feelings and communicating with everyone she met. Her mother exclaimed, 'I thank and bless you for what you did for my daughter.' Interestingly, the positive emotional statements associated with creosote bush are accepting companionship with all life, connecting to my inner source and expressing my feelings.

In counterpoint to the psychoemotional effects of the flower essences, they can also have perceptible effects at the physical and physiological level. One day, when Krebs was first becoming involved with energy healing, he was using a pair of locking pliers and they closed, catching a small piece of his palm. Having worked with tools for most of his life, this was not an uncommon occurrence! As usual, almost immediately a blood blister appeared on his palm—to the sound of expletives. His girlfriend of the time said, 'I'll just go get you some Rescue Remedy.' This elicited nothing but an eyeroll from him. When she returned, she gave Krebs a squirt of Rescue Remedy in the mouth and put a few drops of it on the blood blister and said, 'Rub this in.' To his total amazement, Krebs watched the blood blister disappear in about one minute, something he had never seen before. This use of Rescue Remedy applied to the actual tissue in physical distress appears to have real physiological results.

Reference

1.   Gerber, R 1988, *Vibrational Medicine*, Bear, Santa Fe, p. 154.

Chapter 38

ACUPRESSURE

What is acupressure?

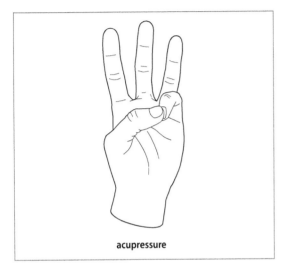

Figure 38.1 Acupressure mode. The acupressure hand mode involves placing the thumb pad on the nail of the little finger. If this mode is held, then an indicator change indicates that an acupressure correction should be applied.

Acupressure is the application of pressure to acupoints, and it actually preceded the use of acupuncture by several thousand years. The practice of acupressure pre-dates written Chinese history, as stone and bone implements used to apply pressure to acupoints have been found in archaeological sites throughout China dating from several thousand years BC. While acupressure is still practiced today in China and Japan, it has been largely replaced by the use of needles, and hence acupuncture as a healing modality.

Acupuncture or acupressure therapy consists of either stimulating or dispersing the ch'i by activation of specific acupoints on the surface of the body. The Chinese propose that ch'i energy is a dynamic force that circulates throughout the body in constant flux but that follows specific pathways and specific rules, and directly affects various specific physiological functions.[1] These pathways are known as *channels* or *vessels* by the Chinese but in the West are usually called *meridians*.

Acupressure can indeed be extremely effective, as there are many acupressure techniques that can be applied in specific circumstances to great effect. A commonly known example is applying pressure to large intestine 4, located between the thumb and index finger, to relieve a headache. While very often fingers or thumbs are used to apply the pressure to the acupoint, there are also more specific methods using blunt probes. One of the most effective is the use of an implement the Chinese call a *tei shin* in Mandarin or a *tai shin* in pinyin. Both finger acupressure and stimulation with the tei shin are standard techniques to stimulate acupoints, with a long anecdotal history of effectiveness.[2]

The tei shin is a blunt probe that retracts into the handle against spring pressure. The tip of the probe is placed on an acupoint and the handle is thrust down toward the skin repeatedly, causing the pressure on the tip of the probe to increase and decrease, resulting in a dent in the skin. As long as this dent persists, there is strong stimulation of this acupoint, so long-term activation of the acupoint can be achieved from relatively short-term tei shin stimulation. In recognition of the effectiveness of tei shin treatments, the Chinese often call this technique 'needleless acupuncture'.

There are two general types of acupressure therapy: 1, the application of pressure to specific acupoints for the treatment of specific conditions; and 2, the application of acupressure to the command points in the Law of Five Elements of acupuncture. Both acupressure and acupuncture have specific advantages in specific applications, even though they may both be used to balance the ch'i flow in the Law of Five Elements.

Through millennia of observation, the Chinese found that stimulation of specific acupoints by either acupressure or needle acupuncture could be used for specific physiological, physical, and even psychoemotional imbalances. Therefore textbooks of Chinese medicine will list an acupoint with its associated clinical conditions. For example, the acupoints bladder 64, 65 and 66 on the side of the foot and little toe are said to be involved in various disorders of vision. Interestingly, stimulation of these acupoints also activates parts of the cortex that are known to be involved in various aspects of visual processing.

Many of these points have association with more than one clinical condition from a western perspective but are often used in conjunction with other acupoints to treat a single western clinical condition. These conditions can range from perturbed physiology (e.g. an upset stomach), to energetic imbalances (e.g. over-energy in tissues, which we in the West term *pain*), to psychoemotional disturbances (e.g. grief or anger).

Using acupressure and acupuncture, the Chinese successfully treat many different organ and gland dysfunctions as well as imbalances within the immune system, the sensory systems, and even the brain.

Acupressure effects on brain function

In animal studies, Zhongfang and colleagues showed that the stimulation of specific acupoints using electroacupuncture could activate or inhibit the electrical activity of specific neurons within the amygdaloid nucleus, the subconscious emotional control center of the brain, resulting in increasing and decreasing rates of neuronal discharge.[3] They also found that electroacupuncture stimulation of different acupoints caused either consistent but different responses in the discharge rate of a single group of neurons in the amygdala or no effect on these neurons. Thus stimulation of specific individual points caused highly specific patterns of discharge in this deep brain structure. Zhongfang and coworkers also found that stimulation of sham points produced no detectable change in neuronal firing rates in the amygdala.

Traditional acupuncture techniques are stated to be helpful for strengthening cerebral function and improving intelligence.[4] In human subjects, Abad-Alegria and colleagues demonstrated that acupuncture stimulation of the acupoint heart 7 produces long-lasting increases in the P300 wave, a late evoked electroencephalographic potential that has been associated with cognitive activities.[5] Stimulation of another acupoint, large intestine 4, did not change the P300 wave, suggesting that this cortical response to acupoint stimulation is highly specific.

A recent study showed that a common acupuncture technique eases blood pressure by stimulating specific receptors in the central nervous system,[6] while Bucinskaite and coworkers found that electroacupuncture increases levels of various neuropeptides in the rat brain, with significant increases in the hippocampus, a limbic structure directly involved in short-term memory.[7] Also, a decrease in neuropeptide Y, along with a decrease in the depression subscale score of the Comprehensive Psychopathological Rating Scale was noted in five out of six patients suffering from major depression who were treated with electroacupuncture in a pilot study by Pohl and Nordin.[8]

Using functional magnetic resonance imaging (fMRI) scanning, researchers have shown that specific acupoint stimulation causes specific patterns of neuronal activity in the cerebral cortex that correlate with traditional Chinese medicine's treatment for visual disorders.[9] Even though the acupoints were on the side of the little toe and the side of the foot, stimulation of these points activated specific and unique areas of the occipital cortex. Each of the acupoints stimulated is associated in traditional Chinese medicine with a specific type of eye or vision disorder, providing a strong correlation between acupoint stimulation and relevant cortical activation.

Another fMRI study showed that needle acupuncture stimulation of large intestine 4 causes activation of the limbic system and subcortical structures associated with reward and punishment as well as emotional and behavioural regulation.[10]

Again, specific acupoints activated highly specific limbic and subcortical areas. In these studies, as in the study of Zhongfang and colleagues,[11] stimulation of non-acupuncture sham points had no effect on cortical or subcortical activation.

Recent fMRI studies substantiate the specificity of brain area activation by specific acupoint stimulation and the lack of activation of the brain by sham acupoint stimulation in human subjects. Pariente and coworkers demonstrated that acupuncture treatments produce real effects beyond placebo by using a retractable needle so that the subjects did not know when they were receiving real or placebo treatments.[12] Zhang and colleagues showed that stimulation of acupoints on the same spinal segment activates unique and highly specific areas of the brain, and that each point stimulates different brain areas.[13]

Several other studies have substantiated this specificity of acupoint stimulation with brain areas.[14] Yan and colleagues demonstrated that acupuncture of liver 3 and large intestine 4 each activate unique brain areas relative to sham acupoints.[15] They concluded that these observations reveal that acupuncture of specific acupoints induces unique patterns of brain activity specific to each acupoint, and that these patterns may relate to the therapeutic effects of acupuncture. For excellent reviews of the effects and specificity of acupoint stimulation on brain areas, you are referred to the review by Dhond and coworkers.[16] However, other recent studies have produced less specificity between brain area activation and acupoint stimulation using electroacupuncture, so the exact nature and degree of acupoint–brain area specificity remains unclear at this time.[17]

Acupoint stimulation in the acupuncture studies discussed above was either traditional needle acupuncture, in which a needle is inserted into an acupoint and then manually activated, or electroacupuncture, in which a small electrical current is applied to a needle inserted into an acupoint. However, using fMRI to monitor the effects on cortical activation Jones and coworkers have recently shown that the effects elicited by conventional needle acupoint stimulation are indistinguishable from those produced by highly

focused pulses of ultrasound directed to acupoints over a wide range of ultrasound parameters.[18] Therefore what appears to be important is that the acupoint is sufficiently stimulated, not the specific type of acupoint stimulation.

Acupressure has a number of advantages over traditional acupuncture, as it is non-invasive, not painful, and well tolerated by children. Also, the problem of sterile needles and bleeding are eliminated. Most importantly, acupressure corrections can provide multipoint sequential stimulation, something very difficult to do with needles and not part of traditional acupuncture theory. However, this multipoint acupressure stimulation is capable of powerfully stimulating specific brain structures and resynchronizing brain function and normalizing neurotransmitter levels, as evidenced by the profound changes in people's performance on standardized psychological tests and in the classroom following treatment.

While the mechanism of how these multiacupoint mode combinations activate or access specific subcortical and cortical structures and functions remains unknown, the recent scientific evidence of highly specific activation of cortical and subcortical structures by specific acupoint stimulation discussed above provide at least a plausible mechanism for acupressure therapy.

Unique contributions of Energetic Kinesiology to acupressure theory
Identifying acupoint imbalances

The Chinese developed their acupressure and acupuncture theory based on millennia of observations in clinical practice. Through millennia of observation, the Chinese associated many specific acupoints with a specific clinical condition or conditions, as a single acupoint may be involved in several different physiological conditions, either singly or in various combinations. However, there are many other issues or complaints for which there may be no traditional acupoint association. The Chinese would use their traditional methods of assessing these unique imbalances, such as pulse diagnosis, to establish which meridian energy or energies had become imbalanced.

In contrast, using muscle monitoring, if a person has a generalized complaint of pain in a particular body region, or even a specific emotional problem, muscle monitoring can provide direct access as to the nature of the problem and exactly which acupoints are associated with the problem. Once the issue is in pause lock, all you need to do is hold acupressure mode and an indicator change indicates that a specific meridian has an energetic imbalance that is a part of or underlies this issue. By then circuit locating the alarm points, an indicator change will identify the meridian that has an acupoint that is directly involved with or related to this imbalance. To locate the specific acupoint on that meridian, you need only circuit locate each acupoint in turn. The acupoint (or acupoints) giving a priority indicator change is (or are) the point (or points) to be treated for this particular condition in this specific context.

However, kinesiology cannot only locate the specific acupoint to be treated; it then identifies the specific therapy needed to treat this condition. Once the acupoint has been entered into circuit, the practitioner need only use various hand modes and specific indicator points to identify the specific type of acupressure therapy to apply for resolution of this imbalance. Furthermore, once the therapy has been applied the muscle biofeedback can assess whether the treatment was indeed effective or if more of the same therapy or another therapy should be applied to completely resolve the issue. So instead of having to wait to see if the treatment was effective for the client, you can determine whether additional treatment is required for complete resolution of the presenting issue.

As discussed in chapter 6, one of the ways the Chinese knew of the acupoints and ch'i flows was by developing the ability to actually 'see' the acupoints. For instance, Krebs's Zen monk friend Rob, who could actually see the flow of ch'i, had noticed something he did not understand. Normally, when he needled an acupoint he could see the ch'i just shoot through the point. However, sometimes when he needled acupoints the ch'i would just trickle through the point, for reasons that he did not understand. He had also noticed that when there were reduced ch'i flows through the acupoint, these treatments were less effective. So clearly, blocked acupoints appeared to have a negative effect on treatment outcomes, but why?

This has to do with the dynamics of acupoint function. Normally, they are like mini chakras oscillating in alternating clockwise and counterclockwise directions, yang and yin from the Chinese perspective. This oscillation is part of the function of the acupoint, which is to regulate ch'i flow through the meridians, with each acupoint acting as a valve. Obviously, a valve needs to be able to open and close in order to regulate flow. When acupoints become blocked, they often can only open or close but they cannot operate in both directions. These are called frozen yin or yang acupoints, depending on which spin is blocked. In highly compensated cases, the acupoints have very limited ability to open or close and are largely stuck in a fixed position and are hence frozen yin and yang. Their inability to regulate ch'i flow often then leads to chronic physiological conditions.

Because these frozen acupoints cannot be seen by even highly sensitive individuals, and only their effects can be seen, how are we to know of their existence? By the use of muscle biofeedback, it is relatively easy to detect these blocked acupoints and then apply acupressure treatment to release the blocks and return the acupoint to its normal function. This in turn can lead to resolution of the associated chronic physiological condition. This is something that cannot be done in traditional Chinese acupuncture and may account for times when acupuncture treatments are less effective.

Identifying frozen acupoint imbalances

As stated above, the concept of frozen acupoints is not part of traditional Chinese acupuncture but was developed by Utt and Krebs within Applied Physiology. Utt used muscle biofeedback to locate acupoints that could not be sedated or tonified using the north or south poles of a magnet, respectively. For example, the spin of the magnet field of a magnet is clockwise for the south pole, and counterclockwise for the north pole, as viewed from behind the magnet.

Indeed, the spin of the magnetic field associated with the north and south poles can be easily visualized. Just turn on an old, not-flat screen, black-and-white television. Then take a strong magnet (e.g. 3000 gauss) with the north pole facing the television screen, and move this toward the screen. As the north pole approaches the screen, the image will be rotated counterclockwise. Reverse the magnet with the south pole approaching the screen, and the image will now be rotated clockwise. WARNING! Do not do this on a flat screen or colour television or you will be sorry, as the results will not be pleasing and will be expensive to rectify!

Utt would bring a magnet directly downward over an acupoint while monitoring an indicator muscle, something the Chinese did not have access to, and observe what happened. Because the acupoints are continually oscillating first clockwise and then counterclockwise, when in balance the sudden powerful increase in the clockwise or counterclockwise magnetic flow should cause an indicator change, as the normal oscillating flow is disrupted by the magnetic flux. Therefore an acupoint in balance will show an indicator change when either the north pole or the south pole of the magnet is brought toward the acupoint, because of the extreme clockwise or counterclockwise magnetic fields of the magnet.

However, Utt discovered that sometimes there would be no indicator change when one or even both poles of the magnet were brought down onto the acupoint. From his perspective, it was as if the acupoint was frozen, unable to respond to even strong magnetic fields that always caused an indicator change with balanced acupoints. Interestingly, when the stressors underlying the frozen acupoint were located and resolved using kinesiology acupressure techniques, the acupoint would now return to balance and once more give an indicator change whenever the north or south pole of the magnet was brought down onto the acupoint. Of even greater significance, physiological or even psychoemotional imbalances associated with the acupoint were also normalized.

But what was actually happening when an acupoint was frozen? This was elucidated by Krebs's monk friend when he watched Krebs demonstrate acupressure corrections while teaching. In his own clinical practice, the monk would see the ch'i shoot through the acupoint on needling the acupoint, especially when his needle grabbed the ch'i, with the skin literally twisting around the needle. And then during the session he observed unobstructed ch'i flow, which accelerated every time he stimulated the acupoints by spinning the needle in the acupoint. However, at other times, even though the monk needled the acupoint in the same way, he could see only just a trickle of ch'i moving through the point, which would sometimes actually stop between needle activations. He also noted that the observation of ch'i trickle was associated with chronic conditions and less successful outcomes from his acupuncture treatments.

It was not until Rob reported his observations to Krebs that a more comprehensive understanding of frozen acupoints was developed. Remember that the acupuncture system is predominately expressed in the etheric energies of the body, the interface between our physical and physiological being and the higher astral and mental levels. This is why it responds not only to physical level inputs, such as electricity and magnetism, as well as purely etheric flows of ch'i in the acupuncture system, but also to fluctuations in our emotions and thoughts at the astral and mental levels.

Krebs and many other Applied Physiologists repeatedly observed that when acupoints were frozen, consistently the causal issues were predominately emotional and/or mental issues, not etheric imbalances. And when these emotional and mental issues were resolved, the acupoints returned to a balanced state, and treatments using these formerly frozen acupoints were now successful and produced long-lasting effects.

Krebs hypothesized that while his monk friend could clearly see that the acupoint demonstrated a state of etheric imbalance, the restricted ch'i flow, his auric vision did not extend into the astral and mental frequencies of the aura, and therefore he could not see the underlying issues that actually resulted in this restriction. However, muscle biofeedback can detect imbalances at all levels of the aura, including the emotional and mental levels, and then direct the practitioner to an effective acupressure treatment or another energetic technique to resolve the emotional or mental issue(s) underlying the frozen acupoint. Once these underlying issues have been resolved, the acupoint returns to a balanced state, and it can now be effectively stimulated to rebalance ch'i flows via the Law of Five Elements to produce long-lasting corrections.

Identifying priority pathways in the Law of Five Elements

Another unique contribution of Energetic Kinesiology to the use of acupressure theory is how to apply the rules of acupressure. Indeed, it is called the Law of Five Elements because the rules and principles by which is works is constant and invariable, just like the law of gravity. The primary rule is that energy, like electricity, always seeks the shortest route, but what do you do when you have two equally short routes, both of which follow the Law?

For example, you may remember that there are two types of pathways in the Law of Five Elements: the Sheng cycle and the Ko cycle. If there is an under-energy in liver and an over-energy in spleen, there are two equal length pathways by which the over-energy may move to the under-energy: 1, via the Sheng cycle to lung and then via the Ko cycle to liver; or 2, via the Ko cycle to kidney and then the Sheng cycle to liver. Both these pathways are exactly the same length, so which one should you use? The Chinese follow a rule that says use the pathway that is effective *most* of the time from millennia of observation. However, in those cases when that is not the most effective pathway the treatment is much less effective. Using muscle monitoring, it is easy to determine which pathway is priority and will yield the best results.

Seven Element Acupressure Therapy

Another unique contribution of Richard Utt to both kinesiology and acupressure was the development of the Seven Element Acupressure Theory. Traditional Chinese medicine recognized five elements: Fire, Earth, Metal, Water and Wood.

Each element was represented by two meridians, or channels, that distribute the ch'i energy throughout the body, except for Fire, which was represented by four meridians. The heart and small intestine meridians formed the element Sovereign Fire, while pericardium and triple heater formed the element Ministerial Fire.

The *Nei Ching*, the *Liu Xing*, or the six phases recognized that the Fire element of traditional acupuncture, although represented as a single element with four meridians, actually represents two quite separate and different elements: 1, Sovereign Fire, comprising heart and small intestine meridians; and 2, Ministerial Fire, comprising pericardium and triple heater meridians. In fact, in the Liu Xing school of acupuncture, six elements are indeed used even today.

In the esoteric components of the Nei Ching, there is also reference to a seventh element, Governing Fire, composed of two of the eight extra meridians, Governing and Central Vessels. These are the only two of the eight extra meridians that have their own unique acupoints. They form a core energy circuit called the Celestial or Heavenly Circuit to indicate their importance, as they represent the primary polarity of the maximum yang of Governing and the maximum yin of Central interacting, with each creating the other. This is the great *Tai Ch'i*. Adding Governing Fire to the six-element model gives seven elements represented by 14 meridians.

In Seven Element Acupressure Theory, the Governing Fire element represents universal unmanifest energy that enters the meridian system via Governing Vessel 20 (Heavenly Gate) as spirit, leaving it at death. This energy enters the original cavity of spirit (the pituitary gland) and crystallizes as a seed of *Yuan Ch'i*; being the source of Governing Fire prenatal ch'i. This element regulates and nourishes the Ministerial Fire element, which then controls the Five Element movements of energy and spiritizes matter. According to these ancient sources, Governing Fire can be thought of as being the seat of the spiritual self.[19]

In the traditional esoteric Chinese theory, Governing Fire contacts what they call 'clear light mind' or the void, the realm of pure and absolute values. In Bohm's theory this would be the implicate order, the realm of all frequencies and all possibilities. Energy flowing from the void or clear light mind would be the holomovement of the implicate order into the explicate order of the individual. Clear light mind from the yogic perspective is called the *logos* and in Christian tradition it is called the *divine*. In the yogic tradition, Governing Fire would represent the monadic and atmic levels of form being manifest from energy, while in the Christian tradition it would represent the soul.

Thus in a sense the Governing Fire represents your connection to all there is or God, hence the soul of Christian belief. When this connection is strong and stable, you have a strong sense of self because God is always OK and if you are part of God you are also OK. When this connection is more tenuous, the little self or ego feels insecure and seeks approval from others to feel OK. This is indeed another unique contribution to acupressure therapy, as you can now directly balance Governing Fire and thus the relationship between the higher self and the ego self. See Figure 38.2.

Applying the Seven Element Acupressure Theory

Seven Element Acupressure Therapy utilizes all the traditional points of Five Element Acupressure plus points on the Central and Governing Vessels that are not part of the traditional Five Elements. In the Five Elements, the pattern of the five elements is represented again by five element points on each meridian: in the microcosm is the macrocosm (see Figure 6.6). For each meridian, there is a Fire point, an Earth point, a Metal point, a Water point and a Wood point. These are called the command points, as they command the flow of energy between the meridians of the different elements.

Because Governing and Central Vessels are not included in the traditional five elements, they do not have traditional command points. However, there are Governing and Central points that indeed do connect to each of the meridians of the five elements, even though they are not part of the traditional five-element flow. These points do, however, influence the flow within the five

elements. Richard Utt added these points into the six elements already included in the Five Element chart, as well as separating Sovereign Fire and Ministerial Fire as individual elements. These two changes were made in creating his Seven Element Acupressure therapy.

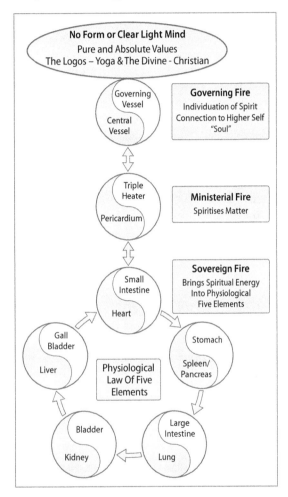

Figure 38.2 The Chinese esoteric Seven Elements. In the esoteric Chinese tradition, there are seven elements that represent their whole cosmology and by which matter is spiritized. What is now called the *vacuum* or *zero-point field* in physics or the *implicate order* by Bohm, the realm of all possible frequencies, was called *No Form* or *Clear Light Mind* by the Chinese. Man's contact with this realm was through the integrated flow of Central and Governing meridians they called Governing Fire, and this essence of spirit was stepped down via the non-material Ministerial Fire meridians of triple heater and pericardium to spiritize matter.

This therefore provides another type of acupressure correction that can be used in treatment. Once an imbalance has been entered into circuit and acupressure shows as a correction, you need only hold hologram mode as well as five-element mode with deep touch (this is the seven-element mode) to determine if seven-element acupressure is required. A priority indicator change indicates that the application of seven-element acupressure will be the most effective technique to treat this specific imbalance. This technique involves finding two meridian alarm points sequentially, the hologram coordinates, then going to the seven-element chart to see which acupoint needs to be treated. Further muscle biofeedback will then guide you to what type of acupoint imbalance is present and which treatment is most appropriate for the imbalance.

In kinesiology, acupressure therapy has been taken beyond overt physical stimulation of the acupoint using normal pressure to include acupoint activation via vibrational sources. These treatments can include the application of light, sound, flower essences, homeopathics, and essential oils or a combination of these. For example, the same holographic coordinates that identified which acupoint to treat are also associated with a specific flower essence, a specific sound and a specific colour. Therefore you may apply a flower essence to tuning forks that are then directed at the acupoint or apply a specific homeopathic to the acupoint and then shine a laser onto the point.

Jones and colleagues have shown that acupoint stimulation by highly focused pulses of ultrasound are indistinguishable from those elicited by conventional needle acupuncture.[2] Indeed, pulses of focused ultrasound are a type of acupressure. In a sense, light is just a far more subtle vibration than sound and application of light, especially pulsed lasers, is now a very subtle form of acupressure.

References

1. Porkert, M 1974, *The Theoretical Foundations of Chinese Medicine*, MIT Press, Cambridge, pp. 43–76.
   Kaptchuk, TJ 1983, *The Web That Has No Weaver: Understanding Chinese Medicine*, Ryder, London.
   Maciocia, G 1989, *The Foundations of Chinese Medicine*, Churchill Livingstone, Edinburgh, pp. 15–34.
   Xinnong, Cheng, chief ed. 1987, *Chinese Acupuncture and Moxibustion*, Foreign Language Press, Beijing, pp. 1–2.
2. Jones, JP, So, CS, Kidney, DD & Saito, T 2001, Evaluation of acupuncture using f-MRI and ultrasonic imaging, in *20th Annual Meeting of the Society for Scientific Exploration*, La Jolla.
   Helms, JM 1995, *Acupuncture Energetics: A Clinical Approach for Physicians*, Medical Acupuncture Publishers, Berkeley, pp. 26–27.
   Maciocia, G 1989, *The Foundations of Chinese Medicine*, Churchill Livingstone, London, pp. 15–34.
3. Zhongfang, L, Qingshu, C, Shuping, C & Zhenjing, H 1989, Effect of electro-acupuncture of 'Neiguan' on spontaneous discharges of single unit in amygdaloid nucleus in rabbits, *Journal of Traditional Chinese Medicine*, Vol. 9, No. 2, pp. 144–150.
4. Qian-Liang, L 1989, Research on strengthening cerebral function and improving intelligence, *International Journal of Oriental Medicine*, Vol. 14, pp. 227–232.
5. Abad-Alegria, F, Galve, JA & Martinez, T 1995, Changes of cerebral endogenous evoked potentials by acupuncture stimulation: a P300 study, *American Journal of Chinese Medicine*, Vol. 23, No. 2, pp.115–119.
6. Li, P, Tjen-A-Looi, S, Longhurst, J & Li, P 2001, Rostral ventrolateral medullary opioid receptor subtypes in the inhibitory effect of electroacupuncture on reflex autonomic response in cats, *Autonomic Neuroscience*, Vol. 89, pp. 38–47.
7. Bucinskaite, V, Lundeberg, T, Stenfors, C, Ekblom, A, Dahlin, L & Theodorsson, E 1994, Effects of electro-acupuncture and physical exercise on regional concentrations of neuropeptides in rat brain, *Brain Research*, Vol. 666, pp. 128–132.
8. Pohl, A & Nordin, C 2002, Clinical and biochemical observations during treatment of depression with electroacupuncture: a pilot study. *Human Psychopharmacology*, Vol. 17, No. 7, pp. 345–348.
9. Cho, ZH, Chung, SC, Jones, JP, Park, JB, Park, HJ, Lee, HJ, Wong, EK & Min, BI 1998, New findings of the correlation between acupoints and corresponding brain cortices using functional MRI. *Proceedings of the National Academy of Sciences of the United States of America*, Vol. 95, pp. 2670–2673.
   Li, G, Cheung, RT, Ma, QY & Yang, ES 2003, Visual cortical activations on fMRI upon stimulation of the vision-implicated acupoints, *NeuroReport*, Vol. 14, pp. 669–673.
10. Hui, KK, Liu, J, Makris, N, Gollub, RL, Chen, AJ, Moore, CI, Kennedy, DN, Rosen, BR & Kwong, KK 2000, Acupuncture modulates the limbic system and subcortical gray structures of the human brain: evidence from f-MRI studies in normal subjects, *Human Brain Mapping*, Vol. 9, pp. 13–25.
11. Zhongfang, L, Qingshu, C, Shuping, C & Zhenjing, H 1989, Effect of electro-acupuncture of 'Neiguan' on spontaneous discharges of single unit in amygdaloid nucleus in rabbits, *Journal of Traditional Chinese Medicine*, Vol. 9, No. 2, pp. 144–150.
12. Pariente, J, White, P, Frackowiak, RS & Lewith, G 2005, Expectancy and belief modulate the neuronal substrates of pain treated by acupuncture, *Neuroimage*, Vol. 25, pp. 1161–1167.
13. Zhang, WT, Jin, Z, Luo, F, Zhang, L, Zeng, YW & Han, JS 2004, Evidence from brain imaging with fMRI supporting functional

specificity of acupoints in humans, *Neuroscience Letters*, Vol. 354, pp. 50–53.

14. Cho, ZH, Chung, SC, Lee, HJ, Wong, EK & Min, BI 2006, Retraction: New findings of the correlation between acupoints and corresponding brain cortices using functional MRI, *Proceedings of the National Academy of Sciences of the United States of America*, Vol. 103, p. 10527.

    Hu, KM, Wang, CP, Xie, HJ & Henning, J 2006, Observation on activating effectiveness of acupuncture at acupoints and non-acupoints on different brain regions [in Chinese], *Zhongguo Zhen Jiu*, Vol. 26, pp. 205–207.

15. Yan, B, Li, K, Xu, J, Wang, W, Li, K, Liu, H, Shan, B & Tang, X 2005, Acupoint-specific fMRI patterns in human brain, *Neuroscience Letters*, Vol. 383, pp. 236–240.

16. Dhond, RP, Kettner, N & Napadow, V 2007, Neuroimaging acupuncture effects in the human brain, *Journal of Alternative and Complementary Medicine*, Vol. 6, pp. 603–616.

17. Kong, J, Kaptchuk, TJ, Webb, JM, Kong, JT, Sasaki,Y, Polich, GR, Vangel, MG, Kwong, K, Rosen, B & Gollub, RL 2009, Functional neuroanatomical investigation of vision-related acupuncture point specificity—a multi-session fMRI study, *Human Brain Mapping*, Vol. 30, pp. 38–46.

18. Jones, JP, So, CS, Kidney, DD & Saito, T 2001, Evaluation of acupuncture using f-MRI and ultrasonic imaging, in *20th Annual Meeting of the Society for Scientific Exploration*, La Jolla, California.

19. Anonymous 1979, *Chinese Medical Classics. The* Nei Ching (Su Wen *and* Ling Shu) *and* Nan Ching. The Study Materials of the Occidental Institute of Chinese Studies Alumni Association, Miami, pp. 188.

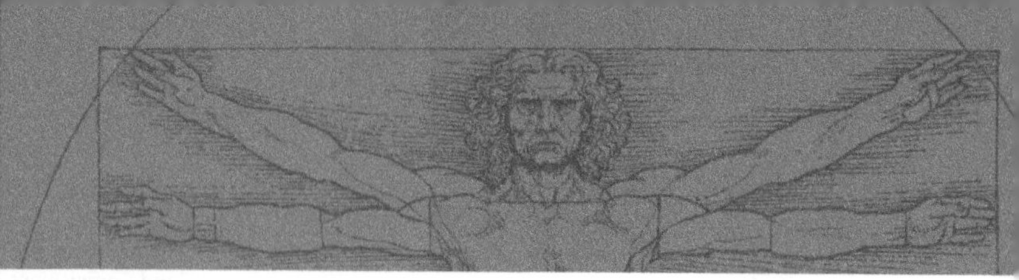

Chapter 39

FIGURE 8 ENERGIES

Development of the use of figure 8 energy flows in kinesiology

The use of figure 8 flows in kinesiology has several possible origins which are discussed in more detail in Robin Brown Frossard's recent paper.[1] Apparently, Dr Alan Beardall, one of the original Dirty Dozen Applied Kinesiology chiropractors, was inspired by a picture in a book in his private library of Tibetan art. This led him to develop the concept of the figure 8 flows in the early 1970s, and he associated these flows with a Tibetan origin. Another member of the Dirty Dozen, Dr Sheldon Deal, confirmed that he had indeed learned of the figure 8s from Dr Beardall, even though, according to practitioners in Beardall's office at the time, he may not have used them in his clinical practice.

There appears to be a second possible link through which the figure 8 energy flows may have entered kinesiology, perhaps independently of Dr Beardall. Dr George Goodheart cited a 1974 book by Dr William McGarey, *Acupuncture and Body Energies*,[2] in which Dr McGarey mentions the figure 8s, with references to both Japanese acupuncturists and Edgar Cayce. Dr McGarey reported that Edgar Cayce described a flow of energy, vibratory in nature, in and through the human body in the form of a figure of eight in many of his readings. Furthermore, Cayce stated that these flows were related at a deep level to the health of the body, and that they appeared to be a healing influence on the body. Goodheart was apparently influenced to investigate these figure 8 flows.[1] According to Dr Paul Sprieser, by 1978 Goodheart was using muscles to test for the presence of figure 8 flows of the trunk by 'sweeping the hand from the upper left costal margin down to the lower right superior iliac spine, as well as in the opposite direction'. However, Goodheart linked the figure 8s with the gait patterns rather than overall bodily functions.

Whatever the actual origin of the figure 8s entering the field of kinesiology, it appears that Dr John Thie had included the figure 8 energies in his 1979 manual of *Touch for Health*, and Dr Deal introduced the figure 8 flows into Applied Kinesiology in the mid 1970s. Deal also showed these figure 8 flows to Richard Utt, and he and Utt experimented with them. Utt then developed the figure 8s further in his Applied Physiology system. From their Applied Kinesiology and Touch for Health origins, the figure 8 energy system spread rapidly into a number of developing kinesiology systems.

There were apparently only six figure 8 flows initially recognized in kinesiology by Deal and Thie in 1975, one over each major body segment, front and back. Deal brought these figure 8 energies into Applied Kinesiology in 1975. Gordon Stokes, the instructor trainer for Touch for Health through the 1970s and cofounder of Three In One Kinesiology, then incorporated the figure 8 flows into the Three In One Kinesiology system in the early 1980s. Dr Bruce Dewe, founder of the Professional Kinesiology Practice system, then added a single figure 8 flow that covered the whole front and back of the body, which was incorporated in the Professional Kinesiology Practice Tibetan Energy Workshop.[4] In the early 1980s, Richard Utt further developed these flows, as his research showed that there are additional figure 8 flows over the side of each body segment, as well as one over the head and one under the feet.

Detecting figure 8 imbalances

The original way to detect figure 8 imbalance in kinesiology was to stroke the hand across each

Figure 8 energies   293

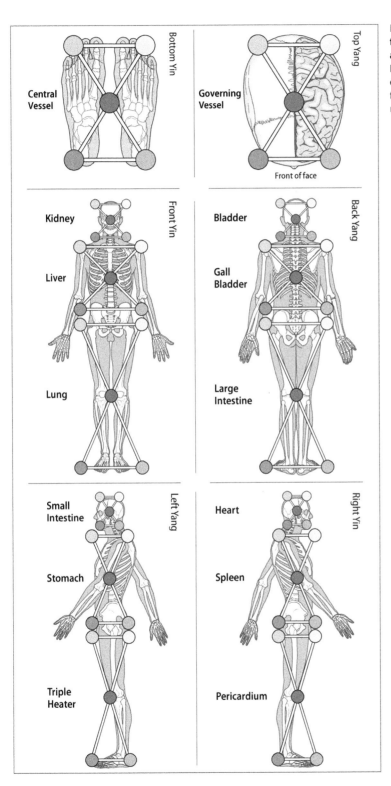

Central
Vessel

Bottom Yin

Governing
Vessel

Top Yang

Front of face

Kidney

Front Yin

Liver

Lung

Bladder

Back Yang

Gall
Bladder

Large
Intestine

Small
Intestine

Left Yang

Stomach

Triple
Heater

Heart

Right Yin

Spleen

Pericardium

Figure 39.1 The Seven Element figure 8 energy flows and their associated meridians. In the Applied Physiology Seven Element Hologram, each of the 14 major figure 8 energy flows is associated with a specific meridian flow.

segment of each figure 8 in turn while monitoring an indicator muscle. An indicator change following stroking across a specific segment indicated an imbalance within that particular segment. Because constriction of flow is normally only in one direction, when the sweep of the hand 'pushes' more energy into the constriction, it rapidly increases the resistance to flow, causing the indicator change.

Gordon Stokes, cofounder of Three In One Concepts, developed a technique that he called the *fuzzy glove* to quickly check for any figure 8 imbalances on any body surface. He would just stroke his hand in a waving motion from the head to the feet of any surface, for example from the face down the trunk to the front of the legs and feet, while monitoring an indicator muscle. If there was an indicator change, he knew that one of the segments of the figure 8s on that surface had an imbalance. Then, by merely fuzzy gloving the head, trunk and front of legs, he could quickly locate which segment had a figure 8 imbalance. Once this segment had been located, he then knew where to apply the correction.

However, if there was an indicator change when only an individual segment was challenged, this indicated that there was a single segment of that body region's figure 8 with an imbalance. For instance, if fuzzy gloving the front of the body from head to feet gave an indicator change, then each body segment would be challenged separately, with the segment showing an indicator change being the body segment with a figure 8 imbalance. Then each part of the figure 8 flow for that body

segment could be challenged individually to investigate in exactly which component of this figure 8 there was a constriction of energy flow.

For instance, the fuzzy glove might show the front trunk to have a figure 8 imbalance. Therefore the monitor would then sweep their hand from the right shoulder to the left hip and monitor, and repeat this procedure back for the left hip to the right shoulder, to check for clockwise and counterclockwise imbalance. If there is no indicator change in either direction, then this segment of the figure 8 flow is in balance. This procedure would then be repeated for each of the other figure 8 flow segments until the segment with constricted or blocked flow is indicated and entered into circuit.

In 1989, Utt found that there are actually 14 figure 8s, not just six, covering every surface of the body. With 14 figure 8s, the method of stroking of each segment became a rather lengthy process, so Utt developed a method to quickly locate any figure 8 energy imbalance. He realized that there could be a pairing of a specific figure 8 energy flow and a specific acupuncture meridian alarm point, as there are 14 major figure 8 energy flows and 14 meridian alarm points (Figure 39.1). Utt then researched this alarm point–figure 8 energy flow relationship, assigning a specific meridian alarm point to each figure 8 flow. Furthermore, Utt discovered a specific indicator point for identifying general figure 8 energy imbalances. This point is spleen 21 on the left side of the body (see Figure 39.2). If spleen 21 on the left gives an indicator change when challenged, then there is always a

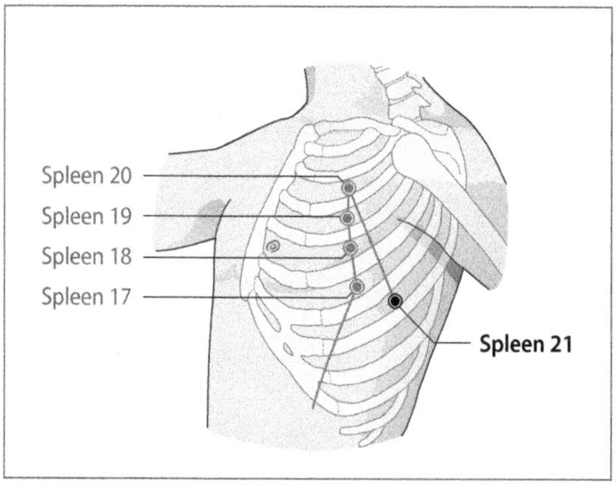

Figure 39.2 **Indicator point for the figure 8 energy system (spleen 21 on the left side).** The specific indicator point for figure 8 energy imbalance is a challenge to spleen 21 on the left side; thus when the monitor circuit locates spleen 21 left, there is an indicator change, but when the client touches their own spleen 21 left and there is no indicator change, this verifies that the imbalance in circuit is associated with a figure 8 energy imbalance. Once spleen 21 left has indicated a figure 8 energy imbalance, the resulting indicator change is entered into pause lock and the meridian alarm points circuit located; an indicator change on a specific meridian indicates that the associated figure 8 energy flow has an imbalance.

Spleen 20
Spleen 19
Spleen 18
Spleen 17
Spleen 21

Figure 8 energies 295

figure 8 energy flow imbalance over some segment of the body. In a challenge, there is no indicator change when the client touches their own spleen 21 on the left side, but there is an indicator change when the monitor touches this same point.

Now there was a direct pairing of a meridian alarm point with a specific figure 8 energy flow, locating a figure 8 energy imbalance was as easy as challenging the specific figure 8 indicator point, spleen 21 on the left side. If this gives an indicator change, then there is a figure 8 imbalance in one of the 14 major figure 8 flows. Then by circuit locating the alarm points, the figure 8 flow associated with the alarm point causing an indicator change would indicate the specific figure 8 with an imbalance. The specific segment of the figure 8 flow, and whether the flow imbalance is in a clockwise or a counterclockwise direction, can quickly be determined by the procedure discussed above.

Once the figure 8 imbalance is located, then some type of correction technique must be applied to rebalance this energy system. In different types of Energetic Kinesiology, there are various systems for correcting these imbalances. We will describe only the more commonly used techniques.

Balancing the figure 8 energies
Correcting general figure 8 energy imbalances

As discussed in chapter 7, the figure 8 energies have an oscillating flow, alternating between a clockwise direction and a counterclockwise direction. Therefore one of the most common figure 8 imbalances is when the energy flows too far in the clockwise or too far in the counterclockwise direction. To correct this imbalance requires some mechanism of increasing the flow in the deficient direction and decreasing the flow in the excess direction.

To apply the correction, you first need to know in which direction to apply it. The monitor simply strokes the figure 8 in first the clockwise direction, then monitors for an indicator change. If there is no indicator change, the monitor strokes the figure 8 in the counterclockwise direction, then monitors for an indicator change. If the flow is in balance, this movement of the hand and its associated

electromagnetic flux will only momentarily disturb the oscillation, which will be quickly re-established as the hand departs the figure 8 flow, therefore there will be no indicator change.

If, on the other hand, the figure 8 flow is already circulating more clockwise than counterclockwise, and you move your hand clockwise through the figure 8 flow, this will augment the incipient imbalance causing an imbalance in the figure 8 long enough that it will be clearly detected on muscle monitoring. However, movement of your hand counterclockwise (against the direction of imbalanced flow) will reinforce the weaker flow and momentarily rebalance the figure 8, therefore no indicator change is observed.

Correction of imbalanced figure 8 flows can therefore be accomplished by stroking the figure 8 pattern in the direction of the weaker flows until it balances the stronger flow, once again creating an even oscillation of flows. It is then necessary to challenge spleen 21 on the left side or fuzzy glove all the figure 8s once more to check for any other figure 8 imbalances. The procedure is complete when there are no further indicator changes on challenging spleen 21 on the left side or with the fuzzy glove technique.

In addition to the traditional correction of tracing the figure 8 flow with the energy of your hand, you may also use tuning forks or light to balance these energies by tracing the figure 8 in the direction of weaker flow. It is also possible to put the figure 8 imbalance into circuit and then balance using hand modes, specific indicator points, challenges and verbal questioning to address the underlying factor(s) creating these disturbances, as there are often psychoemotional components to figure 8 imbalances.

In order to correct the figure 8s, you need to take into account the following factors: 1, where the imbalance is located (the whole figure 8 or only a segment); 2, the direction in which to correct (clockwise or counterclockwise); 3, the type of correction technique to be applied (swooshing with the hand, sound, or light, or entering the figure 8 imbalance into circuit); and 4, the amount of time or number of times to apply this correction.

Five Element figure 8s

In a stroke of insight, Utt realized that the figure 8–meridian association could be extended to a Law of Five Element relationship. Indeed, Figure 39.3 shows how a figure 8 can be represented as four distinct corners (A, B, C and D) and the intersection point in the middle €. In the Law of Five Elements, each meridian has five command points. Utt then found that each corner plus the center intersection point of the figure 8 represents a specific command point. The Fire element point was found to be located at the intersection point in the middle, and each corner represents one of the other four elements. Going clockwise around the Five Elements, A is Wood element; B, Earth element; C, Metal element; and D, Water element.

To identify a Five Element figure 8 imbalance, Utt used a variation on the standard figure 8 indicator point, spleen 21 on the left side. By holding Five Elements mode while challenging spleen 21 on the left, an indicator change indicates that there is a Five Element figure 8 imbalance. To locate which figure 8 has an imbalance, the monitor checks each alarm point, with the alarm point giving a priority indicator change the figure 8 out of balance. Then to locate the segment of restricted flow, one has to stroke from command point to command point and find which segment and in which direction gives an indicator change, then enter this into circuit. Now the monitor only needs to circuit locate the two command points on each end of the stressed segment and check for the priority to correct.

If the segment of the figure 8 goes to the center Fire point, then you would need to challenge the segment from the corner command point to the Fire point in the middle, then from the Fire point to the corner command point on the opposite end of that segment. Once the specific segment with restricted flow is identified, the monitor needs to circuit locate the command point associated with that segment. This command point can be entered into circuit and a correction performed.

If acupressure shows as the priority correction, the monitor would then determine the type of acupoint imbalance, as there are two primary types of acupoint imbalances. One is a temporary imbalance in the acupoint which can be corrected by applying acupressure to the acupoint. The second results from blockages within the acupoint itself which have an underlying cause that cannot be rectified by simple acupoint stimulation. This second type of imbalance is known as a *frozen acupoint*, which must be corrected before acupoint stimulation (see chapter 6 for a description of frozen acupoints). After treatment, the previous imbalanced command point is rechecked for its state of balance. No indicator change when circuit locating this command point indicates that this segment of the figure 8 is now in homeostasis, and its associated physiology and psychoemotional states can now normalize.

In correcting the Five Element figure 8s, you need to take into account the following factors: 1, finding the priority command point to pause lock; 2, the type of correction technique to apply (e.g. acupressure, sound or light, or putting it into circuit and balance); and 3, the amount of time to apply this correction, if the technique has a time component (e.g. acupressure, sound and light). While figure 8 energy imbalances may not be as common as other imbalances, they can be an important and effective correction for many types of physical, physiological and even psychoemotional issues.

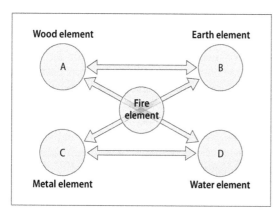

Figure 39.3 The Law of Five Elements figure 8 energy flows. If spleen 21 left gives an indicator change, then you may check for a Five Elements figure 8 energy flow imbalance by simply holding spleen 21 left and then holding the Law of Five Elements hand mode (thumb pad on the distal crease of the little finger); if this gives a reciprocal indicator change, then a blocked or imbalanced command point of the Five Elements associated with this figure 8 energy flow underlies the figure 8 energy imbalance.

Figure 8 energies 297

References

1. Brown-Frossard, R 2013, Tibetan Figure Eights, *International Conference on Kinesiology and Health*, Vienna, Austria.
2. McGarey, W 1974, *Acupuncture and Body Energies*, Gabriel Press, Phoenix.
3. Thie, JF 1979, *Touch for Health*, De Voross & Company, Marina del Rey, California
4. Dewe, B & Dewe J 1992, *Tibetan Energy and Vitality: Timeless Ways to increase Your Energy and Vitality*, Professional Health Publications International, New Zealand.

Chapter 40

HOLOGRAMS

The holographic concept

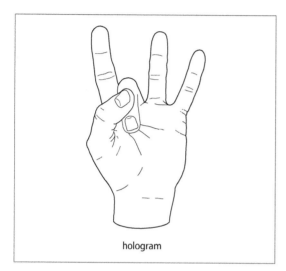

hologram

Figure 40.1 Hologram mode. The hologram hand mode involves placing the thumb pad over the first knuckle of the middle finger. If this mode is held, then an indicator change indicates that a hologram correction should be applied.

Research in Applied Physiology went beyond the simple muscle–meridian energetic interface developed in Applied Kinesiology by incorporating holographic principles into its concepts and applications. Indeed, recent advances in the fields of physics, mathematics and physiology have led to the development of the holographic paradigm. Today, this paradigm is providing a versatile interpretive metaphor for many traditional holisms, such as palmistry, iridology and acupuncture, whose energetic claims have never dovetailed comfortably with conventional western medical models.[1]

The holographic paradigm was originally founded in a technical development in optics. In 1947, Dennis Gabor discovered the mathematical principles to describe a potential three-dimensional

photography, which he termed *holography*, based on the equations of Gottfried Wilhelm von Leibniz, developed in the late 1700s. However, Gabor could not demonstrate the properties of holograms predicted by his equations until the development of lasers, and therefore was not awarded a Nobel Prize in Physics for this discovery until 1971. Indeed, it was not until the 1960s that Leith and Upatnieks developed the first successful hologram using newly invented lasers.

What are holograms?

The hologram is a special three-dimensional picture created by frequency interference patterns. Holography uses laser light which is a very special type of light known as *coherent light*, and a holographic plate.[2] Figure 40.2 shows the components of holography.

1. A laser beam is sent through a beam splitter, creating two laser beams from the one source.
2. The *reference beam* passes through a diffusing lens and is directed by mirrors to the holographic plate.
3. The *object beam* passes through another diffusing lens and illuminates the object being photographed, then the light reflected by the object falls on the holographic plate.
4. The unaffected reference beam meets the reflected object beam, creating an interference pattern.
5. This interference pattern is encoded within the holographic plate as a two-dimensional pattern, either light and dark lines or ridges and valleys.
6. When a laser of the same frequency is shone on the holographic plate at the same angle as the original laser, the original object is perceived to hover above the holographic plate as a three-dimensional image.

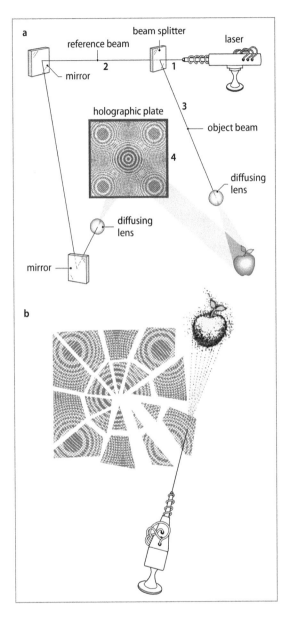

Figure 40.2 How holograms work.

a, A laser beam is split into an object beam and a reference beam, with each directed by mirrors into two pathways. The object beam goes through a diffusing lens, striking the object and reflecting light onto a holographic plate. The reference beam goes through another diffusing lens and is directed to meet the light waves reflected from the object as they hit the holographic plate. The object and reference beams create a holographic interference pattern on the holographic plate.

b, The information of the object is stored as the holographic interference pattern is distributed throughout the plate. If the same frequency laser is shone onto even a small piece of the plate, light waves reflected from the plate will interact to create a light image of the whole object seemingly floating above the holographic plate—the hologram.

If a hologram is illuminated by incoherent light, i.e. normal lightbulbs, no hologram can be seen. However, if it is illuminated by coherent light of the same frequency, a truly three-dimensional hologram of the object appears. Some holograms even permit people to walk all the way around them.

The amazing part of this process is that if only a small piece of the hologram is cut away and illuminated by laser light of the same frequency, it still creates the *whole object*; it is just a less distinct version.

The hologram is a frequency interference pattern, and within this pattern every piece contains the whole. This principle 'every piece contains the whole' can be seen in the body's cellular structure, where every cell contains the master DNA blueprint with the information to make an entire human body.

The holographic concepts of the universe and Man were first expressed by the Chinese principles of yin and yang, the dynamic opposite qualities that create the universe and are expressed in the structure of Man. A totally holographic principle is the Chinese concept that 'in the macrocosm lies the microcosm, and in the microcosm lies the macrocosm.'

Holographic supertheory

The hologram has several key features that make it immediately useful as an extended metaphor, if not model, of reality. First, holograms have an enormous capacity to store information in a small space; something like 10 billion bits of information can be encoded in one cubic centimeter of film. Second, the information is distributed throughout the system, such that if the holographic plate is shattered, a single fragment will regenerate the original image with only a little loss in quality. Third, by changing the angle at which the laser light strikes the holographic plate, multiple images can be layered on the same surface like interpenetrating or overlapping realities. The hologram excels at encoding and decoding wave pattern frequencies and acts like a lens to translate the *frequency blur* into coherent images.[3]

Dr Karl Pribram, a researcher in neurophysiology at Stanford University, was the first to propose that the brain stores and retrieves information or memory holographically, not locally.[4] Shortly after, physicist Dr David Bohm of London's Birkbeck College (now Birkbeck, University of London) rejected the randomness of quantum mechanics and postulated a holographic universe that he called the *implicate order*. The implicate order is the frequency domain, or blur of wave patterns, that enfolds everything: time, space, past,

present, future—all opposites. The apparent world of our senses from Bohm's perspective is a holographic regeneration, or unfolded *explicate order*, of this primary frequency realm. The dynamic movement between these two frequency realms he termed *holomovement*.

The explicate order can then be considered merely an interference pattern of primary frequencies of the implicate order translated into a hologram through the lens of our sensory perception. When other frequency lenses are used to regenerate the hologram from the same implicate order, for instance etheric frequencies of the acupuncture meridians, different explicate orders arise. In keeping with the Zen worldview, our apparent reality is nought but illusion generated by the limited lens of the narrow electromagnetic spectrum perceived by our senses.

The holographic paradigm or worldview, including the concept of a holographic universe, arose from the creative fusion of Pribram's and Bohm's ideas in the mid 1970s to create the holographic supertheory. The theories of Pribram about the brain and Bohm about the holographic universe were radical, and still are in many circles, and very much against the grain of classic scientific models. This holographic paradigm has generated great interest in the application of holographic concepts to our understanding of consciousness and the universe. 'Thus, a new holographic model is being developed which emphasizes the interdependent, parallel, and simultaneous processing of events,' rather than the more linear processes usually focused on in science. This new model has profoundly altered the way the dynamic interactions between the brain–mind and body are viewed. The chronology of the holographic supertheory is presented in Table 40.1.

Table 40.1 Chronology of holographic supertheory and background to the Seven Element Hologram

Year	Event(s)
1794	• Gottfried Wilhelm von Leibniz, discoverer of integral and differential calculus, proposed that a metaphysical reality underlies and generates the material universe. The space–time, mass and motion of physics and transfer of energies are intellectual constructs.
1902	• William James proposed that the brain normally filters out a larger reality.

Year	Event(s)
1905	• Albert Einstein published his theories on mass, time and energy.
1907	• Henri Bergson stated that the ultimate reality is vital impulse comprehensible only by intuition. The brain screens out the larger reality.
1929	• Alfred Whitehead, mathematician and philosopher, described nature as a great expanding nexus of occurrences not terminating in sense perception. Dualism, such as mind versus matter, are false; reality is inclusive and interlocking.
	• Karl Lashley published a great body of research demonstrating that specific memory is not to be found in any particular site in the brain but distributed throughout.
1947	• Dennis Gabor employed Leibniz's calculus to describe a potential three-dimensional photography: holography.
1965	• Emmett Leith and Juris Upatnieks announced their successful construction of holograms with the newly invented laser beams.
1969	• Karl Pribram proposed that the hologram is a powerful model for brain processes.
1971	• Physicist David Bohm proposed that the organization of the universe may be holographic.
1975	• Karl Pribram synthesized his theories along with Bohm's in a German publication on gestalt psychology.
1977	• Karl Pribram speculated on the unifying metaphysical implications of the synthesis.
1992	• Richard Utt developed a healing technique based on the holographic supertheory premised on Bohm's model of the enfolding, unfolding nature of existence and Pribram's theory that the brain stores memory like a hologram. The technique utilizes vibrations of tuning forks and flower essences to unfold stressful memory from the primary realm into manifest order for therapy by transmutation of negative emotions, thoughts and vibrations to universal love, utilizing affirmations to enfold the lesson back into holomovement (the primary realm), stimulating change, healing and growth of consciousness for the individual.

The implications of the holographic paradigm for holistic healing are vast and exciting. Every aspect of the universe seems to be part of some larger, grander being, and more comprehensive system. Psychologist Ken Dychtwald stated, 'Each particular aspect has the ability to be intimately knowledgeable about every other aspect within the master hologram.' Indeed, the ancient Chinese concept of 'In the macrocosm is the microcosm' appears prescient.[5]

In the holographic brain and body then, there is an instantaneous cross-correlation between all the interacting systems comprising the individual. Holographically, every system of the body is capable of being cross-referenced to every other system. Indeed, it appears that the organ systems of the body are represented over and over again in the acupuncture meridian system; microacupuncture systems of the ear, hand, nose and face; the iris of the eye (the basis of iridology); and the palms of the hands and the soles of the feet (the basis of reflexology).

Development of the holographic techniques

Incorporating these holographic concepts into Applied Physiology, Utt developed a unique healing system that he called the *Seven Element Hologram Technique*. Access to the holographic body was provided by his realization that each meridian-related muscle could provide a readout of the whole acupuncture system. Indeed, holographic muscle monitoring allows you to access the neurological–energetic interface, with specific muscle responses giving a readout of specific energetic imbalances. Because the energetic hologram of the Chinese acupuncture system then interfaces with the other frequency holograms of the subtle bodies (e.g. astral, mental and spiritual), holographic muscle monitoring provides direct access to the human hologram in all its dimensions.

The body can be likened to a holographic plate that stores the stresses and stories of our life. In fact, stresses and stories are stored in the body on a continual basis. In the holographic technique, the monitor uses alarm points to first locate the *object* meridian (analogous to the object beam) and second the *reference* meridian (analogous to the reference beam). This is like shining the laser beam onto the holographic plate, but instead of bringing forth Princess Leia as R2D2 did in Star Wars, it brings the buried stresses and stories of the person's life into consciousness.

The object and reference meridians found via the alarm points are referred to as *coordinates*. This is similar to the coordinates found on the earth called latitude and longitude. Just as a boat lost at sea can be located by establishing its latitude and longitude coordinates, so too can the buried stresses and stories of a person's life.

In this holographic technique, the first priority alarm point, for example stomach, gives the object frequency pattern and identifies the location of the stress within the stomach muscle–organ/gland–meridian matrix. The second alarm point, for example gall bladder, gives the reference frequency, whose interaction with the object frequency generates a unique interference pattern. This interference pattern represents the qualities of stomach meridian as it is modulated by the qualities of the gall bladder meridian, at all levels within the person.

The interaction of the object and reference meridians can create either a coherent harmonic interference pattern or a less coherent disruptive interference pattern, which will be reflected at all levels within the hologram of the body. In the absence of active stressors, the coordinate interference pattern will be coherent and sustaining to the functioning of the person as a whole. However, in the presence of active stressors the coordinate interference pattern can be disrupted and cause various imbalances at many levels within the person.

For instance, when there is an active stressor affecting the stomach and gall bladder coordinates, this may be expressed at the physical level of muscles by altering the function of stomach-related muscles, for example pectoralis major clavicular (PMC) in position 4 of contraction. Alternatively, it may be expressed at the etheric level as a specific acupoint imbalance, in this case stomach 43; at the emotional level as a specific emotional state, i.e. feeling discontented; at the mental level as a specific thought form, i.e. thoughts of animosity; or at the spiritual level as a specific attitude, i.e. expecting the worst from others.

In this holographic model, there is a matrix of the 14 meridians of acupuncture, each of which interacts with every other meridian. This means that there are 196 different possible meridian coordinates, each with its own unique set of frequency patterns expressed at all levels of the being. That is, every coordinate can represent imbalance within a specific muscle position, acupoint, emotion, thought form and attitude.

Indeed, Utt would say that the stress of people's lives is stored in various stress holding patterns that reflect the imprint of various stresses in their life at many different levels. The stress holding patterns are not just held in one dimension of our being but rather distributed throughout all dimensions of our being. Clearly, they may be consciously expressed in one particular domain, for example muscles or emotions, but they will be affecting all domains of our multidimensional being. These holographic stress holding patterns can be found within all levels: anatomy, physiology, cells, muscles, organs, the acupuncture meridian system, the chakra–nadi system and even the more esoteric figure 8 energy systems.

Many people think that stress can be compartmentalized into one part of their being and will not affect other areas of their functioning or life, for example, 'I leave my stress at the office.' In reality, stress at every level affects all the other levels of our being: physical structures, emotional reactions, mental thoughts and processing, and spiritual development, at least to some degree. However, many of these stresses manifest in ways that are below the level of conscious awareness, and hence their effects are often not connected to the cause.

Fourteen-position holographic muscle monitoring

Although the Chinese 14 major meridians are thought of as being surface flows of ch'i, traditional Chinese medicine recognized that all the primary meridians are also interconnected by numerous secondary vessels that interpenetrate the body. Taken in total, all the meridians and their associated secondary vessels create a three-dimensional energetic matrix encompassing the body. To this Utt brought a holographic perspective of the body and saw the muscle–meridian relationship as one representation of this hologram. He integrated the Chinese meridian system and its interactions as represented by the Law of Five Elements, with muscle balancing and holographic principles evolving at that time to create Holographic 14-Position Muscle Monitoring.

Applied Physiology research has revealed that each muscle, besides its primary meridian relationship, also has a direct energetic relationship via these secondary vessels to every other meridian in the body. For example, while PMC can indicate the balance of stomach energy, it can also give a readout of its relationship to the energetic balance between stomach meridian and any of the other 13 meridians in the body (the 12 regular meridians plus governing and central). The normal contracted position for monitoring PMC gives a readout of stomach energy in relation to stomach energy. There are, however, 13 other positions that PMC can be monitored in, each of which gives a readout of the stomach energies' relationship to another specific meridian.

How Utt discovered these relationships is an interesting story. In 1986, Utt was having photographs taken to demonstrate the contracted and extended position of the meridian-related muscles to be balanced in Applied Physiology. He had the photographer take pictures of the muscle in several positions in between fully contracted and fully extended, so that students would clearly understand the full range of motion of the muscle. When looking at these photographs, he suddenly had the thought, 'What is the muscle doing in each of these positions?'

Clearly, if he monitored the muscle in each of these positions it would be a type of contraction monitoring, but what exactly was being monitored?

To research this, Utt would take a meridian-related muscle into what he designated position 1, the normal fully contracted position. He would then sedate each of the alarm points one at a time and remonitor the muscle. Sedation of the alarm point causes a dispersion of the energy in the associated meridian, resulting in a momentary under-energy of the meridian as a whole. This is reflected in the meridian-related muscle as an under-facilitated or unlocking response.

Using this technique, Utt found that PMC in position 1 unlocked only when he sedated the stomach alarm point, thus confirming position 1's direct relationship to the stomach meridian. Then he moved the PMC a little into extension, again he sedated each of the alarm points one at a time, and following each sedation he remonitored the PMC in this new position. He was surprised to find that now it was not the stomach alarm point that caused the PMC to unlock but rather the large intestine alarm point!

As he continued to move the PMC further into extension, sedation of different alarm points caused the PMC to unlock each time. Then he repeated this process with the PMC starting in full extension, designated position 8, and began moving gradually back toward full contraction. Again he found the same thing: each position was unlocked by sedation of a different alarm point. After repeating this process for each of the 16 primary muscles of the Applied Physiology system, he had a lot of data that appeared random. It took him almost two years to make the seminal discovery that there is a coherent relationship uniting the alarm point–muscle position pairs.

By the end of 1987, Utt had researched the 14 positions of all 16 Applied Physiology muscles for their respective meridinal relationships. However, they appeared to be almost randomly distributed with no obvious pattern. Several times he had tried to plot them on the superficial energy flow, the Chinese meridinal wheel. This is an orderly progression of the peak energy as it moves from meridian to meridian across 24 hours. But no matter how he tried to do this, it made no sense, so in frustration he put this research away.

In 1988, while looking at a Law of Five Elements chart and referring back to the data for the PMC, Utt had a flash of insight: 'My God! If stomach is position 1 in the Law of Five Elements, large intestine is the next meridian in the Sheng cycle and indeed this is the meridian I found as the next position.' He looked again and found that bladder meridian was the next meridian in the Sheng cycle *and* the next meridian alarm point that unlocked the PMC as he moved from contraction to extension. Now he understood why there were seven alarm points in contraction monitoring and seven alarm points in inhibition monitoring.

Indeed, in the Five Elements the flow of energy is always in a clockwise direction and one of the primary flows is called the *Sheng* or *promotion cycle*, with each meridian receiving energizing flow from the meridian that proceeds it in that cycle. Reverse flows are considered to be perverse flows, because they inhibit the ch'i flow in its proper direction. What Utt actually observed was that the first seven positions are all energy flowing in accordance with the Sheng cycle and energizing, which would be analogous to active contraction in a muscle. In contrast, the seven positions from extension to contraction are related to inhibition monitoring, analogous to the reverse or inhibiting flows in the Five Elements.

Using 14-Position Muscle Monitoring

Utt discovered that monitoring through the full range of contraction and extension of the prime mover provides the energetic relationship between the primary meridian related to that muscle and all the other meridians of the body. He found that there are seven distinct segments over which the prime mover is facilitated between the contracted and extended positions (facilitation monitoring). Likewise, there are seven distinct segments over which the prime mover may inhibit its antagonists between the extended and contracted positions of the muscle (inhibition monitoring). Each segment

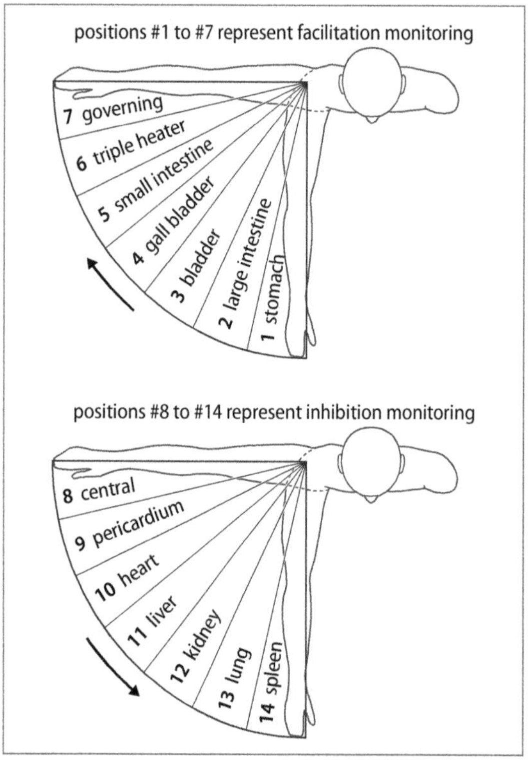

Figure 40.3 The muscle hologram: object and reference positions. Choice of meridian-related muscle determines the object meridian of the muscle hologram. Position 1 is the holographic relationship of the meridian-related muscle to itself, with positions 2–7 each representing a reference meridian to that object meridian following the Law of Five Elements flow in a clockwise direction; positions 7 or 8 are always Central or Governing depending on whether the object meridian is yin or yang. Positions 8–14 represent the reference meridians in the reverse flow of the Five Elements, so that position 14 is the coupled meridian of the object element (e.g. Earth element: stomach object 1, spleen reference 14).

of the range of facilitation or inhibition monitoring responds to stimulation of only one of the 14 alarm points, indicating an energetic relationship between the meridian associated with the muscle being monitored and the alarm point of the meridian being stimulated.

Closer inspection revealed that the most contracted position, the position usually monitored in most other types of kinesiology, always responded to the alarm point of the meridian associated with that specific muscle. The next six positions in facilitation monitoring were each related to another meridian of the same polarity as the meridian-related muscle being monitored. Using PMC as an example, positions 1–7 would all represent yang meridian relationships to the yang stomach meridian energy. The seven positions of inhibition monitoring from extension to contraction would each represent yin meridian relationships to the yang stomach meridian energy (see Figure 40.3).

While position 1 always represents balance of the primary meridian associated with the muscle to itself (e.g. PMC 1 = stomach energy to stomach energy), Utt discovered that positions 7 and 8 always represent governing or central meridians. Whether governing meridian is represented by position 7 or 8 depends on whether the muscle being monitored is related to a yang or a yin meridian. For instance, if PMC (a yang meridian muscle) is being monitored, then governing meridian would be represented by position 7 and central meridian by position 8. Likewise, if a yin meridian–related muscle is being monitored, then position 7 would be central and position 8 would be governing.

Not surprisingly, position 14 represents the complementary meridian in each element to that of position 1. For example, if position 1 represents stomach, then position 14 represents spleen, the complementary meridian of the Earth element. The other positions represent the meridians going clockwise around the Law of Five Elements. For instance, if position 1 is stomach, position 2 is large intestine; position 3, bladder; position 4, gall bladder; position 5, small intestine; position 6, triple heater; and position 7, governing. In contrast, after position 7, the energy flows to the opposite polarity meridian and then flows retrograde back to the original element. For instance, if we continue our example with PMC, position 8 is central; position 9, pericardium; position 10, heart; position 11, liver; position 12, kidney; position 13, lung; and position 14, spleen.

It should be noted that position 1 begins with the most contracted position for that muscle and ends at one-seventh of the full range of motion of the muscle moving toward extension. Position 14, on the other hand, begins at the end of position 1 and ends at the starting point for position 1. Likewise, position 7 begins one-seventh of the distance before the end of the full range of motion for that muscle, while position 8 begins at the full range of motion and ends one-seventh of the distance back toward position 1 (see Figure 40.4).

Note that the position numbers in each element always add up to 15. Thus, if you want to know what meridian is represented by position 11, you just count clockwise from position 1 to position 4: the other meridian in that element has to be position 11. For instance, if stomach is position 1, then gall bladder is position 4 and then liver would have to be position 11.

After working out all the muscle positions and the meridians related to them, in 1988 Utt suddenly realized that this relationship represents a hologram. Each meridian of the body is not an independent structure but is a reflection of its interaction with all the other meridians of the body, each with its own unique perspective of the body. So if stomach meridian is the object meridian, then the other 13 meridians are references to this object. Position 1 would be stomach energy *referenced* to stomach energy, position 2 would be stomach energy *referenced* to large intestine energy, and position 3 would be stomach energy *referenced* to bladder energy, etc. And positions 7 and 8 are stomach energy *referenced* to governing energy and central energy, respectively.

The importance of 14-Position Muscle Monitoring

Via its primary and secondary energetic relationships to the complete meridian system, every muscle can now give a readout of the

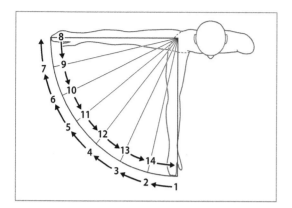

Figure 40.4 Holographic muscle monitoring positions.
Position 1 begins in the most contracted position of the object meridian-related muscle and extends one-seventh of the way to the end of the range of motion. Thus, in contraction monitoring, position 1 ends where position 14 begins in extension monitoring, and likewise position 7 of contraction monitoring ends at full extension, which is the beginning of position 8 in extension monitoring.

three-dimensional energetic matrix of the body. The neurology activated by monitoring the meridian-related muscle in each position provides the physical or neurological interface with the energetic systems of the body. Indeed, it is in these three-dimensional neurological energetic matrices that our stress holding patterns are truly held. Therefore 14-Position Muscle Monitoring provides a mechanism to investigate and unravel these stress holding patterns and release these from the physical and energetic matrices of the body.

Of equal importance, 14-Position Muscle Monitoring also provides an explanation for why the same muscle may need to be rebalanced again and again; indeed, why the correction does not hold! If the PMC is balanced only in position 1, it is in balance only with respect to stomach energy. There may still be one or more positions that are imbalanced. For example, imbalances may remain between stomach energy and bladder energy such that bladder meridian is constantly borrowing energy from stomach meridian to make up for a deficit in bladder energy flow. This small but constant drain on stomach energy will eventually unbalance stomach energy, causing the PMC to monitor out of balance once more.

Alternatively, the PMC when monitored in position 1 may always appear in balance, yet stomach problems may persist because each position has a specific physiological effect. Physiological disturbances related to PMC imbalances in other positions may result in persistent digestive imbalances even though overall stomach function, as reflected in position 1, appears normal.

Likewise, virtually all kinesiologists have been amazed or perplexed by balancing, say, a psoas muscle related to the kidney meridian and then having the person report improvement in a lung or large intestine condition. This is perfectly understandable once the full energetic matrix is appreciated, as the imbalance in kidney energy may have been the cause of the lung or large intestine condition via these energetic interconnections between the meridians. For instance, kidney meridian may have been pulling or borrowing energy from the lung meridian via the direct secondary vessel between the lung and kidney meridians in the Law of Five Elements. Thus, once the problem creating the imbalance in the kidney meridian was resolved, ending the compensatory borrowing of energy from the lung meridian, so the lung meridian was able to re-establish its own balance.

By being able to investigate the relationship of stomach energy to all other meridian energies and balance each position showing an imbalance, PMC will generally remain balanced for far longer than if the PMC is balanced only in position 1. Thus, 14-Position Muscle Monitoring provides a means of balancing both the physical and energetic systems to a greater depth than was previously possible.

Utt's a priori choice to use the Law of Five Elements as the centre piece of Applied Physiology and its reflection in the Holographic 14-Position Muscle Monitoring was a brilliant concept. The Five Element relationships open access to all levels of our being: physical, emotional, mental and spiritual.

Other holographic techniques

While the muscles are the most tangible and accessible component of our multidimensional body, as you can just grab hold of one, the body also interfaces directly with all the other dimensions. Thus, imbalances in muscle function, which are observable, may indeed be the expression of imbalances within the more subtle energy dimensions of our being.

For instance, the PMC having an under-facilitated state in position 5 could be caused by a fairly physical or physiological problem, for example spindle cells or Golgi tendon organs that have become unset. Or it may be a reflection of an energy state in the meridian system caused by a blocked acupoint. Or it may be a reflection of an emotional or attitudinal state in the higher subtle bodies, but one that is now manifest at the level of the physical muscle, which is observable.

Indeed, the holographic concept has been extended through all levels of our multidimensional being. Not long after developing the Muscle Hologram in 1988, Utt then developed the Flower Essence Hologram in 1990. Because flower essences predominantly represent the psychoemotional and psychospiritual states of our emotions, thoughts and attitudes, the same muscle responses that may represent a muscle imbalance at the physical level can also represent a psychoemotional imbalance at the astral or mental levels.

Utt continued his development of the holographic aspects of our being with the development of the Acupressure Hologram and Organ Hologram. Using the 196 different muscle–meridian coordinates, he researched which particular anatomical structures and functions are associated with each muscle–meridian coordinate. Finally, he developed the Cell Hologram, which gives references not only to individual types of cells but also to the organelles contained within the cells. Thus, an imbalance in a particular muscle position could indicate stresses from the cellular level to the spiritual level of our being.

The key to using all these different holograms is, of course, context. The same muscle response in the same position can relate to a cell organelle, a muscle, a specific organ structure or function, an acupoint, or an emotional or a mental attitudinal state. This context is provided by which hand mode or acupressure format is activated before locating the holographic muscle–meridian coordinates.

The last two holographic components are the chakra and figure 8 energy holograms. Utt did not develop a chakra hologram; however, he did develop a figure 8 energy hologram that uses the Seven Element coordinates to determine both the specific figure 8 that is imbalanced and the dimension of this imbalance. The development of the chakra hologram was undertaken by one of Utt's most prolific protégés, Hugo Tobar, together with his colleague Kerrie McFarlane.

After developing the chakra holograms with Kerrie McFarlane, Tobar went on to develop holograms for many aspects of the human being. For example, he has developed the Biochemical Hologram, Nutritional Hologram, Hormonal Hologram, Bone and Muscle Holograms, Brain Hologram and many different Neurological Holograms in his Neuroenergetic Kinesiology system.

References

1. Leviton, R 1988, The holographic body, *East West*, Vol. 18, p. 42.
2. Gerber, R 1996, *Vibrational Medicine*, Bear, Santa Fe, pp. 45–51. Brennan, BA 1993, *Light Emerging*, Bantam Books, pp. 37–38.
3. Talbot, M 1991, *The Holographic Universe*, Grafton Books, London.
4. Weber, R 1982, The enfolding–unfolding universe: a conversation with David Bohm. In: Wilber K, ed. *The Holographic Paradigm*, Shambhala Publications, Boston, pp. 83–84.
5. Kaptchuk, TJ 1983, *The Web That Has No Weaver: Understanding Chinese Medicine*, Ryder, London, p. 80. Rodgers, C 1986, *An Introduction to the Study of Acupuncture: The Five Keys*, Acupuncture Colleges Publishing, Sydney, pp. 2 & 6.

Chapter 41

CHAKRAS

Balancing chakra energies has been an integral part of many healing modalities because of their multi-dimensional effects within the human body, mind and spirit. The chakras penetrate every layer of the aura, and they therefore have an effect at every level of our being. Imbalances in chakra energies can thus have effects at many levels simultaneously.

Because the chakras were first described several thousand years ago, a number of healing techniques have been developed to balance chakra energies and function. Traditionally, these involved more intuitive approaches, such as visualizing the chakras and sending energy into them via the hands, symbols, crystals and other sacred objects.

Development of the use of chakras in kinesiology

One of the first Energetic Kinesiology modalities to incorporate the balancing of chakras was John Barton in his Biokinesiology. Because of Barton's Bible-based background, he chose not to use the word *chakra*, which is Sanskrit and has given rise to our English term 'wheel'. Instead, he chose the more neutral term *energy centers* and related them

to the nerve plexuses, such as the solar plexus. He identified 10 major energy centers, each controlling a major system in the body, such as the nerves, meridians, ligaments and hormones. He used emotions and acupuncture points, as well as reflexes on the feet, ears and head, both to confirm the identity of the imbalanced energy center and to balance them.[1]

Following treatment from an Applied Kinesiologist and then learning Touch for Health, Richard Utt began to study the energy systems of the body in great depth. After two years of traditional acupuncture training and considerable reading about the chakra systems, Utt had a series of dreams in which the blueprint of the matrix between the acupuncture system and the chakra–nadi system was revealed. It then took him almost two years to research and develop this blueprint into what he called the Seven Ch'i Keys, a kinesiology technique to balance the chakras by using acupoint stimulation in specific patterns. Balancing the chakras via the acupuncture meridian system only was totally unique and had never been done before.

In 1984, Richard Utt developed the hand mode for chakras to assist in locating chakra imbalances that he could now correct using the Seven Ch'i Keys. This mode involves placing the index finger on top of the thumbnail, as shown in Figure 41.1. Once the chakra mode was developed, it was then taken into many of the other developing Energetic Kinesiology modalities. These other modalities developed their own chakra balances. These early chakra techniques include Professional Kinesiology Practice, scanning the chakras, finding an emotion and then correcting with Emotional Stress Release points; Kinergetics, scanning the chakras and

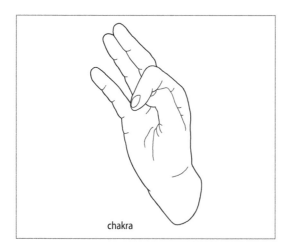

chakra

Figure 41.1 Chakra mode. The chakra hand mode involves placing the index finger on top of the thumbnail. If this mode is held, then an indicator change indicates that there is a chakra imbalance that needs to be addressed.

sending healing energy to correct them; Three In One Concepts, defusing the blockage and infusing chakra power via Emotional Stress Defusion and imagery techniques; and Transformational Kinesiology, scanning the chakras, finding the auric level of disturbance and then using imagery techniques to clear the imbalance.

Balancing the chakras

Applied Physiology's Seven Ch'i Keys

While the template for the Seven Ch'i Keys came from a series of dreams, its realization took several years of further investigation and considerable clinical research with several gifted psychics who could actually see chakra structures. From Richard Utt's reading, he understood that there are different types of chakra imbalances, and he worked out acupressure corrections for nine individual types of major chakra imbalances. The psychics would then inform him of what they actually saw when he applied these techniques, and normally this confirmed the efficacy of his correction techniques.

Of course, the idea of a clinical technique developing from a series of dreams seems totally unscientific. However, some of the greatest discoveries in science originated in dreams. The structure of the aromatic carbon ring in organic chemistry was first envisioned by Friedrich Kekulé, a 19th century organic chemist. After years of studying the six carbon ring structure, he and other scientists could not work out where the double bonds were located, as every time they measured them they seemed to be in a different position. One night in a dream, Kekulé solved this problem when he saw a snake suddenly grab its tail and begin to spin faster and faster until it was just a blur. His insight was that there was a new type of electron orbital called the phi orbital, in which the electrons were above and below the plane of the molecule and basically constantly changing their positions. The basis of organic chemistry was based on a dream![2]

The major chakra cones are made up of a number of smaller cones, each of which oscillates clockwise then counterclockwise. The number and color of these cones varies with each chakra. By *color*, we mean how they are perceived by people who can see them. Clearly, they are not a color in the normal visible spectrum or we would all see them! What they appear to be are supraharmonics of the colors in the visible light spectrum. Thus, for people who can see in this frequency range the supraharmonic of red light at 478 nanometers can best be described as red by them. And so on for the other colors.

The chakra cones come in two primary types: colored cones and white cones. The white cones relate to the metaphysical aspects of our being. In contrast, the colored cones are associated with specific physiology that is expressed through the endocrine or autonomic functions associated with that chakra. The smaller colored cones actually come in all seven colors of the visible spectrum, but in each chakra a primary color dominates, hence the association of a specific color with each chakra in most traditional systems: base chakra, red; sacral chakra, orange; navel chakra, yellow; heart chakra, green; throat chakra, blue; brow chakra, indigo; and crown chakra, white. The reason the crown chakra appears white is because it has even numbers of each of the different colored cones, which when taken together are seen as white.

Utt discovered that each primary chakra cone is associated with two of the primary meridians: the yin and the yang meridian of a specific element in Chinese acupuncture. He hypothesized, and the psychics he worked with confirmed, that there are secondary vessels from the yin and yang meridians from the associated elements that appear to support the structure and function of each major chakra cone. Therefore stimulating the acupoints on the associated meridians could affect chakra structure and function.

The five chakra imbalances are density imbalances, spin imbalances, projection imbalances, broken cone imbalances and hooked cone imbalances (Figure 41.2).

Density imbalances

The smaller cones may be uniformly distributed throughout the overall chakra, which indicates that the chakra density is in balance. Or they can become densely packed in some areas and only

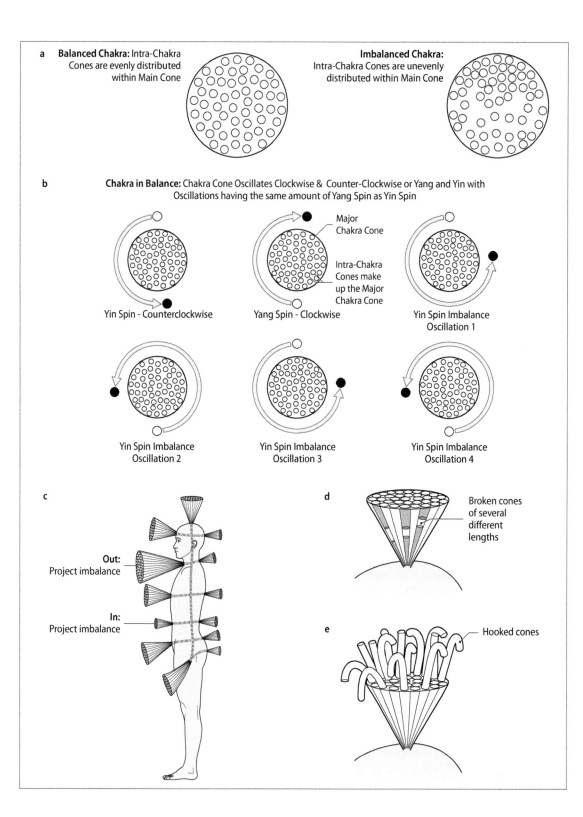

a   **Balanced Chakra:** Intra-Chakra Cones are evenly distributed within Main Cone

Imbalanced Chakra: Intra-Chakra Cones are unevenly distributed within Main Cone

b   **Chakra in Balance:** Chakra Cone Oscillates Clockwise & Counter-Clockwise or Yang and Yin with Oscillations having the same amount of Yang Spin as Yin Spin

Yin Spin - Counterclockwise

Major Chakra Cone

Intra-Chakra Cones make up the Major Chakra Cone

Yang Spin - Clockwise

Yin Spin Imbalance Oscillation 1

Yin Spin Imbalance Oscillation 2

Yin Spin Imbalance Oscillation 3

Yin Spin Imbalance Oscillation 4

c   **Out:** Project imbalance

In: Project imbalance

d   Broken cones of several different lengths

e   Hooked cones

sparsely distributed in other areas of the chakra. This is a chakra density imbalance and may have overt physiological and psychoemotional effects. When balancing the density of a chakra, you are directly affecting the colored cones and hence its physiology and psychoemotional aspects, not the metaphysical aspects.

Utt worked out that there are 12 specific acupoints that control the distribution of the smaller cones within the chakra. The number of acupoints that are imbalanced indicates the degree of chakra density imbalance. When only one or two acupoints are imbalanced, then only four of the other acupoints need to be stimulated. If six or more acupoints are imbalanced, then all 12 acupoints are stimulated sequentially. Stimulating these acupoints in the proper order results in the cones becoming evenly distributed throughout the chakra once more, eliminating the density imbalance and usually normalizing the associated physiology. The most common physical imbalance associated with density imbalances is pain.

The 12 acupoints involved in balancing density are combinations of the acupoints that regulate

Figure 41.2 Types of chakra imbalance. Each of these types of chakra imbalance and their associated effects on the different levels of your being are discussed above and only briefly summarized below.

a, Density imbalances. These are represented by an uneven distribution of the smaller cones within the primary chakra cone.

b, Spin imbalances. These involve the progression further in one clockwise or counter-clockwise direction on each oscillation so that the chakra cone as a whole slowly progresses in the direction of the dominant spin.

c, Projection imbalances. All chakra cones should project approximately the same distance from the physical body when in balance, and thus if the cones are too far out, or too far in, this affects chakra function.

d, Broken cone(s) imbalances. Smaller cones should be continuous from the body all the way to the higher spiritual levels of the chakra, but they may develop breaks or gaps in one or more of these smaller cones.

e, Hooked cone(s) imbalances. The secondary meridians associated with stabilizing the chakra cones are destablized because of blocked entry or exit points on these meridians, resulting in the smaller cones within the chakra hooking back on themselves.

energy flow in acupuncture: command points, luo points, horary points, Yuan points, source points and accumulation points. Because there are 12 acupoints needing to be stimulated in a sequence, Utt arranged them in a clock and termed this a *chakra clock imbalance.*

Spin imbalances

One of the most common chakra imbalances is a *spin imbalance.* Remember that chakras are not actually spinning per se but rather progressing in either a clockwise or counterclockwise direction. So a spin imbalance is represented by the chakra rotating more in one direction than in the other, and if many of the individual cones are all spinning in one direction the chakra as a whole will appear to be spinning in that direction. Clearly, a chakra can have a clockwise spin imbalance or a counterclockwise spin imbalance. Balancing spin imbalances clarifies the color of the chakra. For instance, the tint may become brighter or less muddy, and it may also bring about a change in hue. Spin imbalances are also associated with physiological and psychoemotional imbalances.

As spin imbalances represent the yin and yang aspects of chakra function, they tend to be expressed as under-activity (yin) or over-activity (yang) of the associated physiological and psychoemotional states. For example, the throat chakra is associated with both thyroid function and verbal expression. Therefore a yin spin imbalance in the throat chakra may be expressed as hypothyroid tendencies and an inability to speak out, while yang spin imbalances may be expressed as a tendency toward hyperthyroid and talking too much.

In Applied Physiology, spin imbalances can be corrected by using various combinations of the luo and horary points for the two meridians related to that chakra.

Projection imbalances

Another common chakra imbalance is projection imbalances. Each major chakra cone projects a certain distance from the physical body. When the chakra system is in balance, each chakra cone projects the same distance from the body. For instance, the brow, throat, heart, navel and sacral chakras would all project similar distances from the physical body.

Projection imbalances are of two types: an in imbalance or an out imbalance. If the chakra is not projecting as far out as the other chakras, this is termed an *in* imbalance. On the other hand, if the chakra is projecting further out from the body compared with the other chakras, this is termed an *out* imbalance. These imbalances represent under- and over-energies in chakra function. In addition, within a chakra, one or more of the smaller cones may project further out or in than the majority of the other cones. This would cause a more specific physiological or psychoemotional imbalance related to the properties of that chakra.

For instance, the navel chakra is associated with expressing your personal power in the world. If there is an in imbalance that affects the whole chakra cone, it is usually expressed as an inability to bring your personal power into the world and may be experienced as introversion. However, if only some cones of this chakra are in relative to the others, then this may be not a personality-wide imbalance but rather indicate an inability to express your personal power in specific situations, for example when confronted with a person you see as an authority figure.

Again, in Applied Physiology there is a sequence of acupoints that when stimulated will balance the degree of projection of a specific chakra. This will bring its projection from the body back in line with the other chakras and bring all the smaller cones back in line with the primary cone.

Broken cone imbalances

Normally, the individual chakra cones are continuous from sushumna, the central channel, to the face of the cone. It can happen that because of the shocks and traumas, an individual cone may break or have a gap along its length. The nature of the disturbance, both physiological and psychoemotional, depends on the level within the chakra cone that the gap or break occurs, as each chakra layer has a predominant theme. The degree of disturbance will depend on the number of individual cones that have broken.

The erratic energy pattern caused by a broken cone is compensated for by energy flow from the chakra's associated meridians. Thus this leads to imbalances within those meridians. Therefore to correct broken cones, instead of a sequence of acupoints, the association points of the meridians associated with the chakra are stimulated. This stimulation reconnects the cones and re-establishes normal functioning of that chakra.

Hooked cone imbalances

A *hooked cone imbalance* in a chakra is just what it sounds like: one or more of the individual cones of the chakra hooks or bends back on itself. This imbalance is caused by a blockage of energy flow in the secondary vessels from the yin or yang meridians that stabilize the overall cone structure. Hence the smaller cones begin to wave about, disrupting normal chakra function, and those that can see them say they appear to wave about and continually hook back on themselves.

The source of this imbalance is a blocked entry or exit point within one of the associated meridians. If an entry point of a meridian is blocked, then the cones of the associated chakra will hook in. Alternatively, if an exit point of a meridian is blocked, then the cones will hook out. At the physiological level, these blocked acupoints have an effect on the organ energy and meridian function.

Stimulation or balancing of the blocked entry or exit points normalizes both chakra function and the related meridian function. At the psychoemotional level, hooked cones are associated with hesitancy, self-sabotage and procrastination.

Use of the Seven Ch'i Keys

The Seven Ch'i Keys has proven to be an effective treatment for a number of different levels of imbalance and is a broadly applicable correction technique. In fact, there is almost no more effective technique for reducing acute pain than the application of the Seven Ch'i Keys. For example, one of Krebs's students who had learned the Seven Ch'i Keys had a daughter who had fallen and broken her ankle. The mother knew that the ankle was broken, and the child was in extreme pain, so she merely did one Seven Ch'i Key chakra correction after another with her *tei shin* until the child was no longer experiencing pain.

When she brought her daughter to the emergency room, she told the doctor that the child had broken her ankle and needed an X-ray. The doctor refused, saying 'It's not possible for her to have a broken ankle and not be in pain!' The mother replied, 'I heard the ankle break and I know it's broken; you have to do an X-ray. The reason she isn't feeling pain is because I did an acupressure technique that eliminates acute pain.' This was not convincing to the doctor, who still refused to do an X-ray because nobody could have a broken ankle and not be in pain! The mother almost had to result to physical force to get the doctor to X-ray her daughter's broken ankle. On looking at the X-ray, the doctor exclaimed, 'Oh my God, it's broken!' To which the mother replied, 'I told you it was broken!' Clearly, this pain-free state would not last long while the break remained untreated, and she was grateful for the skill of the doctor in casting the ankle so that it could truly heal.

In addition to balancing physical pain and muscle imbalances, the Seven Ch'i Keys are a broadly applicable technique for correcting a number of other imbalances, including glandular, hormonal, psychoemotional and psychospiritual states.

Neuroenergetic Kinesiology's chakra holograms

Another kinesiology approach to balancing chakras is through their holographic relationships to all levels of our multidimensional being. This concept was developed by two of Krebs's former students, now colleagues: Kerrie MacFarlane and Hugo Tobar.

While the Seven Ch'i Key technique balances the major chakras on the etheric level via the acupuncture meridian system, as discussed in chapter 5 the chakras actually exist on all levels of the human aura. The chakra system can also be perceived from a holographic perspective, as indeed each chakra has individual associations that are expressed on all levels. Like the acupuncture system, in which every meridian contains a representation of the whole meridian system, each

chakra contains a representation of every level of your aura: physical or etheric, emotional, mental and spiritual. Each individual chakra thus represents a particular perspective on the whole being.

Using the meridian–chakra relationships originally established in Applied Physiology, Kerrie and Hugo applied the hologram concept of meridian coordinates for each chakra. In this case, the object beam is represented by one of the two meridians associated with a particular chakra and the reference beam relates to a specific level of the aura. To locate a particular chakra imbalance, the monitor merely holds chakra mode at the same time as double-hologram mode (two hologram modes held simultaneously). This provides for two references: 1, primary auric layer, for example etheric, astral or mental; and 2, the sublayer within that primary layer.

To locate the chakra with an imbalance, the monitor circuit locates the alarm points, and the first alarm point to give a priority indicator change is the object chakra. The second alarm point to give an indicator change identifies the layer in which the specific chakra imbalance is located. The polarity of the first reference, yin or yang, also indicates whether the imbalance is in the front (yin) cone or the back (yang) cone.

In the traditional yogic literature, each primary auric layer is further divided into seven sublayers, hence the microcosm within the macrocosm. To reference these sublayers in the chakra hologram system, you locate a third alarm point, called the *second reference*, which indicates more specifically in which sublayer of the aura the imbalance is located. The sublayer of the imbalance would indicate whether the imbalance is affecting a physical structure; a physiological function; or an emotional, mental, or spiritual state.

Because the chakra hologram deals equally with each layer of the chakra and the layers above the etheric become progressively more metaphysical, the chakra hologram therefore deals in far greater depth with the metaphysical aspects of chakra function. In contrast, the Seven Ch'i Keys deals extremely effectively with issues at the physical and etheric levels and less directly with higher psychoemotional and spiritual imbalances.

MacFarlane and Tobar then extended this chakra hologram concept to the minor chakras of the body. Every major joint and a number of major acupoints on the head are associated with smaller chakra cones called the minor chakras. The minor chakras tend to innervate the physical body through their direct organ contact, for example splenic chakra, or the area of the body on which they are located, for example palm chakra. There are also six minor chakras on the head that relate more to the psychospiritual aspects of our being.

Interestingly, two of the primary corrections for chakras involve the use of sound being broadcast or light being shone into the chakra cone. Thus, these physical level vibrations can interact with the supraharmonics of these vibrations in the chakra structure. Surprisingly, clients receiving a sound or light correction directed into the chakra cone, even when the source is held 30 centimeters (a foot) or more from the body, often experience real sensations in their physical body.

References

1. Topping, WW 2000, *Energy Centers*, Topping International Institute, Bellingham, Washington.
2. Translated into English by Wilcox, D & Greenbaum, F 1965, *Journal of Chemical Education*, Vol. 42, pp. 266–267.

Chapter 42

SOUND

Sound is one of the most powerful types of vibration in the universe. In the beginning was the Word, and hence sound is an essential part of creation. As with all vibrational patterns, the degree of coherence and frequency of that sound determines its effect. Coherent sound vibrational patterns can be soothing and healing, while incoherent ones are aggravating and annoying, for example symphony versus cacophony (random noise).

For thousands of years, shamans and priests have used the effects of rhythmic sounds to create mind-altering and brain wave entrainment effects. In the 1960s, experiments on the effects of drumming on electroencephalographic patterns found that rhythmic beating dramatically altered brain wave activity. Other researchers of shamanic rituals found that the theta wave frequency range predominated during initiation procedures. Likewise, the Gregorian chants were used to establish synchronous brain wave patterns to induce deep meditative states among the chanting monks.

Development of the use of sound in kinesiology

Tuning forks

Richard Utt began to investigate the use of sound as a healing technique within the field of kinesiology in the late 1980s. At first, he worked with an audiometer, a device that creates pure tones, and then he hit on the idea of using tuning forks that produce physical vibrational patterns matched to the energy of different meridians. He researched this by first balancing a meridian then creating an imbalance in the meridian and testing tuning forks of different frequencies until he found which one would bring the meridian back into balance.

In the late 1990s, an English kinesiologist, Alan Sales, basically repeated this research using a sound laboratory and Utt's original procedure. He would take a balanced meridian, create an imbalance within it, and then use a sound generator to find which frequency would rebalance the meridian. Sales's findings largely corroborated Utt's original frequencies for each of the meridians. In fact, he found the same frequency for many of the meridians as Utt had, and those frequencies that differed were less than 10–15 hertz, which is less than differences between the various musical scales.

Utt also researched the type of material the tuning fork needed to be made from to have the highest healing qualities. Utt initially looked at stainless steel and aluminium tuning forks, the two most commonly available. While these produce pure tones, he found that these did not produce very reliable results in healing. He then researched a special type of aluminium that at that time was used predominantly in the construction of antiballistic missiles. This alloy of aluminium, copper and tin gives the vibrational patterns a rich set of overtones. Utt discovered that it was indeed the overtones, not the pure frequency, that were associated with the best healing outcomes. It should be noted, therefore, that the less expensive tuning forks available on the market are almost always stainless steel or pure aluminium and therefore lack the richness of overtones needed for effective healing.

Tuning forks cause physical vibrations of the air, which cause vibrations in the body's tissues and energetic structures. These vibrational patterns can entrain tissues and energetic structures to higher levels of coherence, reflecting more homeostatic states of function. Tuning forks can be used singularly or in combination. When a single tuning fork is used, for instance directed at an acupoint or held in a chakra, that frequency will entrain that structure to vibrate in a more harmonious way.

However, when tuning forks are used in combination, the sound frequencies of each fork now combine to create a unique interference pattern that has its own harmonic structure that is different from that of the individual forks. This interference pattern, which is represented by a unique waveform, may also entrain tissues and energetic structures into more homeostatic patterns of function.

Other sound techniques

While tuning forks are currently the most common method for incorporating sound into kinesiology treatment, there are a number of other possibilities. Any sound source can be used as a therapeutic treatment in a particular context. Treatment may include, but is not limited to, the use of a chromatic tuner, an audiometer, CDs (e.g. those of The Listening Program), computer-generated sounds, Tibetan bowls, musical instruments or even the human voice.

To illustrate the variety of possible sound sources, Krebs was working with a client in his country house and sound mode came up as the priority correction. However, Krebs did not have his tuning forks with him and therefore just entered sound mode into pause lock again to see if there was another correction that could be used instead. But sound mode came up again as the priority correction, indicating that it was indeed the priority correction the body wanted for this imbalance.

While he was standing there thinking 'Now what can I do?', there was suddenly a dinging sound in the background from the wind chime on the front porch. Krebs decided to challenge for using the wind chimes for a correction and the muscle biofeedback indicated 'yes'. So he got the wind chimes and then dinged each tube in sequence until he found out which chime to ding and for how long to balance the circuit. To his surprise, the correction was long lasting.

Applying sound in treatment

Sound mode is a way to set the context for using sound as a balancing technique within Energetic Kinesiology. It is an assigned hand mode with the thumb pad over the first knuckle of the index finger, as shown in Figure 42.1. Once sound mode gives an indicator change within any particular context, it indicates that a specific frequency or frequencies of sound are an important part of the context of that imbalance. Thus, whenever there is an imbalance in circuit and sound mode produces an indicator change it may indicate two different types of application.

The first is that a particular sound may provide

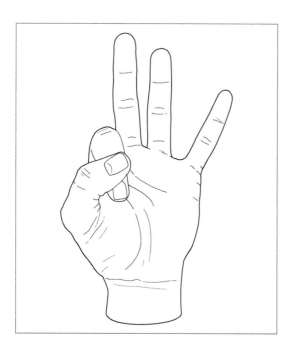

Figure 42.1 Sound mode. The sound hand mode involves placing the thumb pad over the first knuckle of the index finger. If this mode is held, then an indicator change indicates that sound therapy should be applied.

a mechanism for entering more information into the circuit. For instance, sounds are strongly associated with specific psychoemotional events, therefore the hearing of a specific sound or even a single specific frequency may activate subconscious emotional or mental programs permitting this information to be added to the circuit. Second, once the full context of the circuit has been established sound can then be used as a very effective correction technique.

With so many sound options available, how do you know which one is most appropriate in a particular context? This is the role of muscle biofeedback. Once sound mode has given a priority indicator change, then it is only a question of locating the priority sound source to be applied therapeutically. Once the source is identified, there are two additional factors that must be determined: 1, the location for applying the sound; and 2, the length of time to apply the sound. For example, the sound may need to be applied only to the left ear for two minutes.

Applying tuning forks

There are a number of ways you may apply tuning forks in a healing context; the most common are to use single forks or combinations of forks. A number of different types of tuning forks may indeed be used as single-frequency resonators with specific effects. In fact, this is the most common way in which tuning forks have been used in healing. Examples of this include Ohm forks, specific chakra forks, specific meridian forks, specific organ forks, forks to balance individual muscles and even forks that are said to resonate at the frequency of DNA.

A unique application of tuning forks was developed by Richard Utt in which the meridian alarm points are used to indicate which tuning fork or fork combinations match a particular frequency of imbalance. This imbalance may be at the physical, etheric, emotional, mental or even spiritual levels. An additional application utilizes the concept of holographic sound balancing by locating an *object* meridian and a *reference* meridian via the alarm points. When these two meridian tuning forks are then rung together, they create a unique interference pattern that can bring discordant energetic or physical systems into greater coherence, the basis of healing. The sound hologram concept is also used within the chakra hologram. In this application, it is not only meridian-associated tuning forks but also specific chakra-related tuning forks that can be applied.

As with all applications of sound in healing, it is important to identify: 1, the location to apply the tuning forks; and 2, the length of time to apply them.

Chapter 43

LIGHT AND COLOR

Development of light and color healing

There are references to light and color and their use in healing from ancient times. In ancient Egypt, sunlight was used for medical treatments and healing temples were built at Heliopolis that had colored crystals in the walls and were specially aligned with the sun's rays to heal. The Greeks knew that light could be beneficial to health, and their light therapy was known as *heliotherapy*. The Chinese also recognized the value of color for diagnostic purposes in the *Nei Ching*, which is over 2000 years old.

In 125 AD, Apuleius experimented with a flickering light stimulus produced by the rotation of a potter's wheel and found that it could be used to reveal a type of epilepsy. Around 200 AD, Ptolemy noted that if he produced flickering sunlight, the patterns and colors could produce a feeling of euphoria. Plateau discovered that healthy people were able to see separate flashes of light at much higher flicker speeds than people who were sick. Then, in recent years, studies using light sources such as a tachistoscope to provide rapid light flashes have revealed that long-term meditators are able to see discrete flashes of light at much higher flicker rates than non-meditators.

In the 19th century, the Danish physician Niels Finsen was awarded the Nobel Prize in Physiology or Medicine for his achievements using light therapy. Finsen created the first device to generate technically synthesized sunlight and demonstrated the beneficial effects of various wavelengths in the treatment of tuberculosis. This same technology has proven to be effective in the fields of dermatology, neurology and physiotherapy.

Light therapy has also been used for the treatment of skin disorders, sleep disorders and some psychiatric disorders. Light therapy that strikes the retina of the eyes is used to treat circadian rhythm disorders such as seasonal affective disorder.[1]

Other medical applications include pain management, accelerated wound healing, hair growth, improvement in blood properties and blood circulation, and sinus-related disorders. Many of these use low-level laser therapy and red light therapy in the 620- to 660-nm range.

There is growing scientific evidence that light can be a powerful healer affecting many conditions and many levels of our being. To quote the biophysicist Dr. Fritz-Albert Popp: 'We know today that Man is essentially a being of light. And the modern science of photobiology ... is presently proving this. In terms of healing ... the implications are immense. We now know, for example, that ... light can initiate, or arrest, cascade-like reactions in the cells, and that genetic cellular damage can be virtually repaired, within hours, by faint beams of light. We are still on the threshold of fully understanding the complex relationship between light and life, but we can now say emphatically that the function of our entire metabolism is dependent on light.'

Use of light and color in kinesiology

In 1988, Richard Utt developed the hand mode for light–color as a way to set the context for using light or color as a balancing technique. It is an assigned hand mode with the thumb pad being placed over the proximal knuckle of the middle finger, as shown in Figure 43.1.

The use of color in kinesiology

In traditional Chinese medicine, each element was observed to resonate with a particular color. The Fire element is traditionally red; the Earth element, yellow; the Metal element, white; the Water

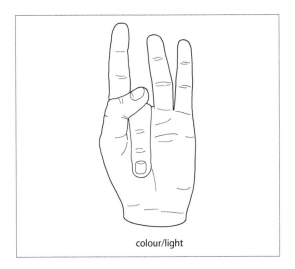

colour/light

Figure 43.1 **Light and color mode.** The light and color hand mode involves placing the thumb pad over the proximal knuckle of the middle finger. If this mode is held, then an indicator change indicates that light or color therapy should be applied.

element, blue; and the Wood element, green. There is also evidence that the Chinese used these colors in various aspects of healing.

In Chinese medicine, these colors were considered diagnostic, in that your reaction to certain colors would indicate which elements of the five elements were imbalanced. Once the imbalanced elements had been identified, then other Chinese medicine techniques, such as acupuncture, cupping, moxibustion or the use of healing herbs, would be applied to address the imbalance.

These traditional element-related colors were brought into Touch for Health by Dr John Thie. He developed a color balance based on these traditional Chinese color–element associations. Muscle monitoring was used to determine which elements and muscles were imbalanced and therefore which colors may have therapeutic value to correct these imbalances.

Two other applied kinesiology chiropractors, Dr Stoltenberg and Dr Franks, investigated the color–meridian relationships further using applied kinesiology muscle biofeedback and more sophisticated color-generating devices. They discovered that there are two distinct forms of color associations with the elements. The first is the traditional Chinese association that certain colors were diagnostic of imbalances within certain elements. The second is the association of specific colors as a healing technique for those elements.

In contrast to the traditional Chinese colors for diagnosis, Stoltenberg and Franks discovered that the healing colors are still red for Fire, yellow for Earth and green for Wood, but blue for Metal and violet for Water. Richard Utt took these healing colors into Applied Physiology. He also recognized that the traditional Fire element of the four meridians is actually two elements fused together, and that each has its own healing color. Instead of the Fire being four meridians that are all red, he divided it into its traditional subelements: Sovereign Fire, which is red, and Ministerial Fire, which is orange.

Each element has a yin meridian and a yang meridian, and traditionally yin is the dark side and yang is the light side. Thus Utt found that indeed the yin meridians responded most strongly to a dark shade of the meridian-associated color and that the yang meridians responded more strongly to a light shade. Therefore, in the Applied Physiology model the healing colors of each element are Sovereign Fire element, the heart meridian, which is dark red; small intestine meridian, a lighter red; Ministerial Fire element, the pericardium meridian, a dark orange; and triple heater meridian, a lighter orange. For the Earth element, the spleen or pancreas meridian is a dark yellow and the stomach meridian a lighter yellow. For the Metal element, the lung meridian is a dark blue and the large intestine meridian a lighter blue. For the Water element, the kidney meridian is a dark violet and the bladder meridian a lighter violet. For the Wood element, the liver meridian is a dark green and the gall bladder meridian a lighter green.

Utt created a holographic color balance based on the healing colors of the seven elements. This could be used in both a kinesiology and a non-kinesiology format. It consisted of using a set of cards, one in each of the meridian healing colors as listed above, the holographic flower essence manual and various other holographic charts, for example neurolymphatic, neurovascular and Seven Element Acupressure.

In a non-kinesiology format, a person would think deeply about an issue in their life and then look at each of the meridian-related colored cards and select the one that 'jumps out' at them. Then they would think about their issue again and repeat the process to select a second colored card. The first card represented the object meridian and the second the reference meridian. Then they would read both the negative and positive statements of that particular flower essence and consider how this related to their specific issue. They could then go to the chart book and stimulate the related neurolymphatic reflex, neurovascular reflex and related acupoint, etc.

In the kinesiology application, the client's issue would be entered into circuit and if light–color mode gave a priority indicator change, then the client would look at each meridian-related colored card one at a time. The first card giving a priority indicator change represents the object meridian, and the second card represents the reference meridian. The monitor can then balance the circuit by determining whether the related flower essence, neurolymphatic reflex, neurovascular reflex and/or acupoint need to be stimulated or whether other information was required. This process can be done as part of the information-gathering phase or it can be done as the correction technique to balance the circuit.

The use of aura soma in kinesiology

A modern, although more esoteric, form of color healing was developed in 1984 by Vicky Wall, who was a practicing chiropodist, pharmacist and herbalist. At the time, Vicky was 66 years old and clinically blind. In a series of recurring meditative visions, Vicky was given the same message repeatedly: she was told to 'Go and divide the waters.'

She said she had no idea what she was doing when she found herself in a small laboratory formulating a mixture comprising different layers and colors of natural ingredients. Vicky later reported that 'other hands guided her own', because she could neither see the beautiful combinations of colors she had created nor understand their intended purpose. However, this marked the birth of *Equilibrium*, her original set of aura soma bottles. Over time and through interaction with her clients, Vicky intuited the properties of each of these Equilibrium bottles. From these discoveries, the aura soma therapy developed, and it is now taught worldwide.

Kinesiology practitioners have also been able to utilize the aura soma system in their clinical practice by using muscle biofeedback to select the appropriate aura soma bottle for the presenting condition of their client. These can be used as a direct therapy, whereby muscle biofeedback is used to determine where to apply the aura soma oils and how often they should be used. These oils may be applied to acupoints, to reflex points or to other areas of the body. This can be used as either part of the information-gathering phase or as a correction technique. In addition, you can challenge to see if the client needs to take the aura soma with them and continue the therapy at home.

Another use of aura soma in kinesiology was developed by Kerrie MacFarlane and Hugo Tobar in the chakra hologram. They determined the association between the different chakras and various aura soma colors. When light–color mode shows within the context of a chakra hologram, the appropriate aura soma colors can be rapidly determined using muscle biofeedback. The important considerations are: 1, the location for applying the aura soma oils; 2, the length of time to apply the aura soma oils; and 3, whether the therapy needs to be continued at home.

The use of colorpuncture in kinesiology

Scientists are now discovering that light is actually an important medium by which cells communicate, and it is the basis of many body functions. Through over 25 years of intensive empirical research, the German scientist and naturopath Peter Mandel developed *colorpuncture*, a unique color-healing system. In colorpuncture, frequencies of colored light are focused on the skin using a handheld aculight tool with specially designed handmade interchangeable glass rods that emit different colors of light through a focused tip.

According to this model, as the light is absorbed by the skin and transmitted along meridians, it stimulates intracellular communication, supporting healing. While colorpuncture can be applied to any area of the skin, it is commonly applied to specific acupoints, as through their meridian–organ or gland connections these points have a more direct effect on our physiology than other points on the skin.

Colorpuncture has also been effectively employed by many kinesiologists around the world. This is because muscle biofeedback provides an effective mechanism to determine: 1, the specific light frequencies to be applied; 2, the acupoint(s) or other points on the body to which these frequencies should be applied; and 3, the length of time to apply these frequencies.

Other light techniques in kinesiology

Above, we have discussed the most common light and color therapies that have been employed in kinesiology. There are, however, a number of other forms of light and color therapy that have been used in healing. In these other forms of light–color therapy, the choice of the color, the form of the color (e.g. gem, crystal or light), the frequency of the light, the location at which to apply the light (e.g. chakra or acupoint) and the length of time to treat are usually determined intuitively. In contrast, kinesiology provides a direct means of using muscle biofeedback to determine each of these steps or phases to effectively employ any light or color therapy.

Reference

1. Lam, RW, Levitt, AJ, Levitan, RD, Enns, MW, Morehouse, R, Michalak, EE & Tam, EM 2006, The Can-SAD study: a randomized controlled trial of the effectiveness of light therapy and fluoxetine in patients with winter seasonal affective disorder, *American Journal of Psychiatry*, Vol. 163, pp. 805–812.

SECTION VIII

Concluding sessions

Once the kinesiology balance has been completed, it is essential to check a number of factors before finishing the session. First is whether the balance has created any transitory subtle energy imbalances in the client's energy systems. If these are addressed, this will allow the client to establish an integrated state of balance more rapidly. This is sometimes termed *balancing them to the balance*. Second is whether the corrections applied have actually resolved the presenting issue, which is determined by challenge, that is, re-entering the initial context of the balance. Third is whether the client reports feeling spacey or light-headed, which is resolved by grounding the client to bring them back into a normal state of feeling. Each of these post-balance checks and their application will be discussed in greater detail in this section.

The ways in which you can support your client after their kinesiology session are also discussed in this section. These include being available for ongoing treatment, responding to client reactions, promoting client self-responsibility and providing them with practical techniques to maintain good health.

Chapter 44

COMPLETING BALANCES

Stabilizing the client's energy system

One of the observations that is quite common, particularly after a very deep balance, is that while no more corrections are needed to address the original issue, the very act of balancing may have created subtle energy imbalances in one or more of the client's energy systems. This is partly because of the fact that the energies of the body are not like electricity. These flows do not travel at the speed of light; rather, they are much more like flows of water. Thus, when there is an energy imbalance represented by over-energy in one part of the system, just initiating energy flow via the correction does not lead to instantaneous change in all systems. Instead, there is often lag time as the energy actually flows, but like water it will automatically seek its level of balance over time once there are no blocks to its flow.

In this transitory process of changing energetic flows immediately following the correction(s), the more subtle energy systems may actually demonstrate new states of imbalance caused by the correction. Therefore it is useful to challenge each of the primary energy systems for their state of balance following the correction phase of the session. Richard Utt termed this process *balancing the balance*. The most common imbalances are found in the chakra system, the meridian system, the figure 8 energy system and the body's centering mechanisms.

Attending to these transitory subtle energy imbalances allows the client's overall energy system to more rapidly establish an integrated state of balance.

Challenging the original context

Once the balance is complete, it is necessary to see if the corrections that were applied have actually resolved the initial issue put into circuit.

This procedure is called *challenging* the circuit.

At the end of a balance, it is important to go back and re-evaluate the client's progress toward their original goal or intended outcome. This involves returning to the original context set at the beginning of the session. To effectively challenge a circuit, it is best to first close the circuit, which involves closing pause lock on both the monitor and the client to erase all information that was being held in circuit, and then re-enter the original imbalance.

If a pre-activity was used to set the context, then this activity will need to be repeated at the end of the session to evaluate the changes that have been achieved. If a goal was set at the beginning of the session, this goal will need to be challenged after the balancing is complete. For instance, if there was a negative emotion involved that created stress for the client, they would then need to address this same negative emotional context while being monitored to demonstrate that the correction is truly complete. No indicator change on the challenge, more modes, circuit modes or suppression mode indicates that the balance has been successful.

If the client's presenting complaint was a physical pain, it is important to have the client benchmark the pain both before and after balancing. By having the client rate their pain on a scale of 0–10, as discussed previously, it will help them notice the change that has occurred. This is particularly true of pain, as it is never supposed to be there. So if you do not make a note of the actual level at the beginning, unless it disappears totally the client may only notice that they still have pain, with no awareness that it has changed location or quality or has even been greatly reduced.

You then need to have the client perform the same action that initially generated the pain, for example move the arm into a particular position, apply pressure to a particular part of the body or focus on where the pain was located and the nature of that pain (shooting, throbbing, aching, etc.). While they are reactivating the original physical pain, it is important to monitor an indicator muscle to see if the pain has been resolved at both conscious and subconscious levels. While it may feel OK now and therefore there is no conscious pain in the moment, the presence of subconscious stress would suggest that the pain will return, as there is still an unresolved subconscious component that needs to be addressed. This needs to be explained clearly to the client, and they need to be encouraged to book a follow-up session in the near future to clear the unresolved components.

Grounding clients

Following a kinesiology session, some clients may experience light-headedness or feel spacey. Normally, even with no treatment, these feelings will resolve themselves within a short period of time. However, if this spacey, light-headed feeling is not addressed, clients may feel somewhat uncomfortable and even somewhat dysfunctional during this time.

Rather than having your client leave the clinic in a disoriented state, you can apply the following types of grounding procedures to help bring the client back to the present time and into a normal state of feeling. To assess for this ungrounded state, for example feeling spacey or light-headed, first have the client sit up and then monitor supraspinatus bilaterally. If it monitors under-facilitated, then perform one of the techniques outlined below. Second, once there is no indicator change when monitoring supraspinatus sitting, have the client stand up and remonitor the supraspinatus bilaterally. If it monitors under-facilitated, perform one of the techniques outlined below until supraspinatus is bilaterally in homeostasis when both sitting up and standing up:

- Hold kidney 1 or Governing Vessel 20 and monitor. If there is a priority indicator change, then hold the acupoint that gave the indicator change and circuit locate the other point. A reciprocal indicator change indicates that these two sets of points need to be held until a pulse is felt. The person should hold Governing Vessel 20 on top of the head while the monitor holds the kidney 1 points bilaterally on the soles of both feet until a pulse is felt.
- Have the client hold one palm facing their brow chakra, the glabella, or over the top of their head, Governing Vessel 20, while the practitioner holds one palm facing the root chakra and monitors the client for an indicator change. If there is a priority indicator change, the monitor holds their palms facing this pair of charkas until they feel a pulse.
- Check for figure 8 energy imbalance by using the methods discussed earlier: fuzzy glove method or challenging spleen 21 on the left. If there is a priority indicator change, correct the figure 8 energy showing imbalance.
- Circuit locate the heart self points, as discussed previously, and if there is a priority indicator change, perform this procedure.

After completing all necessary grounding procedures, clients often report feeling 'more centered and present' or 'not light-headed anymore'. It is always beneficial to have the client leave your clinic in a positive state.

Chapter 45

CLIENT SUPPORT

Ongoing treatment

The end of a session is the time to discuss future bookings with the client and any recommendations you may have. It is important to be clear and confident when finishing sessions so that clients will leave feeling positive and confident about the treatment.

After completing treatment, you must evaluate the client's need for ongoing and/or additional balances and then communicate this honestly and clearly to the client. You should discuss how many sessions you believe the client will require to achieve their desired outcomes. If clients are clear about what to expect from the start, they will be more likely to continue with the treatment over a period of time. Then you need to evaluate progress each session and inform the client if they are likely to need more or fewer sessions than previously negotiated.

Future sessions need to be clearly explained to the client, including time of next session, possible content of next session, estimated number of future sessions needed to reach desired outcomes and how long the client should have between sessions. For example, 'To fully resolve this physical pain, I recommend you have four sessions each one week apart. After the four sessions, we will re-evaluate how you are feeling and I am confident that you will have seen a significant improvement.'

When clients first come to you for treatment, they will most likely have a set of symptoms that they want to work with and/or overcome (symptoms may be physical, emotional, mental, energetic or spiritual). Once those symptoms have been cleared, the client will most likely feel much better, but those symptoms are just the outer layer. Once the client is out of crisis, you will then be able to start working on the true cause(s) of disharmony in their lives.

If your clients are going to achieve lasting results from their kinesiology treatment, it is important that these deeper underlying issues be dealt with. The focus may then shift to what they really want to achieve or change in their life and how you can assist them to go about achieving this change. There are many years of compensations and suppressions that build up in all of us, and a client will not overcome them in just a few sessions.

It is important to discuss this process in an honest and caring way with each client so they will not be disappointed if their whole life does not change after one or two sessions!

Client reactions

It is possible for clients to experience some reactions after receiving kinesiology balancing. Generally, these are nothing to be alarmed about; however, it is still important to ask all clients to monitor their reactions and contact you if they are concerned. Sometimes clients will worry unnecessarily or even decide not to return for further balancing because they have had unexpected reactions. It is best to prepare clients for any reactions that could occur following the balancing techniques you have provided.

Reactions may include:

- changes in emotional state
- movement of pain and/or discomfort
- muscular spasms
- changes in energy levels (i.e. feeling tired or energized)
- ongoing mental, emotional, physical or energetic changes.

How you respond to clients when they report reactions is important. The client may need to return within a relatively short time frame if these issues continue. Depending on the specific reaction, you may suggest that they could benefit from a follow-up session to address this issue. Alternatively, it may just be a normal reaction following the treatment they have received and you can let them know that it will pass in a short time and suggest activities to help this process.

When a client reports reactions following kinesiology treatment, you must record these reactions in the client's case notes, and it might be necessary to adjust the balancing you provide in subsequent sessions. If a client's reactions are not a normal response following kinesiology balancing, you should consider whether to seek advice from another healthcare professional or whether to refer the client to another healthcare professional to investigate these reactions further. Make sure you act quickly and access the appropriate services to assist your client if you feel their safety and/or health is in danger.

Client self-responsibility

You can help your clients create change, but you cannot do it for them! Therefore it is important to encourage your clients to be independent and responsible for their own lives and health.

Ways in which you can promote client independence and responsibility include:

- listening carefully to everything clients say
- taking your questions from exactly what the client has said, *not* from your interpretation of what they have said
- ensuring each goal is the client's goal in their own language
- giving clients the responsibility of setting their own goals so the changes will be something *they* want
- encouraging clients to see the benefits of them making changes in their life
- discussing any positive changes you notice with the client
- encouraging clients to continue making changes that they are benefiting from.

Practical techniques to maintain optimal health

To help promote client independence and responsibility, it is important that you educate your clients of techniques that will help them promote and maintain optimal health. The improvements they experience from kinesiology sessions will be much greater if they are implementing strategies for themselves outside the clinic.

Practical techniques that promote and maintain optimal health may include postural improvement strategies, simple follow-up activities or strategies to work on between sessions, activities or tasks to avoid, stress management techniques, advice on lifestyle modifications, exercises, or discussing the causes of their condition and suggesting prevention strategies.

You can provide resources to assist your clients in taking responsibility for their lives and maintaining optimum health by having literature and information materials available for clients to take home with them. You should also know of information sources that you can refer clients to should they require further information. This information could, for example, relate to stress management resources, environmental toxins or the client's condition. Always discuss thoroughly any alternative sources you recommend to a client, for example a website, including what information they can expect from this resource and how it might benefit them.

In order to promote client independence, you should be able to provide them with advice on how they can better care for themselves. This may include directing them to resources that will assist in self-care, providing details to fully inform them of their condition, current literature and/or research regarding their condition, and additional products that may be of benefit.

All recommendations you make to a client need to be recorded fully in the client's case notes at the end of every session.

SECTION IX

A model for energetic healing

To truly understand how Energy Medicine or Vibrational Healing works, one must first have an understanding of both our current physics model and the newer models of physics that incorporate both the physical and the metaphysical worlds. Until recently, only the classical model of physics prevailed, a world ruled by the laws of motion first articulated by Sir Isaac Newton in the 17th century. These laws were altered by the advent of Einstein's model of relativity, and then again more recently by their probabilistic expression of the workings of our world in quantum mechanics.

In many ways, quantum mechanics reduces our physical world to a world of relative vibrational frequencies, not the solid 'stuff' most people still believe in, which more closely matches the world experienced by our five physical senses. The solid atoms, the building blocks of the Newtonian world, are replaced by a plethora of subatomic particles such as quarks, leptons, muons and neutrinos. But these subatomic particles appear more as vibrational frequencies with charge than solid matter, and they are actually measured in electronvolts rather than the more typical units of mass, such as grams.

Not only does the matter of our normal physical world give way to insubstantial subatomic particles, but the behavior of these particles is equally bizarre. Repeated observations support a view of a world where two states of matter, a particle and a wave, may coexist, a state called *superimposition*. This seemingly impossible superimposed state is resolved only when the particle–wave is actually measured. This 'collapse'

of this superimposed state creates the world we observe. And how you, as the experimenter, choose to measure it actually determines what it becomes: a particle or a wave! Another quantum quirk, non-locality or Bell's theorem, states that non-local effects are not only possible but predicted. That is, an event on one side of the universe can actually affect an event on the other side of the universe at the same time, and is hence non-local. To quote Deepak Chopra, 'Quantum mechanics is not only stranger than you think it is, it is stranger than you can think!'

However, with all its ability to accurately describe our physical world, there are several problems with this current worldview. One thing this model does not explain is something that is observed daily by people using Energy Medicine to heal. How can insubstantial inputs, such as holding acupoints or shining a colored light into a chakra, result in profound healing? What is the physics of healing? Why does simply stimulating specific acupoints on the skin alter pain and resolve muscle- and organ-based problems, normalizing the function of very real physical and physiological systems?

There is a new model of physics with a sound mathematical basis that not only provides answers to these questions but also provides a mechanism by which human intention may interact with the physical world. It is, in fact, a model by which human intention may alter the function of the physical world. Once this new model has been understood, it provides a cohesive view of Energy

Medicine. But without a comprehensive understanding of the structure and function of the energy systems of the body, how you might apply this new model to healing is unclear.

The concept of homeostasis and the stages of stress of the generalized adaptation syndrome, when combined with the principles of chaos theory and the Tiller–Einstein model of positive–negative space/time, offer a new model of healing based on the subtle energy flows of the universe. The stages of stress of Hans Selye's general adaptation syndrome result from the need to maintain physiological homeostasis in a constantly varying environment to avoid crossing the phase transition boundaries of the homeostatic limits, which when crossed generate distress. To prevent distress and bring the physiological parameter in distress back within the homeostatic limits, the body generates a series of compensations. If the stressor causing the distress remains unresolved, it leads to long-term chronic physiological compensations resulting in a new compensated homeostasis, but one further from optimum function.

As homeostasis represents a complex set of dynamically interacting dynamic equilibria, chaos theory best describes this new self-organized system. Once self-organized, the new compensated homeostasis resists change, and unless decompensated and driven into chaos by crossing the phase transition of the compensated homeostatic limits, it cannot change. However, once the system goes chaotic, what causes reorganization to move closer to optimal homeostasis? In the model proposed, based on the Tiller–Einstein model of positive–negative space/time, deltronic flow, in the form of love and compassion from negative space/time and directed by human intention, provides the organizational information to 'push' the reorganization toward optimum function, a process called *healing*!

In order to understand this new model for energetic healing, we first need to present a brief overview of the standard model of quantum mechanics, plus chaos theory, and how it relates to biological systems.

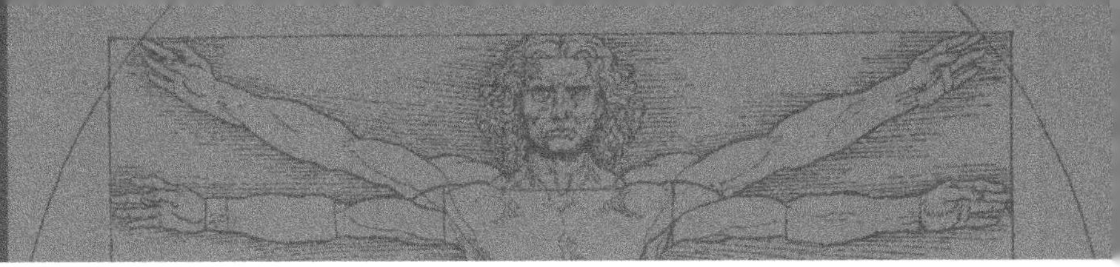

Chapter 46

THE STANDARD MODEL OF QUANTUM MECHANICS

Fundamental particles of matter

Solid physical matter is made up of atoms, the original fundamental particles propounded initially by the Greek philosopher Democratis. Until early in the 20th century, the atom, as understood by the Bohr model, with a solid nucleus of positively charged protons and neutral neutrons circled by tiny negatively charged electrons, was believed to be the fundamental particle of matter (see Figure 46.1).

Then it was discovered that atoms are composed of subatomic particles called *fermions*. While fermions do not have solidity in the normal way we think of matter having, they possess mass and are represented by various vibrating particles measured in electronvolts. Fermions and their force particles are summarized below.[1]

- Fermions are the subatomic particles: quarks and leptons (electrons, neutrinos, muons and tau particles). Quarks come in six types or *flavors*: up, down, strange, charm, top and bottom.
- Fermions exert forces on each other by exchanging force particles called *bosons*. These differ from fermions in how much they spin: fermions have a spin of ½ and bosons have a spin of 1.

- Quarks attract each other by exchanging gluons, the bosons that carry the strong nuclear force.
- This powerful attraction binds three quarks together to form baryons (protons and neutrons) or mesons (made up of a quark and an antiquark).
- Negatively charged electrons bind to the positively charged nucleus (of protons and neutrons) by exchanging photons, the bosons carrying the electromagnetic force.
- Weak nuclear force is carried by massive W and Z bosons, which cause a type of radioactive decay, but they get their mass from the Higgs bosons that flash into and out of existence anywhere in space and *drag* on the W and Z bosons to give them their mass.[1]

- The nature of the quantum universe is a vacuum or void, not empty but rather seething with a chaotic sea of virtual particles that pop into and out of existence, borrowing energy from the vacuum, called vacuum energy or zero-point energy, which is enormous. (See Lynne McTaggart's book *The Field*[2] for a readable explanation of zero-point energy.)

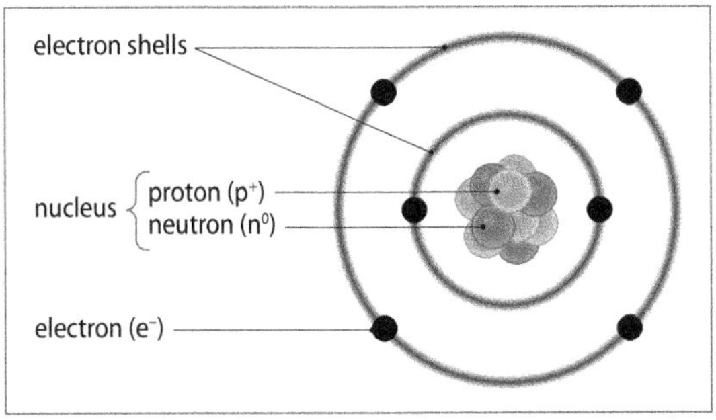

electron shells

nucleus { proton (p⁺)
neutron (n⁰)

electron (e⁻)

Figure 46.1 The Bohr model of the atom. There is a dense nucleus of positively charged protons and neutral neutrons that are orbited by negatively charged electrons. The number of protons equals the number of electrons. The electron shells, or orbitals, are set at fixed distances from the nucleus or quantized as calculated using Planck's constant. Energy absorbed by the atom is released by the electrons jumping to higher orbitals and then dropping back into their original orbital by emitting a photon, a quantum of light.

Four fundamental forces

There are currently four fundamental forces recognized in physics, and each force is believed to be carried by an identified or a hypothesized boson. These forces and their bosons are summarized below.

1. *Electromagnetism*, carried by bosons called photons between negatively and positively charged particles, and *magnetism*, carried by hypothetical bosons called magnetons.
2. *Strong nuclear force*: carried by bosons called gluons between quarks to create three-quark particles (protons and neutrons).
3. *Weak nuclear force*: carried by W and Z bosons, which get their mass from Higgs bosons, which blink in and out of existence.
4. *Gravity*: carried by hypothetical bosons called gravitons.

The strong nuclear force overpowers the electromagnetic force, which is why positively charged protons can be packed tightly together in the nucleus despite electromagnetic repulsion. The electromagnetic force overpowers the weak nuclear force holding atoms together, which is why atoms, especially massive atoms such as uranium, persist over time and decay only slowly over long periods. And all three of these forces overpower gravity.

Magnetism is considered a special case of the electromagnetic force from the framework of the earth where magnetism appears to be a fifth separate force because it can exist separately from electricity. However, from the perspective of space, the earth's magnetism is also electromagnetic, as the spinning iron core cutting through the lines of magnetic flux creates the earth's electromagnetic fields. But from the perspective here on earth, electricity can never exist separate from magnetism (hence *electromagnetism*), but magnetism can exist completely separate from electricity. For instance, a magnet can have a magnetic field without creating electricity.

Whenever there is a flow of electrons, called electricity, immediately and reciprocally a magnetic field is generated perpendicular to the direction of flow of the electrons. This is the electromagnetic field of electricity and the reason why electrical appliances, high-power lines and mobile phones may affect your health (see Figure 46.2).

Because of the movement of electrons in the body, every living organism generates electric flows, and these flows have corresponding electromagnetic fields. These fields, such as the electroencephalographically recorded brain waves and electrocardiographically recorded waves of the heart, are measured and used in diagnosis in western medicine. Indeed, it is precisely because the body produces electricity and electromagnetic fields that external electromagnetic fields *must* affect the body's fields, perturbing its function. It is just a question of whether or not this perturbation is large enough to be damaging.

Our knowledge of our physical world is largely dependent on and limited by our ability to measure the electromagnetic energies of the electromagnetic spectrum (see Figure 46.3). Before the advent of electronic instrumentation, our knowledge of the electromagnetic spectrum was limited to the spectrum of visible light, a tiny slice in the range, between

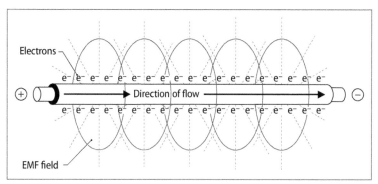

Figure 46.2 Electricity and electromagnetic fields. Electricity is the flow of electrons along a conductor from an area with excess electrons (the negative electrode or cathode) to an area deficit in electrons (the positive electrode or anode), from negative to positive. The instant an electron moves along a conductor, it generates an electromagnetic field perpendicular to the direction of electron flow. EMF, electromagnetic force.

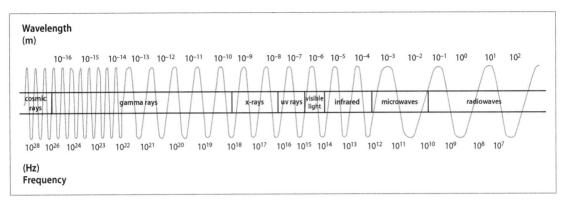

Figure 46.3 The electromagnetic spectrum. The electromagnetic spectrum is the distribution of electromagnetic field frequencies from extremely long radio waves, through microwaves and infrared, to the tiny slice of this extensive spectrum we can know about by our sense—the visible light frequencies perceived as color—into the ultraviolet (uv) rays, to x-rays, gamma rays and highest frequency of all, cosmic rays. The wavelength is measured in meters and the frequency in hertz or cycles per second.

about 400 nanometers and 800 nanometers (that is, 400 to 800 billionths of a meter). But the development of electronic instruments has expanded this limited physical perception to now include knowledge of cosmic rays at one end and extremely long radio waves at the other end of this extremely broad spectrum. In fact, every time an instrument capable of measuring higher or lower frequencies is created, new frequencies are discovered.

Primary properties of the physical world

The primary properties of the physical world are as follows.

- The realm of physical matter is made of atoms and their subatomic particles.
- The primary energy flow is electricity.
- Electromagnetic fields are always created by the movement of electrons (electricity).
- Electromagnetic waves are measured as frequency, that is, the number of peaks or troughs per second. Hence they always include time and polarity, as a peak represents (+) and a trough (−), and the frequency is the time between the peaks or troughs past any fixed point.
- There is the realm of magnetic dipoles: magnets always have a north (−) pole connected to a south (+) pole, such that the two poles or polarities are always linked.

- Positive entropy is the free energy of any system, which increases over time, creating and maintaining the randomness of the vacuum. Stated another way, there is an inherent tendency for disorder to increase with time.
- Velocity of matter is limited to the speed of light (about 300,000 kilometers/second).

The last of these properties is a direct consequence of Einstein's famous equation $E = mc^2$ because energy and mass are related by the speed of light.[3] When speed or velocity is slow, changes to the size of mass are imperceptible, but as you increase your velocity and begin to approach the speed of light, the mass increases proportional to the speed of light. Thus, as the mass becomes larger more energy is needed to move it faster, which only makes it larger, again requiring more energy, so the speed of light can never be exceeded by a body with physical mass (see Figure 46.4).

Dark matter

From observation of stars and other heavenly bodies in distant galaxies, it is now clear that there is not enough observable mass in the universe to account for how the heavenly bodies actually behave following the laws of gravity. To

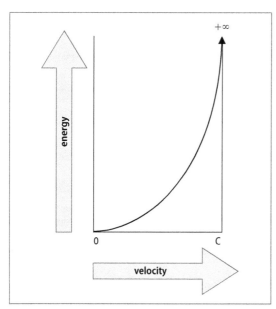

Figure 46.4 The speed of light is constant because of the interplay between matter and energy, as presented in Einstein's famous formula $E = mc^2$**.** The speed of light is the same everywhere in the universe (186,000 miles per second or 300,000 kilometers per second) because photons have a minute mass, and therefore it requires an exponential increase in the amounts of energy to increase its velocity such that the curve reaches an asymptote at this velocity.

compensate for deficit of mass, it has been proposed that there is also dark matter within space and that the amount of this dark matter is such that heavenly bodies behave the way we observe them behaving. This hypothesized dark matter comprises between 70 and 95% of the mass in the universe. Because the universe is known to be expanding, if it were not for this dark matter it would have rapidly dissipated and no longer exist.

But because we can see many bodies out in space, dark matter must exist as their movement exactly follows the laws of gravity. One hypothetical model that has been proposed is supersymmetry. In this way, there would be enough matter for gravity to create the observable universe.

Supersymmetry

This hypothetical model proposes that for every standard fermion there is a heavier yet identical boson, and for every standard boson it proposes a heavier yet identical fermion. In this way, the need for dark matter to make up the invisible mass of the universe is avoided.

These extra particles are known as *superpartners*, which 'live' in and are derived from a sea of virtual particles, the Dirac sea, that constantly blink into and out of existence. In this model:

- the electron partners the selectron
- the top quark partners the stop quark
- the photon partners the photino
- the W boson partners the wino
- the Z boson partners the zino.

Problems with the standard model

The problems with the standard model are as follow.

- While the standard model can explain every interaction between particles of matter, it does not explain the fourth fundamental force, gravity, or explain all the dark matter of the universe, which must make up most of its mass for the universe to behave the way it does according to the laws of gravity.
- While magnetic monopoles are predicted, they have never been observed, even after extensive attempts to find them!
- More importantly, while the standard model explains the evolution of the physical universe, it does not explain life! Life is particularly paradoxical, as it seems to be a momentary violation of the second law of thermodynamics, entropy, the tendency for all matter in the

physical universe to increase in disorder over time.

- Likewise, it does not explain healing, that is, negative entropy in action: disordered tissue becoming 'spontaneously' more organized back to its original state.
- The standard model also does not explain a number of phenomena grouped under the heading of *psi phenomena*, which although relegated to parapsychology have considerable experimental support, for example telekinesis; distance vision; and the ability of focused human intention to change physical parameters such as pH, the rate of enzyme reactions and the growth rate of organisms.[1,2]
- In addition, it cannot explain how homeopathy works, although there is considerable experimental and anecdotal support for its effects on living organisms. (See Lynn McTaggart's book *The Field*[2] for extensive discussions of this issue.)
- The standard model also provides no mechanism for out-of-body or near-death experiences, even though they have been extensively documented, often with corroborating evidence of the experiences observed in these non-material states being true in physical reality.[3]

It should be noted that many of the above phenomena, although extensively experimentally documented at least as rigorously as many accepted results of various scientific experiments, are still rejected out of hand by mainstream scientists. When confronted with quite strong statistical data supporting a potentially psi phenomenon in a review article in *New Scientist* in 2006, a credible scientist made the absolutely 'unscientific' statement, 'I don't care what other explanation you use, it has to be better than psi phenomenon!' In other words, 'Do not bother me with the data; my mind is already made up!'

Indeed, what we accept to be true is controlled by what we consider to constitute proof. In the same review article, they presented two sets of meta-analyses labeled A and B. Inspection of the data clearly showed that data-set B had a higher statistical significance and therefore a higher probability of not being the result of chance and hence true. One data-set was a meta-analysis of all the studies of streptokinase, a drug believed to help prevent heart attack, while the other data-set was of a meta-analysis of studies describing the effects of a psi phenomenon. Quite surprisingly, data-set A, with the least statistical significance, was deemed proof that streptokinase *is* an effective treatment for heart problems. In contrast, data-set B, with a higher statistical significance, was deemed proof that the psi phenomenon does *not* exist.

The author suggested that what constitutes proof is therefore related more to what you already believe, and we would say what you want to believe, than the actual data. Most scientists believe in enzymes, and that they can affect physiological function, but doubt the existence of psi phenomena. Therefore they are willing to accept a much lower level of proof for something they believe than what they consider to be improbable.

References

1. Tiller, WA, Dibble, WE & Kohane, MJ 2001, *Conscious Acts of Creation*, Pavior Publishing, Walnut Creek.
2. McTaggart, L 2008, *The Field*, HarperCollins, New York.
3. Kübler-Ross, E 1997, *On Death and Dying*, Touchstone, New York.

Chapter 47

THE SCIENCE OF METAPHYSICS: A NEW MODEL OF PHYSICS

The Tiller–Einstein model of positive–negative space/time

For the past four decades, physicist William Tiller, professor emeritus, Stanford University, has been working to provide scientific models that explain certain subtle energetic phenomenon such as the flow of ch'i and various psychic phenomena, such as telepathy, clairvoyance and distance or remote healing. He has created a model of reality that finally succeeds in incorporating both the physical domain of the West and the metaphysical domain of the East.

In his book *Vibrational Medicine*, Richard Gerber termed this model the *Tiller–Einstein model of positive–negative space/time*, because its insights are derived from the Einstein equation that relates energy to matter: $E = mc2$.[1] Einstein's equation suggests that energy and matter are interconvertible and interconnected; with subatomic matter considered as a packet of frozen energy. The release of energy from its frozen form is the massive power behind the atomic bomb.

While we normally think of reality as having only three dimensions, Einstein's equations have led to the concept of space/time, which is the fourth dimension in which we exist. Gravity in this model amounts to warping of the fabric of space/time by physical mass. If you feel that this is a difficult concept to grasp, be comforted by the fact that even the physicist Stephen Hawking, in his book *A Brief History of Time*, conceded that he too had problems wrapping his mind around the idea of this fourth dimension.[2]

In this new model, reality can be considered to consist of at least two domains: positive space/time and negative space/time (see Figure 47.1). Each has its own unique properties and is governed by its own particular principles. Although in Tiller's multidimensional model he specifies five important and uniquely different domains, four of them are substructures of the 'vacuum', so for our purposes we will refer to all of them as the negative space/time domain.

For a broader and more detailed understanding, the reader is referred to Professor Tiller's seminal books *Science and Human Transformation: Subtle Energies, Intentionality and Consciousness, Conscious Acts of Creation: the Emergence of a New Physics* and *Psychoenergetic Science: a Second Copernican-Scale Revolution*.

The fifth fundamental force: the magneto-electric force

Tiller proposes that there is a fifth fundamental force, the magnetoelectric force (like supersymmetry, hypothetical at this time), the reciprocal force to electromagnetism, which is carried by another hypothetical particle, the deltron. Deltronic flows allow the magnetoelectric force from negative space/time to interact with matter in positive space/time. Thus deltrons are the bosons of the magnetoelectric force.

In his model, magnetoelectric flows of deltrons between negative or reciprocal space/time (the metaphysical world) and positive space/time (the material world) constitute the subtle energies that bring order into the physical world. These deltron-based subtle energies counteract the effects of the second law of thermodynamics, entropy, the increase in disorder in any physical system over time. Usually stated as the tendency for disorder to increase over time until randomness occurs (think of a nail rusting to random particles of iron oxide from which it was made), these negative entropic flows are best observed in living organisms, as they represent examples of negative

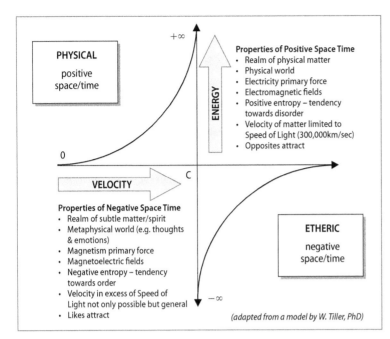

PHYSICAL
positive space/time

$+\infty$

ENERGY

Properties of Positive Space Time
• Realm of physical matter
• Physical world
• Electricity primary force
• Electromagnetic fields
• Positive entropy – tendency towards disorder
• Velocity of matter limited to Speed of Light (300,000km/sec)
• Opposites attract

0

VELOCITY

C

Properties of Negative Space Time
• Realm of subtle matter/spirit
• Metaphysical world (e.g. thoughts & emotions)
• Magnetism primary force
• Magnetoelectric fields
• Negative entropy – tendency towards order
• Velocity in excess of Speed of Light not only possible but general
• Likes attract

ETHERIC
negative space/time

$-\infty$

(adapted from a model by W. Tiller, PhD)

Figure 47.1 Tiller's model of positive–negative space/time. This figure presents and contrasts the properties of both positive space/time, the physical world, and its complement, negative space/time, the domain of subtle energies, mind and spirit—the metaphysical world. The electricity and electromagnetic fields of positive space/time are complemented by the magnetism and magnetoelectric fields of positive space/time, as is positive entropy, a tendency toward disorder, complemented by negative entropy, a tendency toward order. After Tiller WA, 1978, A lattice model of space, *New Directions in the Study of Man*, Vol. II, No. 2, p. 31.

entropy in positive space/time, that is, highly structured physical beings created and maintained over time against the tendency toward disorder in the physical world.

Primary properties of the metaphysical world

The primary properties of the metaphysical world are as follows.

• It is the realm of subtle matter or spirit.
• The primary energy flow is magnetism.
• Magnetoelectric fields are created by deltronic flow.
• It is the realm of magnetic monopoles: pure constant north or south poles exist separately.
• Negative entropy is a decrease in 'free' energy over time, decreasing the randomness of the vacuum; this can be stated as the tendency toward order.
• Velocity in excess of the speed of light is not only possible but general.

Unlike the situation in the physical world, where matter always has mass, the subtle matter, sometimes called *virtual matter*, of negative space/time

has no mass per se but is just a vibrational frequency. Since all subtle matter and particles are massless, there are no limits to the speed at which they may travel; in fact, the equations suggest their speeds approach infinity, that is, there is no time, as they are everywhere at once.

With negative entropy as the guiding principle, taken to its obvious extreme a state of constantly increasing order will eventually lead to perfect order, or 'God'. But this increase in order would be perceived only from the perspective of positive space/time; from the perspective of negative space/time it just 'is'.

Deltronic flows create energy templates, the basis of life

Deltronic flows are the subtle energies of the aura, such as the ch'i flows in the meridians of eastern medicine and pranic energy flows of chakras and nadi channels of yogic science.

Since deltrons carry the magnetoelectric force, they carry organizing energy from negative space/time that interacts with particles or matter in positive space/time. This deltronic flow then provides the energy template that organizes random physical particles into organized matter; in its most obvious form, living organisms. When this deltronic flow is decreased or blocked, the physical structures organized by this flow begin to follow the second law of thermodynamics and become more disorganized over time, resulting in disease, degeneration and decay of physical tissues.

Deltronic flow and healing

Thus, when the stomach meridian energy becomes blocked, the organizing flow of the deltrons comprising ch'i is reduced and the material stomach organ begins to degenerate and may develop organic diseases such as ulcers. Once energetic balancing restores the organizing flow of deltrons, the stomach organ will once again regain and maintain its homeostatic structure, a process called healing!

The healing process of increasing order happens spontaneously once the organizing flow of deltrons are uninterrupted and can deliver their negative entropic magnetoelectric energies to the physical tissues. This may be the basis of the 'healing energy' or *physis* of the ancient Greek Hippocrates.

In the West, these vitalist models have been replaced by the current western medical model that denies any such vital energy, and sees organism, including Man, as only biochemical, biomechanical machines, that if broken obviously need either drugs or surgery. This denial has been partly based on the lack of a possible mechanism for and evidence of the existence of this vital energy. This is why the eastern concepts of ch'i and prana are also denied.

References

1. Gerber, R 1988, *Vibrational Medicine*, Bear, Santa Fe.
2. Hawking, S 1996, *A Brief History of Time*, Bantam Books, New York.

Chapter 48

CHAOS THEORY AND BALANCING BIOLOGICAL SYSTEMS

Introduction to chaos theory

Chaos theory has its origins in the work of the great French mathematician Henri Poincaré, who in 1899 published the mathematical equations underlying chaos theory. However, because of the reiterative nature of these equations they could not be computed at the time. Indeed, the world was to wait until the 1960s for further development of his equations. It was only with the development of modern computers that there was sufficient computational power to actually solve his equations. Poincaré also laid down the mathematical basis for holography, and even relativity, but again could not solve these equations at the time.

Following the development of fractal geometry, first by Lorenz, the principles of chaos theory evolved over the next decade. Fractal geometry and the theory underlying chaos theory were then put on a firm mathematical basis by the great mathematician and jack of all trades Benoit Mandelbrot. In 1977, Ilya Prigogine received the Nobel Prize in Chemistry for elucidating the finer details of this theory.

While the advent of chaos theory was at first touted as a major breakthrough in understanding complex systems, it soon lost favor in the sciences, especially the hard sciences such as physics, because while extremely descriptive it was not predictive.

Much of the physical description of biological systems, from the structure of the venation of leaves and the structure of fern fronds to the circulatory and respiratory systems of Man, can be accurately and mathematically represented by fractal geometry and the equations of chaos theory. But because of the extreme complexity of the interaction of complex systems, especially biological systems that involve numerous interactions of many complex dynamic equilibria, very small inputs at critical times called *phase transitions*, can reorganize the whole system, and exactly which inputs at which times is unfortunately not predictable. Not surprisingly, Lorenz began the development of chaos theory while trying to predict the weather—a highly chaotic system.

There are some striking, counterintuitive and unusual features of chaos theory that provide an excellent model for healing in general and why the set-up system of Energetic Kinesiology in particular can produce such profound healing outcomes. These outcomes often seem impossible from a more classical mechanics point of view, as such subtle interventions should not produce such robust results. The basic principles of chaos theory are briefly outlined below.

Principles of chaos theory

Chaos theory is the best system Man has yet invented to describe the dynamics of complex interacting systems containing many variables and numerous interacting dynamic equilibria. Biological systems are one of the most complex dynamical systems known.

A *dynamic equilibrium* is a system that continuously varies about some value because of a series of feedback mechanisms. The result of these feedback mechanisms is that the system oscillates about a common value but is almost never actually at that value. For example, heartbeats, while averaging approximately 72 beats per minute, vary second by second from only a handful of beats per minute to hundreds of beats per minute. This is the basis of heart rate variability measurements, which have been shown to be one of the best predictors of morbidity (sickness) and mortality of all physiological variables. This is probably because heart rate variability represents the balance between the parasympathetic (slowing down) and sympathetic (speeding up) inputs, and thus represents the balance of your basic physiological homeostasis.

Perturbations to a dynamic equilibrium result in compensatory feedback that responds to negative disruption of the system by creating new, alternative pathways that tend to either return it to its original oscillatory value or establish a new oscillatory value but one that often requires greater energy expenditure.

When several dynamic equilibria are interacting with each other, a higher-order dynamically interacting system is established in which the variations in one system become perturbations in one of the other dynamic equilibria and vice versa, resulting in constantly changing and fluctuating feedback between the dynamic equilibria involved. Indeed, this is why they are termed *dynamic*!

When complex interacting dynamic equilibria initially interact, because each equilibrium acts as an uncontrolled perturbation to the other, the system as a whole appears chaotic. However, over time these interacting dynamic equilibria then tend to self-organize into a new, stable system, oscillating as a whole around a new, now stable value that, once established, now resist further perturbation.

This behavior was first observed and described by a meteorologist named Edward Lorenz in the 1960s, as he was using the then newly developed computers to attempt to describe and predict the weather—a truly chaotic system made up of endless interacting dynamic equilibria. As he ran the equations of his simplified models, Lorenz discovered that, quite contrary to his intuition and current scientific theory, these systems never reached an equilibrium steady-state value but rather established infinitely varying but self-similar patterns about a relatively fixed point that he called an *attractor*. This type of mathematical equation was then named the Lorenz attractor in his honor (see Figure 48.1).

Benoit Mandelbrot, a mathematical genius working for IBM, then began to further develop modeling of complex interacting systems and recognized that these self-organized self-similar patterns could be defined mathematically by a new type of mathematics called fractal geometry. He developed equations using this new mathematics that generated figures known as a Mandelbrot set, which can be understood only when depicted as a picture, especially a colored picture. One of the primary properties of a Mandelbrot set, besides its beauty, is that the same patterns reappear again and again at many different levels of scale.

Fractal geometry defined the mathematics underlying chaotic systems and showed how relatively complex patterns in nature could be generated by rather simple reiterative equations by computing their complex interactions using powerful computers. Remarkably, many of the structures in biological systems are fractal in nature, for instance the intestinal villi; branching of blood and lymph vessels; branching of the bronchi and bronchioles of the lungs; and many of the structural patterns seen in plants, such as

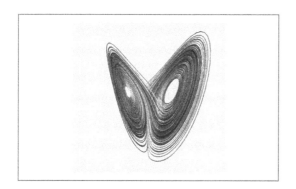

Figure 48.1 A Lorenz attractor. In classic physics, it is believed that all systems will over time achieve a steady state, like a pendulum that at first swings wildly but soon establishes a steady state, retracing the same pathway on each swing. In contrast, in complex interacting dynamic systems with many variables and interlinked equilibria the system generates self-similar patterns about a relatively fixed point, which Lorenz called an *attractor*.

the venation of leaves and the structure of fern fronds (see Figure 48.2).

Once a chaotic system of many interacting dynamic equilibria self-organizes, that is, develops a reiterative set of balancing interactions, it then robustly resists perturbation or further change as more input occurs. This continues until some critical point is reached at which just one more input causes the attractor to break down and the system goes chaotic once more. That critical point at which the system goes chaotic is termed the *phase transition*. However, the chaos following a phase transition over time leads to the development of a new self-organized system around a new attractor, which locks into yet another self-sustaining pattern.

One of the critical features of the phase transition is that because of the complex nature of many interacting equilibria, a tiny input at the critical time can trigger the phase transition and hence reorganization of the whole system. The second critical feature is that there is no *a priori* way of determining: 1, the exact factor that will trigger the phase transition; 2, the new system that will self-organize out of the chaos of the phase transition. So while chaos theory is incredibly descriptive of how biological and other complex dynamic systems work, it is not very useful from the linear perspective of classical physics because it is not predictive.

Within biological systems, the complex interacting equilibria self-organize around homeostasis and then resist perturbations. But as the perturbation increases in strength, the self-organized equilibria representing homeostasis are moved toward its homeostatic limits, the phase transition point for that biological system. If this phase transition is crossed, it will lead to chaotic function in at least some of the interacting dynamic equilibria involved. The chaos created by crossing the homeostatic limit leads to overt distress, which if it continues over time is called *sickness* or *disease*.

Thus, as perturbations push the interacting dynamic equilibria toward the homeostatic limits, compensatory physiological mechanisms are activated to prevent the system from going through a phase transition. If these initial physiological compensations cannot prevent the system from crossing the phase boundary, the system goes into distress.

This distress then initiates a series of further physiological compensations to bring the system back inside the homeostatic limits. However, to do this requires the input of additional energy into

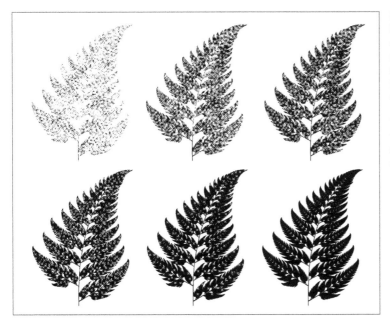

Figure 48.2 Generation of complex biological structures from fractal equations. Fractal geometry is the mathematics underlying chaotic systems and can generate complex patterns from rather simple reiterative equations. Each new point falls randomly, but gradually the complex image of the fern frond emerges from the information encoded in a few simple rules. After Gleick, J 1988, *Chaos*, Penguin Books, New York, p. 238.

the system being perturbed, usually by taking energy from other dynamic interacting equilibria that were supporting other physiological systems or functions, leading in turn to perturbations in these systems, requiring yet another set of compensations. The end result is that the system as a whole goes into a state of balanced imbalance that, while within homeostatic limits once more, is energetically expensive to maintain.

In mathematics, when perturbation causes a phase transition you just go from one relatively self-organized pattern to a new relatively self-organized pattern. But in biological systems, you may go from one self-organized system called *alive* to another, far less interesting self-organized system, at least to the organism involved, called *dead*!

Chaos theory and homeostasis

The principles of chaos theory provide an excellent description of both sickness and health and the transition between the two which we call *healing*. The state of homeostasis is indeed a set of complex interacting equilibria with constant variation around some optimal value for each physiological system and function. If the homeostatic limits are exceeded, this leads to dysfunction and disease or sickness. For instance, the homeostatic limits for the pH of the blood is only ± 0.1 pH unit, for body temperature it is ± 0.5°C and for oxygen levels in the blood it is ± 50–100%. Because the oxygen levels and temperature affect pH, and the pH controls many of the reactions determining the oxygen-carrying capacity of the blood and the body temperature, the interaction of just these three physiological systems can be very complex and is therefore constantly varying over time (see Figure 48.3a).

However, once a biological system has been perturbed over the long term, it establishes a new set of compensated homeostatic limits further from optimum homeostatic values through the

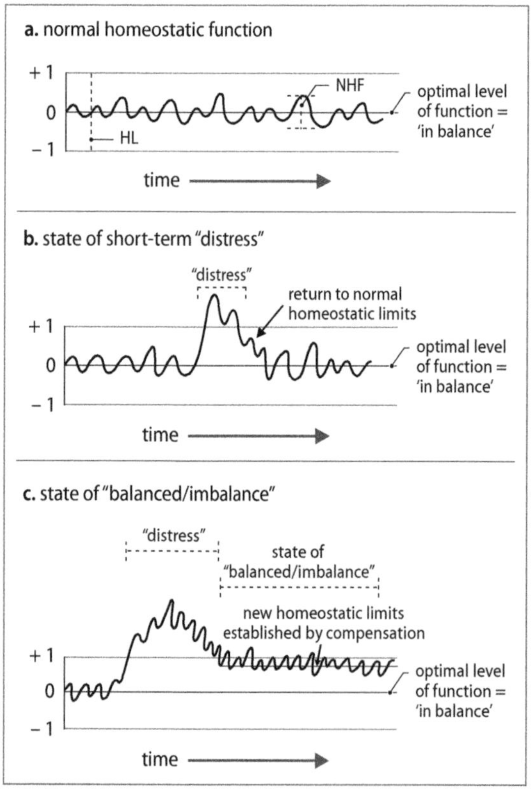

a. normal homeostatic function

+1 — NHF / optimal level of function = 'in balance'
0
HL
−1

time →

b. state of short-term "distress"

"distress" / return to normal homeostatic limits

+1
0 / optimal level of function = 'in balance'
−1

time →

c. state of "balanced/imbalance"

"distress"
state of "balanced/imbalance"
new homeostatic limits established by compensation

+1
0 / optimal level of function = 'in balance'
−1

time →

Figure 48.3 Homeostasis and stress.

a, Normal homeostatic function (NHF). All physiological functions of the body vary around a 'normal' value because of the dynamic interactions of the many negative feedback systems involved in maintaining life. Homeostatic limits (HLs) are the range of fluctuation around this normal value that can be tolerated without disruption of homeostasis, usually denoted by +1 and −1. Movement away from this normal value automatically activates compensations to return the perturbed function to optimum values of homeostasis. This results in a normal degree of variation: NHF.

b, Short-term stress: distress. When a point-in-time short-term stressor has pushed a function across the upper or lower HLs, the systems goes into distress, which institutes immediate compensations to bring this function back inside HLs, ending the distress and re-establishing normal homeostasis.

c, State of balanced/imbalance or compensation. Following a period of ongoing distress, the body develops a series of compensations that bring the perturbed function back within homeostasis but now establishes a new level of homeostasis further from optimum values, either closer to the upper or lower HL because of the presence of an ongoing stressor. This compensated homeostatic state is often called the state of balanced/imbalance and represents ongoing compensation that although functional is energetically expensive.

process of physiological compensation. While this new set of interacting dynamic equilibria now sustain homeostasis, they do it at a cost, and that cost is greater energy expenditure. Yet representing a new self-organized system, this new compensated homeostasis will resist perturbation to return to more optimal homeostatic levels. Therefore to get this system to reorganize closer to optimal homeostasis requires that this compensated system enter, at least temporarily, a state of chaos, as it is only from the chaotic state that reorganization to true homeostasis can occur.

So when an initial stressor acts on a biological system, it will perturb one or more of the interacting dynamic equilibria, resulting is initial physiological stress as that system goes out of balance, disrupting to some degree all the other equilibria with which it is interacting. If this stressor is temporary and not of sufficient magnitude to push the stressed system outside its homeostatic limits, then the system will institute temporary physiological compensations to return the system to its original homeostatic values, thus oscillating once more around some optimum value.

Within a relatively short time, various physiological adjustments are made, returning function to within normal homeostatic limits, and once again normal homeostatic limits are maintained.

Figure 48.3b represents stage 1 stress, the stage of distress, a physiologically chaotic state of function that is resolved after some factor has driven this system outside its normal homeostatic limits. This resolution is achieved by reorganization of this now chaotic system back into its former homeostasis as the original stressor is eliminated.

However, if the stressor goes on too long and the initial homeostatic limits are exceeded, or the stressor is sufficiently strong to drive the system beyond its homeostatic limits, then the system begins to break down and become chaotic, causing physiological distress. At this point, a phase transition occurs as the other physiological systems interacting with the distressed system reorganize to stabilize the distressed system through the process of physiological compensation. While the new self-organized system is now more stable than the state of distress, and the original function has

been brought back inside the homeostatic limits, it is no longer as close to its optimum value and therefore places an energy drain on the organism as a whole (see Figure 48.3c).

But because it is now a new self-organized system that resists change, healing can occur only if this self-organized compensation can be driven back into chaos and then have some factor present to provide a push back toward its original optimal homeostatic value.

Chaos theory and healing

For healing to occur, the compensated system must be decompensated to create a chaotic state from which change to a new self-organized state is possible. Then a force must be present to give that chaotic system a push in the direction of homeostasis and order. Without this push, whether the decompensated system reorganizes closer to or further from homeostasis is up to random chance of other small varying factors happening at the time. Therefore healing requires both decompensation to create chaos and direction for the system to move back toward homeostasis.

Indeed, the role of set-up in Energetic Kinesiology is to destabilize the compensated state to create a decompensated, more chaotic state. As each indicator change is entered into the circuit via pause lock, representing another stressor or distortion of energy flow, the energetic systems enter an increasingly chaotic state. From this chaotic state, reorganization is now possible. However, the degree of reorganization is totally dependent on the degree of chaos created in the system. The greater the degree of decompensation, the more chaotic the system becomes and the greater the possibility of change.

Therefore if a kinesiology set-up creates only a small degree of chaos, the system can reorganize only to a limited degree, while a more complex, multicomponent set-up provides the opportunity for a more profound reorganization of the whole system. Some of the greatest gifts to modern Energetic Kinesiology were from Alan Beardall when he developed both hand modes and pause lock, and Richard Utt's concepts of stacking, acupressure formatting and powers of stress. These tools provide the possibility of greatly increasing the degree of decompensation, and hence chaos, generated by the set-up.

The correction or balance then provides the push back toward the optimal homeostatic value of the unperturbed system, a process we call healing. The balance gives direction to the self-organization that then proceeds automatically by the complex interaction of the dynamic equilibria involved in this particular system. Thus, the system now reorganizes closer to optimal homeostatic values. But what is this push in energy healing?

Whatever the healing technique, the primary factor providing this push in contextual healing systems of energetic medicine is the love and compassion of the practitioner, as this provides a direct source of deltronic flow from negative space/time, bringing with it the organizational energy to heal.

So the source of all healing is activation of this deltronic flow that brings with it the information energy to generate self-organization out of chaos. Whether the practitioner is waving a crystal through the aura, as in crystal healing; poking an acupoint, as in acupressure; needling an acupoint, as in acupuncture; or merely channeling energy, as in Reiki and therapeutic touch, it is the practitioner's intent to heal that activates this healing deltronic flow of energy. This deltronic flow is then transduced via the various energy systems into the physiology of healing.

The second role of the practitioner in energy medicine is to provide a stabilizing force during the process of set-up to allow the client's energy system to experience the chaos of decompensation. Without this stabilizing force, it is not safe for the person to go into the chaos of decompensation, exactly because the compensation was created to end the chaos of distress in the first place! Love and empathetic compassion are the most harmonic forces in nature and are therefore able to stabilize high degrees of chaos as well as provide the push back toward the self-organization of homeostasis.

An example of these phenomena is presented below from Dr William Tiller's recent book *Some Science Adventures With Real Magic*. Dr Tiller and

Dr Krebs undertook a series of experiments in his laboratory in Payson, Arizona, doing different types of set-ups and applying different correction techniques in healing. Dr Tiller's laboratory is a conditioned space, that is, a space in which the energetic domains have been harmonized (for more information on conditioning space, see Tiller's book *Science and Human Transformation: Subtle Energies, Intentionality, and Consciousness*). This allows for more subtle energy effects to be observed more robustly.

The laboratory had a series of pH meters continuously monitoring pH in several different locations to measure changes in the randomness of the void. The void is not really empty space but a seething sea of virtual particles popping into and out of existence. When a virtual particle pops into existence, it withdraws energy from the void, but at the same time its virtual antiparticle also pops into existence and they immediately annihilate each other with this energy, returning to the void. Because the sum of the energy changes between particle manifestation and annihilation is zero, the same amount of energy lost by the void in particle manifestation is then returned to the void by particle annihilation. Therefore there is zero change in energy, so the void is called the *zero-point field*.

From the point of view of modern physics, the void is totally random and hence can be ignored as a factor in experiments. However, Tiller and his group have shown over a number of years that this is true only in the absence of human intent. It is not only Tiller but a number of respected scientists who have shown that human intention plays a significant role in how our physical world operates, and this research is summarized in *The Field* by L. McTaggart.[1]

Human intent can direct informational energy in the form of deltronic flow from reciprocal negative space/time into the positive space/time domain, which momentarily reduces the randomness of the void. This is overtly measurable using the simple physicochemical system of pH. In the absence of human intent, pH will vary randomly about the value of the solution in which the pH electrode is immersed. This value can be set very precisely by the use of buffers to hold the pH stable. However, there are still random variations in pH caused by the noise in the system.

In the pH system, there are only a few variables that account for virtually all the variation in the concentration of hydrogen ions, H^+ ions. This is what pH measures: the H^+ ion concentration or acidity of the solution. A solution with an excess of H^+ ions relative to water is acid, while a deficit of H^+ ions makes the solution alkaline. Only temperature and dissolved oxygen have any significant effect on pH in a closed system, because these factors shift the dynamic equilibria controlling the H^+ ion concentration.

In Tiller's laboratory, there were pH meters continuously recording pH directly into a computer at various locations. In the absence of people in the laboratory, the pH variation is totally random, varying by only ± 0.01 pH unit for days on end, and the pH changes only as the temperature and dissolved oxygen vary according to physical–chemical principles. The pH meters were insulated to reduce the temperature variations, and oxygen content usually varies relatively little in an open environment, rapidly equilibrating with the oxygen content of the surrounding air, resulting in minimal pH variability caused by oxygen variation.

Human intention, when focused and directed, can strongly alter the randomness of the void, which can then change the direction of the pH in a constant direction, perhaps as organizational 'energy' is moved through or from the void. This energy represents information, and in this case not random information but rather directed information, perhaps the basis of the healing energy used in energy medicine! Indeed, in physics today they tend to talk of the information in the system rather than the energy or mass of the system, as information is considered more fundamental.

In Tiller's experiments, Krebs treated several different people with several different conditions, from physical pain to psychoemotional issues to mental problems with decision-making. He initiated the circuit by entering the issue into pause lock, and then continued the set-up. He continued developing the set-up by locating factors creating or altering the stressors causing the presenting

condition using muscle biofeedback in the form of muscle monitoring, discussed earlier in this book. The stressors or factors varied from specific physical imbalances, for example strained tendons, to psychoemotional states.

When he could no longer access further stress in the circuit, he then determined the type of corrective technique to balance the circuit, again using muscle biofeedback. At this point, Krebs stated 'Starting balancing now!' and the technician activated an event recorder that noted this in the pH recorder. As soon as the balance was complete, he stated 'Balance complete now!' and the technician again activated the event recorder.

The next day, when Krebs came into the laboratory, the technician had analyzed the previous day's data and he said, 'Well, I'm a believer!' Interestingly, as soon as Tiller and Krebs sat down in the laboratory the morning before and overtly began to plan these experiments, human intention in action, the pH meters showed a deviation from randomness, but when Krebs stated 'Starting balancing now!' there was a dramatic decrease in the randomness of the void, as the pH began a rapid drop which lasted until he stated 'Balance complete now!' At this time, the pH had returned to the same trajectory of pH decrease as before the correction began and remained on this trajectory until the next correction began, which was again accompanied by a rapid decrease in pH, indicating another decrease in the randomness of the void (see Figure 48.4).

One of the most interesting observations was that the flow of healing energy or organizational information from the negative space/time caused a decrease in the randomness of the void, as measured by a rapid drop in pH with the initiation of each healing event, and a return to the random pH fluctuations at the end of the healing event. All the healing events looked identical, despite the fact that very different healing techniques were employed.

Dr William Tiller made the following comments on the results of these Energetic Kinesiology experiments in his Payson Laboratory in 2001: 'In spite of the different subjects with different issues and different correction techniques employed, the

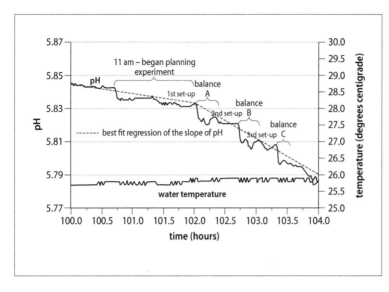

Figure 48.4 Effect of healing on the randomness of the void. Three pH monitors in different locations recorded pH continuously. Each healing event or balance produced an similar pattern: the pH would plateau as Krebs entered information into pause lock, and application of a correction would create a dramatic drop in pH (a deviation from randomness indicating extraction of information from the void) and then pH would plateau once more before the same pattern was repeated with each healing episode. Note that although different healing modalities were used in each balance, the pH response or *healing signature* was almost identical in each case. After William Tiller.

instrument response "signature" was virtually the same. This strongly suggests that the act of "healing" creates an unique "signature" of increasing order in the surrounding S/1 gate reality even at several meters from the "healing event". One could hypothesize that the act of healing initiates a flow of organizing energy (deltronic flow) from the reciprocal space/time into positive space/time, and it is this transfer of "organizing" energy that constitutes or initiates the healing process.'

This suggests that energy flows are merely mechanisms of information flow, and it is information that the organism needs to reorganize and heal.

The role of the healer or kinesiologist

Homeostasis represents a self-organized system derived from the many complex interacting dynamic equilibria necessary to maintain life. Stress initially drives this system toward chaos, but as with all self-organized systems it resists perturbation by generating either short-term compensations (if the initial stressor is resolved) or long-term compensations (if the stress is ongoing). These compensations result in either a return to normal homeostasis if the stressor is resolved, or the establishment of the compensated state of balanced

imbalance if the stressor is ongoing. The compensated state of balanced imbalance, although within the homeostatic limits, is further from optimal homeostasis, and therefore it now requires more energy to maintain this compensated state. Furthermore, in order for this compensation to be maintained it must borrow energy from other systems within the body, creating states of imbalance in other systems.

The set-up procedures in Energetic Kinesiology result in decompensating the balanced imbalance state by releasing the blocked energy; however, this creates an increasingly chaotic state as decompensation proceeds. It is from this chaotic decompensated state that reorganization may occur. The more thoroughly decompensated the system becomes, the greater the chaos and the greater the possibility for a reorganization of the system closer to optimal homeostasis. However, for the system to reorganize closer to optimal homeostasis information or energy is required to bring order into this chaotic disorganized decompensated state. This is a major role of the healer or practitioner.

The role of the healer in the energetic healing process is two-fold: first, to hold the space, that is, provide the energetic stability necessary to permit the system to go into chaos; second, to provide a flow of negative entropic energy, providing the organizational information or energy from negative space/time necessary to push the chaotic, decompensated energy into a new self-organized state, *one that is closer to* optimal homeostasis.

The origin of this organizational information or energy to heal is derived from human intent directing the love and empathic compassion that activates the negative entropic flow of deltrons into the chaotic system, providing the organizing information needed to create a new self-organized state. However, without human intention and loving compassion, the chaotic decompensated state will indeed self-organize but not necessarily closer to homeostasis.

The role of the set-up is to provide information on all levels of the imbalance generated by the stressors causing the current condition. However, direct access to this information, most of which is from subconscious physical, emotional and energetic domains, is not available directly to the person's consciousness. Hence the need for the subconscious feedback from muscle monitoring that appears to interface with all these other subconscious domains.

After Krebs attended his very first evening of kinesiology training, he sat in his office and thought about what he had just experienced. There was one thing he just did not understand: if the mind–body provides information about the nature of the problem at a causal level, and then it directs the practitioner on how to balance or correct this problem, why does the mind–body not just fix the problem? Why is there a need for a healer?

Perplexed, he went to see his friend Rob Crickett, a former Zen monk who had achieved enlightenment, and asked this question of why the mind–body can both know what the problem is, *and* how to fix it, yet not be able to fix it itself? Rob replied, 'Charles, what you say is correct. The being does know what the problem is *and* it does know how to fix it. What you do not understand is that these two parts have lost their connection. That is one role of the healer: to provide that connection. Once established, the body can then immediately heal itself!' Again, the body lacked only the information it needs to heal, but this information was not available because of blocked information or energy flow. No healer actually does the healing;

they only provide the context for healing, the information that was lacking for the person to heal themselves.

This is also true at the physical level for physical, physiological conditions: the body always heals itself, but sometimes it just needs a change of context for the healing to occur. When you have a raging bacterial infection that has overwhelmed a suppressed immune system, which provides the context for the infection in the first place, you may need an antibiotic to reduce the number of bacteria so that your immune system can now bounce back and finish the job of eliminating the remaining pathogenic bacteria and re-establish immune balance. The now balanced immune system then maintains this balance when you stop taking the antibiotics, preventing a reoccurrence of infection.

The antibiotics did not cure you, they merely produced a context—fewer bacteria—for the body's immune system to then heal the infection and then maintain this infection-free state over time. The germ theory is normally incorrectly stated as 'viruses, bacteria and parasites make you sick'. This is not true! The correct statement of the germ theory is this: 'It is the presence of viruses, bacteria and parasites *and* a suppressed immune system that make you sick!'

For personal proof of this statement, think about how often you have been in an office or other workplace with the people around you sputtering and coughing. The air you were breathing contained a sea of pathogenic microbes and flu viruses, yet you did not get sick! However, if you were stressed out, exhausted and/or depressed in the same microbe- and virus-laden environment, you get sick almost every time. Therefore it is the context that determines which types of imbalances or conditions you get and how quickly you will recover from them.

Therefore the true nature of disease and dysfunction is a loss of connection between the part of the body that knows what the problem is and the part of the body that has the information needed to re-establish homeostasis. Indeed, Energetic Kinesiology appears to be an effective tool to both identify the underlying factors creating the problem and then provide the connection and information needed for the body to heal itself.

Reference

1. McTaggart, L 2008, *The Field*, HarperCollins, New York.

RECOMMENDED READING

Cuthbert, S 2013, *Applied Kinesiology Essentials: The Missing Link in Health Care*, The Gangasas Press, Pueblo.

Gerber, R 2001, *Vibrational Medicine, Third Edition*, Bear & Company, Santa Fe.

Goodheart, GJ 1986, *You'll Be Better: The Story of Applied Kinesiology*, AK Printing, Geneva.

Johari, H 2000, *Chakras: Energy Centers of Transformation*, Destiny Books, Rochester, Vermont.

Kaptchuk, TJ 1983, *The Web That Has No Weaver: Understanding Chinese Medicine*, Ryder, London.

Kendall, FP, Kendall McCreary, E, Provance, PG, McIntyre Rodgers, M & Romani, WA 2010, *Muscles: Testing and Function with Posture and Pain Fifth Edition*, Lippincott Williams & Wilkins, Baltimore.

LeDoux, J 1996, *The Emotional Brain: The Mysterious Underpinnings of Emotional Life*, Touchstone, New York.

Levy, SL & Lehr, C 1996, *Your Body Can Talk*, Hohm Press, Prescott.

Sheldrake, R 2009, *A New Science of Life: The Hypothesis of Morphic Resonance.* Park Street Press, Rochester, Vermont.

Swanson, C 2003, *The Synchronized Universe - New Science of the Paranormal, Volume 1*, Poseidia Press, Tucson.

Swanson, C 2010, *Life Force - The Scientific Basis, Volume II*, Poseidia Press, Tucson.

Talbot, M 1991, *The Holographic Universe*, Grafton Books, London.

Tiller, WA 1997, *Science and Human Transformation: Subtle Energies, Intentionality and Consciousness*, Pavior Publishing, Walnut Creek.

Tiller, WA, Dibble, WE & Kohane, MJ 2001, *Conscious Acts of Creation*, Pavior Publishing, Walnut Creek.

Tiller, WA 2007, *Psychoenergetic Science: A Second Copernican-Scale Revolution*, Pavior Publishing, Walnut Creek.

Utt, R 1997, *Stress: The Nature of the Beast*, Applied Physiology Publishing, Tucson.

Walther, DS 1988, *Applied Kinesiology: Synopsis, Second Edition*, Systems DC, Pueblo.

INDEX

Note: Page number followed by f and t indicates figure and table respectively.